Diagnosis and Evaluation in Speech Pathology

Fifth Edition

Diagnosis and Evaluation in Speech Pathology

William O. Haynes
Auburn University-Alabama

Rebekah H. Pindzola
Auburn University-Alabama

Allyn and Bacon
Boston • London • Toronto • Sydney • Tokyo • Singapore

MWB

Executive Editor: Stephen D. Dragin
Series Editorial Assistant: Elizabeth McGuire
Composition and prepress buyer: Linda Cox
Manufacturing Buyer: Suzanne Lareau
Cover Administrator: Linda Knowles
Editorial-production service: York Production Service

Library of Congress Cataloging-in-Publication Data

Haynes, William O.
    Diagnosis and evaluation in speech pathology / William O. Haynes,
Rebekah H. Pindzola. — 5th ed.
      p.   cm.
    Includes bibliographical references and index.
    ISBN 0-205-27212-6
    1. Speech disorders—Diagnosis. 2. Speech disorders—Case
studies. I. Pindzola, Rebekah H. (Rebekah Hand) II. Title.
    [DNLM: 1. Speech Disorders—diagnosis. WM 475 H424d 1997]
RC423.H3826 1997
616.85'5075—dc21
DNLM/DLC
for Library of Congress   97-19808
                                      CIP

Printed in the United States of America

10 9 8 7 6 5 4 3 2   02 01 00 99 98

6/26/01

Contents

Preface

With this fifth edition of *Diagnosis and Evaluation in Speech Pathology* we invite a new group of students and practitioners to consider the complex and fascinating arena of assessment in communication disorders. For almost twenty-five years, this text has introduced diagnosis and evaluation as a *process* conducted in the context of an *interpersonal relationship* between clinicians and clients. This interesting and challenging process is a curious blend of science and art. Assessment is much more than the simple administration of a few tests or scales and the diagnostician is much more than a neutral conduit through which test scores pass. Each case requires the clinician to think, solve problems, form hypotheses, gather data and arrive at conclusions. Often the diagnostic enterprise raises more questions than it answers, and then it becomes important to be a *clinician* rather than just a *technician.* Many readers of the prior editions have commented that they found the book to be both readable and clinically relevant. They have also made insightful suggestions which we have endeavored to include in the present edition. Since the first edition appeared in 1973 the field of communication disorders has gone through many changes. With each successive revision of the text, we have attempted to reflect theoretical, clinical and technological advances that have taken place in the field. The fifth edition is no different. The reader will notice that we have attempted to maintain the strong points of the former edition while including new research and clinical tools.

The authors would like to express appreciation to our students, clients, colleagues and teachers who helped to mold our thinking about the assessment process. We would also like to acknowledge Dr. Lon Emerick who provided the initial impetus for this work over twenty-five years ago. His basic philosophy, sensitivity and enthusiasm still echo throughout the text. We would also like to thank Grace F. Middleton of the University of Texas at El Paso, and Lori Stewart Gonzalez of the University of Kentucky, for reading and commenting on this new edition.

We should never forget that the diagnostic session is our initial contact with clients and we never get a second chance to make a first impression. *Every* evaluation is unique and *each* client deserves the best we can offer in terms of our ability, knowledge, judgment and interpersonal sensitivity. We hope that this text can communicate both the method and the magic of this challenging task.

Chapter 1

Introduction to Diagnosis and Evaluation:

Philosophical Issues and General Guidelines

Speech-language pathology is a wonderfully diverse profession that requires a practitioner to possess a wide range of skills, knowledge, and personal characteristics. A speech-language pathologist (SLP) works as a case selector, case evaluator, diagnostician, interviewer, parent counselor, teacher, coordinator, record keeper, consultant, researcher and student. Because the boundaries between these various duties are not clearly defined, and because the clinician must move continuously from one area to another, it is inevitable that no one person can expect to be equally competent in all areas. The ultimate goal is to maximize one's strengths in all aspects to provide the best possible service to individuals with communicative handicaps.

Diagnosis is one of the most comprehensive and difficult tasks of the speech-language pathologist. The diagnosis of a client requires a synthesis of the entire field: knowledge of norms and testing techniques, skills in observation, an ability to relate effectively and empathetically, and a great deal of creative intuition. Furthermore, because communication is a function of the entire person, the diagnostician must try to scrutinize all aspects of behavior. We must try to remember that we are not simply working with speech sounds, fluency, vocal quality, or linguistic rules but rather with changing people in a dynamic environment. The experienced diagnostician does not look at objective scores of articulatory skill, point scales of vocal quality, or standard scores as ends in themselves, but rather as aspects of an individual's communication ability—we diagnose communicators, not just communication. That revelation is a major factor in the transition from technician to professional clinician.

Because many of our diagnostic tools are imprecise, being largely in the experimental stages, and because communication disorders are by nature complex and perplexing, many of our diagnostic undertakings are incomplete and ambiguous. The lack of absolute and definitive answers to the various questions of diagnosis is often frustrating and demoralizing to the clinician. The ambiguous findings that sometimes culminate a diagnostic evaluation must be dealt with in a fashion that perpetuates the evaluative undertaking rather than closes the door on further probing. Diagnosis is a continuous and open-ended venture that results in answers or partial answers that themselves are open to revision with added information.

Diagnosis and Evaluation Defined

Some clinicians, at first glance, may consider the words *diagnosis* and *evaluation* to be synonymous. It is our intent in this text that diagnosis refer to the classical Greek definition of distinguishing a person's problem from the large field of potential disabilities. The term *diagnosis* in the original Greek means "to distinguish." The prefix *dia-* means "apart," and *-gnosis* translates as "to know." In order to distinguish a person's particular problem from the many possibilities available, we must know the client thoroughly and how he/she responds in many conditions, performing a variety of tasks. Evaluation refers to *the process* of arriving at a diagnosis. Thus, informal probes, trial therapy tasks, and gathering generalization data are part of evaluation. In the *American Heritage Dictionary* (1985) *diagnosis* is defined as "the act or process of identifying or determining the nature of a disease through examination." Our conception of diagnosis, then, includes a thorough understanding of the client's problem and not merely the application of a label. It is relatively simple to call a child "language impaired," but it is a more difficult matter to really understand how this child deals with linguistic symbols in a variety of tasks and situations. *This* is diagnosis in our view. We would also like to expand the notion of diagnosis to include distinguishing the nature of a person's problem at different points in time. Thus, diagnosis and evaluation are ongoing processes. We initially perform evaluation activities to arrive at an initial diagnosis, and we also examine the client repeatedly during the course of treatment. A client's diagnosis often changes over time. For example, a child may initially present with language delay and after a period of language treatment be characterized as primarily demonstrating a phonological disorder. A neurogenic patient may initially be diagnosed with aphasia, but may experience further neurological damage and be rediagnosed with aphasia and dysarthria. Another major thrust of this book is that diagnosis need not be confined to a two-hour block of time in a university setting or a 30-minute period in a medical facility. The competent clinician will continue evaluation activities until the client's performance is understood to the extent necessary for effective treatment.

We perform evaluation tasks with two major goals in mind. First, we evaluate to arrive at a good understanding or diagnosis of a client's problem. Sometimes these evaluation activities will be confined to an assessment period, and at other times they will be performed well into the beginning of treatment. Often we must begin therapy with a client before arriving at a firm diagnosis. This approach is not optimal, but it is justified as long as we realize that (1) *any* treatment approach is experimental to a certain degree in the beginning, (2) most initial treatment goals will generally be "in the ball park" in terms of appropriateness (e.g., we probably would not engage in voice therapy for a stuttering client), and (3) just because we have begun treatment, we have not abandoned our efforts in trying to define the parameters of the client's problem and arrive at a diagnosis. We can always "fine-tune" a treatment program based on an increased understanding of a client's problem and capabilities.

A second major reason to perform evaluation activities is to monitor the client's progress in treatment and describe changes in the communication disturbance. In this use of evaluation activities, we are not necessarily trying to diagnose the problem but to document treatment progress and determine possible changes in the course of treatment. In the chapters of the present text that deal with disorders, we will suggest evaluation tasks often used for these purposes that are not in the formal test category. Formal tests are designed more for categorizing clients as exhibiting certain disorders, while nonstandardized evaluation tasks are used to gain insight into specific client abilities and to gauge treatment progress. We will now discuss some of these purposes of diagnosis and evaluation in more detail.

Diagnosis to Determine the Reality of the Problem

One function of diagnosis is to determine whether the presenting communication pattern does indeed constitute a handicap. Before this is possible, however, it is necessary to have a clear idea of what constitutes a communication disorder. Van Riper's definition of a speech disorder is widely quoted: "Speech is abnormal when it deviates so far from the speech of other people that it calls attention to itself, interferes with communication, or causes the speaker or his listeners to be distressed" (Van Riper and Emerick 1984, 34). Figure 1.1 depicts three components that must be considered in determining a communication disorder.

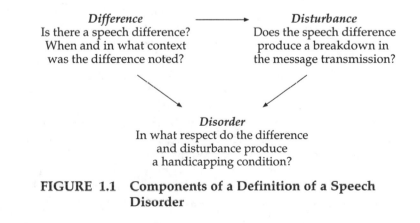

Difference ⟶ *Disturbance*
Is there a speech difference? Does the speech difference
When and in what context produce a breakdown in
was the difference noted? the message transmission?

Disorder
In what respect do the difference
and disturbance produce
a handicapping condition?

**FIGURE 1.1   Components of a Definition of a Speech
Disorder**

1. *Speech Difference.* This refers to whether or not the speech signal calls attention to itself and when this might occur. We can quantify the physical characteristics of the speech signal through recording, measurement, and observation. Computer-assisted spectrographic analyses and pitch measurements are available to help the diagnostician obtain an objective measure of the acoustic nature of the individual's speech. In other words, we must scrutinize the physical characteristics of the speech signal and judge its quality. But these data are of limited value unless it can be determined what *difference* a particular speech parameter makes.

In most areas of communication disorders, the state of the art has not progressed to where we can simply take the quantified data, compare them with established numerical norms, and determine the correctness of the speech sample. Unfortunately, each diagnostician must develop a personal frame of reference. Vocal qualities are subject to individual impressions; and while a clinician may *know* that the voice is awry, evidence of the difference may often elude the sensors and algorithms of our high-tech instrumentation. On the other hand, physicians are able to scrutinize data from a laboratory test and make an immediate diagnosis regarding the normalcy of an individual's blood count. This kind of reference information is not yet available to the SLP. The question of whether the presenting speech difference is different enough to be of concern thus becomes a matter of human judgment. This judgment involves filtering incoming data through the clinician's many synaptic junctions whose thresholds may have been worn thin by bias and experience. An inordinately critical or uncritical ear is a hazard with far-reaching implications.

What constitutes normal behavior? There are several definitions available, but we will discuss only two, representing the diverging philosophies with which each clinician must contend in establishing his or her own concept. The first theory we shall call the concept of *cultural norms.* The assumption is that there are behaviors that society considers aberrant in terms of group characteristics. According to this model, each bit of behavior can be judged against a real or theoretical standard, the nature of which is independent of the individual's personal idiosyncrasies. Thus, even a seventy-year-old person with a hearing threshold of 30 dB in the high frequencies may be thought of as exhibiting a significant hearing loss. The second theory we shall call the concept of *individual norms.* Advocates of this model assume that each individual has made a unique adjustment to life based on previous experiences, physical limitations, and the environment's reactions. Any judgment as to the normalcy of a bit of behavior must be contingent upon individual characteristics such as age, intelligence, and experience. Taken to the extreme, of course, the latter model would assert that each person is normal no matter what he or she does, since the behavior is the end product of all that plays upon the person, and to this extent the concept of individual norms loses meaning. But some case examples may help to clarify and give perspective.

The audiologist who examines the hearing of the seventy-year-old individual referred to earlier and who obtains the typical presbycusic audiometric curve could make a case for the judgment that this person has "normal" hearing. According to personal norms, this is average or normal behavior for a person of seventy; but according to cultural norms, the individual's hearing level is below the average for the total population. Follow-up procedures would be based, then, on the practical matter of getting a more efficient communication system for the individual and also on providing counseling so that the person will understand the nature of his/her hearing. Therefore, both cultural and personal norms play a part in diagnostic judgments and rehabilitative programs. A ten-year-old child with severe cognitive delays and an unstimulable distortion of the /r/ phoneme may not be judged to have seriously defective speech, whereas an eight-year-old presenting a similar speech pattern, but a different intellectual potential, may be recommended for treatment. Such judgments have implications for case selection, and the clinician must reconcile the variances between the physical differences in the sounds involved and the individual variables in conjunction with what is normal for the population as a whole. Each clinician must continually use both concepts of normalcy in diagnostic work.

There are all sorts of ways that a speech signal can call attention to itself and yet be perfectly appropriate. For example, a Black English speaker may alter aspects of speech and language when style shifting between members of one culture and another. While Standard English speakers may notice the differences in Black English, these variations certainly would not be viewed as evidence of a communication disorder. Another example might be when speakers alter their rate, loudness, and vocal quality in order to tell a funny story or relate a particular experience in a dramatic way. Age is another variable. If the speaker is a child of two who exhibits many articulatory substitutions and omissions, does this difference constitute a problem? The answer can only lie in an examination of these errors against the context of normal two-year-old communication. Thus, a difference is not enough to constitute a communication disorder if the context suggests normality. This points out the importance of the SLP's knowing the contextual effects on communication and the contributions of age and the wide variety of cultural, ethnic, and geographical dialects on the speech signal.

2. *The Intelligibility of the Message.* The second component of determining a communication disorder involves the perception of disturbance in the signal that is transmitted. Is the signal distorted or is it intelligibility affected? If the message transmission is adversely affected, there is a high probability of the existence of a problem. Many factors play a part in both the encoding and decoding processes, and the diagnostician must be capable of representing the standard for society when listening and making judgments. The essential judgment to be made is, How well did the intentions of the speaker match the perceptions of the listener, and what are the factors that affect this? Are there attributes of the signal that distract the listener, thus altering the message? Is the signal indistinct, thus allowing only partial transmission of information? Is the signal distinct, but conveying a message other than that intended by the speaker? Is the signal distinct but conveying a message (albeit the one selected by the speaker) that is inappropriate for the context?

We have, in the main, been content with clinical insight and intuitive estimates when we have judged the impact of speech differences upon intelligibility. The speech clinician is able to count the phoneme errors, quantify the number of repetitions or disfluencies per sentence, and establish various quotients of language ability, but as yet we are unable to assess the intelligibility of the transmitted message with any degree of reliability. In most cases the clinician resorts to scaling techniques to mark the impact of the disorder on intelligibility, and we have little way to know specific contributions of individual components of the speech signal or language used on overall signal distortion. Clearly, severe disfluency can interrupt a message, intermittent cessations of phonation and poor vocal qualities can distort transmission, inappropriate phoneme selection or production can lead to unintelligibility, and ambiguous vocabulary or sentence structure can lead to misinterpretations. Whatever the cause of the communication failure, we must document that it occurs. At present, however, we have no widely accepted system to use in this documentation for most areas of communication disorders.

3. *Handicapping Condition.* The final component in defining a disorder involves the determination of handicap in the life of the client. Emerick (1984) suggests:

> *In the final analysis this third aspect justifies the existence of our profession. If the speech difference has no discernible impact on the child's behavior, and ultimately on his adjusting abilities and learning potential, there is little justification for concern on the part of the speech clinician. Although it is not feasible to compile a listing of all of the possible conditions under which a communication difference would become handicapping, it is generally agreed that communicative differences are considered handicapping when: 1) the transmission and/or perception of messages is faulty; 2) the person is placed at an economic disadvantage; 3) the person is placed at a learning disadvantage; 4) the person is placed at a social disadvantage; 5) there is a negative impact upon the emotional growth of the person; or 6) the problem causes physical damage or endangers the health of the person.*

There are numerous examples of famous people who are highly successful and seemingly content with their lives despite manifesting a communication disorder. Some famous personalities have happy, fulfilling lives even though an SLP would have classified them as having a handicap. On the other hand, a minor deviation in a teacher or business executive may mean a significant handicap in terms of credibility and evaluation of job performance. If a person does not view his or her communication disorder as a handicap, it is difficult to justify clinical work or to motivate the client to improve communication skills.

Diagnosis to Determine the Etiology of the Problem

Far too many clinicians view diagnosis simply as a labeling process; however, the actual labeling, or categorizing, is only a small part of the total assessment process. Classification systems within our profession are poor at best, and high-level abstractions (e.g., stuttering) tend to emphasize the similarities within populations rather than the individual differences. The keen diagnostician looks upon classifications as communication conveniences to be viewed with suspicion. Of course, the convenience factor is important, and each clinician who makes a determination of the reality of the problem must be willing to label it. This must of necessity, however, follow an orderly description of the characteristics of the disorder so that it can be clear what route the diagnostician took in arriving at the final classification. A diagnosis that only describes the characteristics of the problem, without judging its type or class, is a dead end. The opposite path is also dangerous; the diagnostician who is willing to begin an evaluation by labeling the problem has reversed the orderly sequence of acquiring knowledge and often effectively closes his or her mind to factors that may later point away from the premature diagnosis.

The notion of "cause" has different meanings depending on its distance from the problem. As you look at a client in a diagnostic session, you search for reasons for the presenting behaviors. In fact, many of these reasons may be buried in the past and can only be revealed by painstaking effort. In many cases, cause and effect may be layered in complex patterns. Not only must we search through the client's past experience in order to uncover events that may help us alter current behaviors, but we must also guard against looking for causes in only one dimension of behavior. A child's brain damage, once identified, is probably not the only etiological factor, because communication is a complicated human function. Social, learning, motivational, and many other factors enter into the total process. Paul (1995) illustrates the complexity of determining causation in an example of babies who were exposed to cocaine because their mothers used the drug during pregnancy:

> *Cocaine was usually not the only risk to which they were exposed. Mothers who abused cocaine during pregnancy also tended to abuse other street drugs, as well as alcohol. Alcohol itself is known to be a serious teratogen and could cause many of the problems thought to be present in these babies, even without any other substance abuse. Further, mothers who abused cocaine and other drugs during pregnancy frequently continued to do so after the child was born. These mothers would not be very available to their infants for either basic care or for social interaction. . . . Finally, mothers who abuse cocaine and other drugs tend to live in poverty. Poverty itself affects both general and communicative development through the tendency for poor children to have been born small and prematurely and to have poor nutrition, inadequate medical care and incomplete or absent inoculation against disease. (95)*

Thus, determining the etiology of a problem is not always straightforward, and we must be cautious about attributing the cause of a disorder to a particular event or factor. Classically, etiology has been defined in terms of predisposing, precipitating, and perpetuating factors. Predisposing factors are generally thought to be important because of their potential link with a third agent. A classic example of predisposing factors is the apparent genetic predisposition to stutter. We know that stuttering tends to run in families; however, it could be that environmental factors cause it to surface. The wary diagnostician must watch for factors that occur with high regularity in association with certain communication disorders. Such data could ultimately be instrumental in uncovering some basic information regarding the nature of the disorder.

Precipitating factors are generally no longer operating and as such may or may not be identifiable. There is a philosophical question of whether we need to search for precipitating factors if they are not still operating, and the point is well taken. Each moment, however, there is created a new set of precipitating factors that, acting as characteristics of the past, perpetuate behaviors of the present. Communication disorders generally are not static entities developed at a given point and perpetuated without modification through time; rather they are ever-changing characteristics that are constantly influenced by intrinsic and extrinsic factors. A child with a language disorder may have begun to lag behind in linguistic development during a period of recurrent ear infections that occurred when language was being learned. If the otitis has long since disappeared and the language disorder remains, it is difficult for the diagnostician to observe or even pinpoint the true cause of the disability. Even if the child did have recurrent bouts with ear infections, it can never be truly substantiated that these infections actually precipitated or played a role in language delay. This is especially true since many children experience frequent ear infections and manage to develop language normally. In many cases the precipitating factors are clear, as in instances of stroke, vocal abuse, structural abnormalities, and certain congenital conditions.

The perpetuating factors are those variables currently at work on the individual. Almost without exception, habit strength is a prime perpetuating factor in many disorders since the client has made various compensations for the problem in terms of cognitive/linguistic strategies and motoric adjustments. Other factors are also crucial, however, and it is the diagnostician's task to uncover the environmental and physical factors that are reinforcing and thus perpetuating the disorder. A hearing loss may be a precipitating and a perpetuating factor in a child's language delay. This child needs a thorough audiological evaluation and a prescription for amplification if indicated, or else the problem will perpetuate. We must always work to identify and, if possible, remove or reduce any factors that maintain a communication disorder.

Diagnosis to Provide Clinical Focus

Although it is important to know the causes of the disorder, it is substantially more important to gain some insight into the possible ways to improve the client's communication. It is at this point that diagnosis and clinical management overlap. This is also where the importance of knowing a host of evaluation techniques becomes significant in the diagnostic enterprise. There is a series of questions that the diagnostician must ask:

1. What do I know about this condition?

   What are the usual etiologies?
   What are the usual effective treatment procedures?
   What is the typical prognosis?

2. What do I know about this person?

   What is the impact of the condition on the person?
   What are the person's strengths and weaknesses?
   How is this person like others I have worked with?
   How is this person different from others I have worked with?

3. What do I know about my own skills in treatment of this disorder and this type of person?

   How have I effectively approached similar problems?
   How have I effectively worked with similar people?

4. What do I know about the services of other professionals available for this person?

   What referrals need to be made?
   What consultations do I need to make?

5. What factors need to be removed, altered, or added to improve the prognosis?

   What inhibiting environmental factors exist?
   What organic factors need alteration?
   What can enhance the person's motivation?

If diagnosis is to be of utmost benefit it must be goal oriented. Diagnosis is an empty exercise in test administration, data collection, and client evaluation if it fails to provide logical suggestions for treatment. Most clinicians would like to believe that for each client, there is a magic procedure that will work to improve communication. In almost every disorder area (fluency, voice, language, articulation), however, there is a multitude of procedures from which to select. Not only are there different types of treatment in terms of philosophy, entry level, and targets trained, but there are differences in the nature of the delivery system (e.g., highly structured, behavioral, client directed, cognitive, etc.). Thus, the SLP is faced with a number of avenues from which to choose in terms of making treatment recommendations. Within the context of the diagnostic session(s), the well-trained and experienced clinician can make some clinical judgments regarding the types of treatment that may be of benefit to a particular client based on his or her performance on evaluation tasks. Sometimes the SLP can make these judgments in a general manner, using overall impressions from the diagnostic experience as a guide. On other occasions, some trial therapy can be performed in the context of evaluation tasks, and actual data can be gathered to support one approach to treatment or another.

This notion of using time in a diagnostic session to gain insight into performance on treatment tasks is known as "dynamic assessment" (Lidz 1991; Olswang et al. 1986; Pena 1996; Wade and Haynes 1989). We feel that dynamic assessment is an important part of any diagnostic venture since it is from these tasks that direction for treatment emerges. Figure 1.2 illustrates salient differences between dynamic and static assessment. Static assessment is like a "snapshot" of a child's performance at a given moment in time. When we administer a standardized test, we are capturing a child's performance at a certain point, and we may characterize this behavior as a number or score. Static assessment, however, does not address how the child may be able to perform more effectively with assistance by the clinician or under altered circumstances. Dynamic assessment relies heavily on Vygotsky's (1978) notion of the "Zone of Proximal Development," which defines a range of performance that a child can produce with assistance from adults or peers. Standardized tests do not allow the clinician to assist a child or ask the client why he or she answered a question in a particular manner. In dynamic assessment we can determine a client's range of performance, given help by the clinician, and can find what types of circumstances result in improved performance. Wade and Haynes (1989) found that investing as little as thirty minutes of an evaluation in trial therapy demonstrated distinct performance differences in the types of cues responded to by children with language impairment.

Almost every communication disorder area has a variety of variables to experiment with during a diagnostic session. We are of the opinion that treatment should be viewed rather like a single-subject experimental design. No one really knows which type of treatment will be effective for a given client or which variables will have the most impact on performance. This is typically learned during the first stage of treatment as the clinician begins to fine-tune the management program. However, the diagnostic session can easily be used to gain some insight into

FIGURE 1.2   Comparison of Static and Dynamic Assessment

Static Assesment	Dynamic Assessment
Passive Participants Child does task without help	**Active Participants** Child participates with adult help; Can ask questions and get feedback
Examiner Observes Scores Test; typically right/wrong responses	**Examiner Participates** Give feedback; help child develop strategies
Results Identify Deficits Test results profile deficits, what child can/cannot do	**Results Describe Modifiability** Results profile how responsive the child is given help; describes strategies
Standardized Administration Given in standardized manner, no deviation from standard format	**Administration Fluid, Responsive** Nonstandardized administration; examiner responses contingent on child's behavior

Adapted from Pena, E., Quinn, R., and Iglesias, A. (1991)

client tendencies and preferences. Clients with aphasia may respond more favorably to certain combinations of cues in word retrieval. Clients with fluency disorders may become more fluent with one particular technique than with a second method. One client may express relief that the clinician is willing to talk about the psychological component of the problem during part of the diagnostic session, which may suggest that this covert dimension should at least be considered as a potential part of the treatment program. A child with a language impairment may respond better to a structured task as opposed to a child-directed one, or vice versa. A person with a voice disorder may be more able to alter vocal parameters by using feedback from certain instrumentation rather than not using this type of monitoring. A nonverbal child may show a marked tendency to learn a few gestures during a diagnostic session than to master vocal productions or words.

We could continue with examples of ways in which the clinician can use a portion of the diagnostic session to learn about the client's response to certain treatment variables. While the diagnostician should never make treatment recommendations based only on hunches, the judicious use of evaluation tasks in the assessment can suggest a reasonable starting point for treatment in many cases. Of course, these recommendations should be treated as working hypotheses and should be stated as such in the diagnostic report. The initial selection of a treatment option is in most cases only an educated guess and is always subject to change based on client performance. This is why we view evaluation as an ongoing process throughout the treatment experience.

Diagnosis: Science and Art

Diagnosis demands a unique blend of science and art (Silverman 1984). The scientific method is applicable to our work as diagnosticians, both in guiding our procedures and in focusing our attitude of operation. The scientific method directs the diagnostician to observe all of the available factors, to formulate testable hypotheses by using clearly stated and answerable questions, to test those hypotheses to determine their validity, and to reach conclusions based on the tested hypotheses. The method demands rigorous adherence to standardized procedures and has as its favorable characteristics objectivity, quantifiability, and structure. The scientific diagnostician tends to rely on tests, test data, and other procedures that lend themselves to quantification. As an attitude of operation, the scientific method implies that the diagnostician has not predetermined the test findings and that there is no bias in seeking the proof or disproof of hypotheses. The diagnostician sees hypotheses as something to be tested rather than something to be defended.

The self-fulfilling prophecy is a lethal but almost universal human characteristic; it must be counterbalanced by a scientific approach to testing. We are familiar with parents of children with language impairment who had traveled all over the country in search of a diagnostic explanation for the linguistic delay. Often these children are victims of the "fat folder syndrome" in which a case file has accrued over the years with reports from various authorities and clinics. Each report often reveals more about the examiner than the child as it cites facts in support of a theory of etiology congruent with the diagnostician's particular specialty. Finding what you want to find is not always in the realm of the scientific method. Diagnosticians often use their pet test instruments, to use a famous saying, as the drunk uses the street lamp—more for support than illumination!

The strict adherence to fact that is demanded by the pure scientific method is often a bit confining. That, in part, may explain why we all practice the art of diagnosis at times. The artistic approach has several specific characteristics. The artist is less dependent on specific observations than on casual and nonstructured scrutiny for the formation of hypotheses. This type of clinician is perfectly willing to disregard formal test results or standard testing procedures in favor of what appears obvious on the basis of clinical experience and expertise. The hunch, or clinical intuition, plays a significant part in such evaluations. The diagnostician will contend that facts can be approached from several directions and that we are capable of assessing the same kinds of behaviors that are measured by formal tests. Such contentions are disconcerting to the test-bound person who has come to expect that the only valid way to gain information is through standardized procedures. One of the emphases in the present textbook is that these informal, nonstandardized evaluation procedures are valuable indeed in defining a client's problem and the potential response to treatment. In many ways these procedures may be more valid than standardized tests, as we will discuss in Chapter 3.

It is obvious that, in the extreme, there are weaknesses in both approaches. The scientist may tend to become so dependent on objective methods of measurement that there is a failure to see the client through the maze of percentiles and standard scores. The whole is greater than the sum of its parts, and every diagnostician must guard against simply measuring the isolated characteristics without getting a full picture of the individual. Do not build altars to any testing device; every objective instrument was once only an idea in someone's mind. The art end of the science–art continuum is just as precarious as the scientific end. The possibility of a diagnostician's projecting more than a modest amount of personal bias into the evaluation is greater when a less-scientific approach is used. Clinical intuitions are often simply clinical biases, and it is very easy to make new evidence fit old categories. The diagnostician must find the proper mixture of each philosophy in establishing assessment procedures (Deutscher 1983; Ringel, Trachtman, and Prutting 1984).

Diagnosis versus Eligibility

As our legal system, medical settings and public school systems have become more complicated, clinicians are faced with increasing pressure to conduct their clinical work within parameters that are set by administrators. The resulting procedures for case selection, testing, and determining eligibility for services many times fall short of the ideal professional criteria used to make these decisions.

A prominent special education attorney of our acquaintance has won cases in almost every state of the union. When asked why his record of litigation was so impressive he replied: "I win cases because schools make important decisions about children based on *administrative* criteria instead of *professional* criteria." We need to continually ask ourselves if we are doing the best thing for the client as dictated by the current state of knowledge in our profession. While we cannot always do everything optimally for a client in certain work settings, we need to be very careful in our decisions to streamline services and not make arbitrary decisions for administrative purposes that undermine our profession.

The influence of administrative decision making on our profession has blurred the distinction between diagnosis, on the one hand, and determining eligibility, on the other. For example, it is not unusual for private practitioners and community clinics to provide services to children who have clear language/phonological disorders but who are ineligible for such services in the local school system. Similarly, it is not unusual for private practitioners and university clinics to provide services to medically involved patients whose insurance carriers will no longer pay for treatment. Ehren (1993) states:

> *Eligibility often shapes caseloads in ways that seem inconsistent with the state of the art. . . . In lieu of making a diagnosis, we ascertain whether the student meets eligibility criteria. Evaluation, then, becomes an eligibility determination process, rather than a process to describe a student's communication status. . . . We need to develop identification procedures that promote clinical decision making. Speech-language pathologists need to return to their clinical roots and employ their diagnostic skills in identifying students with communication disorders. First, we need to make a diagnosis; next, recommend the need for service; then, discuss eligibility. Diagnosis should drive eligibility; eligibility should not dictate the diagnosis. Eligibility criteria should be viewed as the last hoop to jump through in identifying a student. (20)*

The Diagnostician as a Factor

Ultimately, the most important diagnostic tool is the diagnostician. The clients we assess have seldom read the test manual, and the rigid structure of the testing situation may not be compatible with fluid and nonstructured styles of behavior. Tests are abstractions of behavior, and as such they represent only a fraction of the child's total repertoire of responses to the environment. What better measure of an individual's behavior than that behavior itself? Thus, the diagnostician becomes an important aspect of the evaluating situation in selecting measurements, interacting, responding, and assembling information.

What skills are necessary to develop in order to become an effective diagnostician? How do you develop them? There are no easy answers to these questions. Experience in the diagnostic process is an absolute necessity, but experience in number of clients seen is not enough. A pompous clinician once bragged, "I've had over twenty years of experience." The unfortunate thing, however, is that this person had the first year of experience repeated nineteen times, which is altogether a different matter. The diagnostician must be able to gain from new experiences, and this demands *flexibility.* The stereotyped and stagnant diagnostician learns little from increased exposure to people and new situations, but those diagnosticians who use their experience as a pattern to be compared against, rather than as a mold into which all new experiences must fit, will continue to grow and learn. The diagnostician must be flexible enough within the testing situation to shift from predetermined plans to new modes of evaluation as the client presents unpredicted behaviors. The examiner who steadfastly plods through a series of tests even though a client is presenting some interesting new behavior or exhibiting valid instances of communication ability in nontest contexts will miss an important opportunity to gain insight into the problem. It is not atypical for beginning clinicians to panic in the face of an unexpected performance and become intransigent in their application of a series of formal tests because there is a certain degree of comfort in known processes. Continued experience in diagnosis may provide the flexibility needed to move freely to other avenues of information.

Another characteristic of a good diagnostician is a *healthy skepticism* and ability to *critically evaluate* new clinical techniques. Practicing clinicians often eagerly accept new and novel techniques as they become available. As the profession moves into new, uncharted areas of concern, many new materials, tests, and techniques become available. New techniques must not be accepted or rejected carte blanche but rather must be scrutinized for their merit. We must learn to keep up with new developments by participating in an active continuing education program, both personal and professional. On the other hand, the beginning student must guard against the "recent article" syndrome to which we all fall prey upon occasion. Typically, the behavioral pattern goes something like this: You read an article that depicts a particular syndrome and explains the distinctive characteristics of a disorder; for a few weeks thereafter every child you see appears to fall into the pattern described in the publication. The way to overcome the "recent article" syndrome, of course, is to be aware that it exists and to have a thorough understanding of the nature of human perception. With regard to new tests and measurements, techniques grossly foreign to experience tend to threaten and bewilder the inflexible clinician because these are perceived as attacks on trusted and time-proven methods. On the other hand, some clinicians get into the "recent test" syndrome and use the most-popular test of the day simply because it is new. It is possible that training programs that emphasize formal testing, fixed therapy programs, and a focus on materials are more likely to produce an inflexible, nonevaluative clinician than are those programs that emphasize theory, problem-solving ability, creativity, and descriptive assessment techniques.

A clinician must possess many important *interpersonal relationship attributes.* Rogers (1942) speaks of empathy, congruency, and unconditional positive regard as necessary characteristics of the clinician, and they most certainly apply to the diagnostic process as well. In many studies of clinical competence, both supervisors in speech-language pathology as well as adult clients perceive the interpersonal relationship to be a major factor in contributing to successful treatment (Haynes and Oratio 1978; Oratio 1977). Generally these qualities must be nurtured by consistent effort and proper guidance in training programs through analysis by clinical supervisors and review of session videotapes by clinicians in training.

If the term *sensitivity* may be defined as a keenness of sense or a heightened awareness of incoming sensory data, then this term has meaning for the diagnostician. The clinician must be able to detect subtle physical, psychological, or interactional changes in a client's behavior, since these small changes may have significant meaning in the diagnostic process. For further reading in enhancing awareness skills, see the works of Johnson (1972) and others (Buscaglia 1982; Emerick and Hood 1975).

Insight into the meaning and clinical significance of behaviors must be developed from a thorough grounding in the basic processes requisite for communication. Each diagnostician must become so familiar with the normal process of language acquisition and normal communicative functioning that he/she has a built-in set of standards on which to base judgment. The insightful clinician is the knowledgeable professional who is capable of quickly comparing the client's behavior with the norm.

The development of an *evaluative attitude* is often a rather difficult task for the beginning clinician. We are, to a large extent, slaves to our experience; each clinician tends to bring a social attitude into the testing setting. Rather than look upon the client's performance as having meaning for the evaluative process, we consult our own responses and formulate our own points of view in the give-and-take of the conversation. The critical, questioning attitude must be developed so that the clinician looks upon the behaviors in terms of their meaning rather than in terms of the response expected. Social interaction lends itself to superficiality, whereas the flow of the diagnostic interaction must, by design, lend itself to uncovering the meaning of the incorporated behavior. Effective diagnosticians tend to question the surface validity of behaviors and search for motivations, explanations, and interpretations that are not readily apparent.

Closely allied with the concept of the evaluative attitude is the idea of *persistent curiosity*. The diagnostician must develop an inquisitiveness that will make him or her persistent in searching for explanations. Answers are seldom apparent at first, and continuous effort is imperative. Training institutions often foster weakness in this area when they assign clients to students and expect therapy to get under way in a "reasonable" period of time. Additionally, they are so bound to the rigid university timetables that treatment is often discontinuous. In an attempt to give each student a variety of clinical experiences, training institutions often tend to sever clinical undertakings with a client at each semester's end, knowing full well that the diagnostic or therapeutic process is not best served in this way. The student may not always understand that these have been decisions based on program convenience rather than client need and may develop the notion that diagnosis is a temporary therapy-initiating exercise to be completed in an hour or two. The curious and persistent clinician, however, continues to place the client in situations that will permit additional scrutiny. It would be ideal, albeit probably unworkable in training programs, for students to follow their clients over longer periods of time so that the students could see how diagnosis is an ongoing process and an integral part of treatment as the client changes.

Objectivity comes from practicing the art of controlled involvement. The diagnostician must cultivate objectivity because we are all subject to human errors. We must be warm, understanding, and accepting, on the one hand, and objective, evaluative, and detached, on the other. Without some degree of balance between the two extremes, the diagnostician may so severely distort the interaction with the client that little information of value is obtained. Objectivity demands more than simply guarding against undue emotional involvement. To grow as a diagnostician, the examiner must be objective about his or her skills, knowledge, and personal characteristics and must take an objective attitude toward the client.

Rapport may be defined as the establishment of a working relationship, based on mutual respect, trust, and confidence, that encourages optimum performance on the part of both client and clinician. Rapport is developed over a period of time and is not easily established in a single session or during a few minutes at the initiation of one diagnostic encounter. Rapport must not only be developed, it must be maintained, and this calls for continued effort. There is a growing literature in the area of formal tests that indicates that, especially with children, test performance varies with clinician familiarity (Fuchs et al. 1985). In essence, children tend to perform better if they have had an opportunity to become familiar with an examiner. While the reasons for this phenomenon are not totally clear, the concept of rapport is obviously involved.

It is important that our *focus* be on the client as much as possible instead of on our own performance and internal states. Diagnosticians are people too, and we often forget that they occasionally have "a bad day." They too can experience the influence of pervasive personal problems and physical frailties that sometimes make them feel as though they should have stayed at home in bed. The most knowledgeable and skillful diagnostician, however, may fail to achieve adequate results if he or she lacks the inquisitiveness necessary to encourage continuous effort and if there is no professional drive to serve each individual to the maximum potential. Each of us is subject to individual variations in daily behavior (physical problems, depression, stress, etc.) that can have a direct effect on performance; however, it is incumbent upon every professional to control those variations so as to provide each individual with the best service available.

The Client-Clinician Relationship

Although much standardization is possible through strict adherence to test routines, the lowest common denominator in diagnostic evaluations is the examiner. Test results are the product of the subject, examiner, test and test circumstance, each of which has a certain influence. Examinations are clearly selected as a result of the experiences and biases of the examiner. Just as the answers we receive to questions are in part a function of the questions we ask and how we ask them, the diagnostic findings we obtain are in part a function of the tests we administer and the way they are administered. A defective communication pattern may be partially due to a defective testing pattern or a defective tester.

The most-crucial factor in conducting a successful diagnostic session is the client-clinician relationship. When a person works with another, there is always human impact; even when clients are treated by computers, they come to accord human attributes to the machines. No matter how well prepared and rehearsed an examiner may be, if his or her approach to people is poor, failure will ensue. All tests, all examinations, all so-called objective diagnostic procedures are mediated by person-to-person contact.

We can be seduced into grave errors by test norms, percentile scores, and standard examination procedures: A human being is a total functioning unit, and the various tests are multiple and fragmented. Even if the instruments we use are relatively precise (which they are not), and we are deluded into thinking that the client is functioning with the same degree of precision in the testing situation, human elements may disturb the validity of the tests no matter how refined the scoring procedures or how calibrated the machines.

Impersonal, test-oriented clinical examination sessions can also make assessment more difficult since there is no absolute division between diagnosis and therapy. The first contact with a client initiates treatment. During a diagnostic session the client is forming opinions and conceptions about the clinician and the total clinical situation. Barker and his colleagues (1953) have warned that "while to the medical practitioner, diagnosis and therapy are often routine technical jobs, to the patient the situation never has such limited personal meaning. To him diagnosis and therapy are a route to highly important life conditions"(310). Not all clients will require the full impact of this interpersonal dimension. Indeed, some individuals simply want to find out what is wrong and then rectify the situation. The point is, however, that the clinician should be able to discern what the client needs and then adjust his or her style appropriately.

The Client as a Factor: Children, Adolescents, and Adults

Although all age levels present unique diagnostic problems, three groups in particular—young children, adolescents, and to a lesser extent, older or elderly clients—require special effort and expertise. Since the present chapter is generic in nature, we will mainly talk about the general business of relating to the different age groups seen in diagnostic evaluations. The more-specific chapters that follow will provide additional suggestions for dealing with the different age groups in the context of evaluating particular disorders. A major reason for including this generic section is that many readers of the present text are students in training to become speech-language pathologists. It is often difficult for a young person to capture the ephemeral guidelines for relating to people of different ages. It is not as simple as just "being yourself" or talking one way to a child and another way to an adult. There are certain common errors students have made over the years that we can at least alert you to so that you may avoid them. These precepts, of course, are drawn from the experiences of the authors, and there are obviously many more guidelines that could be added.

1. *Young Children.* Preschool and kindergarten children are often difficult to test and examine. Unlike most older children and adults, they just do not see the payoff for all the questioning and prodding. Often a major problem is dealing with

the child's fear of the clinical situation. This apprehension may stem from one or more of the following related factors: (1) inadequate preparation for the examination by parents, (2) uncertainty as to what will be done to or with the child by the clinician, (3) vivid memories of trauma during visits to dentists and physicians, (4) the contagious anxieties and uncertainties experienced by the parents, and (5) stress and conflicts engendered by past listener reactions to the speech impairment. Children confront the clinical examination in a variety of ways, but the two most-trying responses are shyness and withdrawal and, at the other extreme, aggressiveness and hyperactivity.

In many cases with very young children, it is possible to have the parent participate in the interaction, and this avoids any separation anxiety on the part of the child. The parents are typically willing to cooperate, the child is happy, and the parents can often get the child to do many things that the clinician would take several sessions of rapport building to accomplish. Parents can even be used to administer some formal tests that just involve turning picture plates and reading the cues on the backs of the pictures, while the clinician scores the child's responses. We have to choose our battles very carefully, and fighting an obstreperous child in a diagnostic session mainly leads to unsatisfying results for all concerned. In dealing with the children in the birth-to-two age range, *most* of the pertinent information will be gleaned from parents, both from interview data and by observation of parent-child interaction. Not many one-year-olds do well with an unfamiliar clinician, and we need to focus on the parent-child dyad anyway since treatment will doubtless involve the entire family.

There are obviously many other considerations that could be discussed; additional suggestions will be offered in the chapters concerning various disorders. For the present, here are several basic precepts on the management of preschool children in a clinical examination:

a. Help the parents prepare the child for the diagnostic session. They can tell him or her what will transpire, and maybe even bring along some stimulus items favored by the child (toys, picture albums, books, etc.).

b. Play, rather than small talk, is the natural medium of expression for children. This is especially important when dealing with potentially disordered youngsters. While we have all known children in the three-to-five age range that are impressive conversationalists, most children referred for communication disorders are not on this end of the conversational continuum. Try to arrange the diagnostic tasks with this in mind.

c. As a general rule, ask less and observe more. Children usually lack the insight and cooperation necessary to analyze their problem rationally and objectively. Naturalistic observations—assessing a child's behavior in natural environments—yields more useful information.

d. The prospective diagnostician should learn everything possible about normal children in order to provide a baseline for observations of youngsters presenting problems. This can be done by taking courses, studying relevant norms, but most of all by extensive scrutiny and interaction with children in day-care and preschool facilities. The prospective diagnostician should have a good idea of the typical or modal behavior for children at various age levels. One student claimed that a four-year-old client was in grave need of psychiatric appraisal and treatment. We remembered the child and were somewhat puzzled by this recommendation. We demanded a rationale. It seems that the child had an imaginary companion, a wrinkled green elephant that served as a scapegoat and alter ego. We chuckled and then sent the student scurrying to the library to see how common such fantasies are in four-year-olds.

e. Limit the choices you offer a child. Don't ask if he or she would like to go with you, do this or that, unless the alternatives do not conflict with the examiner's goals. The child will invariably say "No!" Also, refrain from saying "OK?" after your utterances ("I want you to name these pictures, OK?"). This question suggests that there is an option available.

f. Be flexible in your use of tests and examinations. If you cannot employ the rigid standardized format for administration, use the test to obtain all the data you can. If the child refuses to name the test pictures or objects, you may be able to get a language sample from other items. Also, if there is no standard order for administration of tests and tasks, go with the items the child appears to be interested in at a particular time. For example, if a test has some objects associated with it and the child is attending to these items, start this examination even if you had initially planned it for later in the session.

g. Absolute honesty and candor is important in working with children. Do not make promises unless you can keep them.

h. The whole assessment does not have to be done in one session; marathon diagnostics tend to be counterproductive. Remember that all we can hope to obtain in one time frame is a sample of a child's behaviors. It is better to terminate (preferably on a pleasant, successful note) than to continue an unproductive session until the child is fatigued and/or upset.

i. Watch your language complexity when talking to children. For obvious reasons, the examiner should avoid sarcasm, idiomatic expressions, ambiguous statements, and indirect requests (Blue 1981).

2. *Adolescents.* Experienced clinicians frequently report that adolescents, the classical teenagers, especially in grades 7 through 11, are often difficult to examine and resistant to treatment. The main problem seems to be getting through to the person. There is no magic formula for this, but we would like to make some suggestions that we have found helpful in guiding our work with adolescent clients:

a. Acquire an understanding of the myriad pressures and changes the teenager is experiencing: rapid physical growth, sexual maturity, conflicts between dependence and independence, the development of self-confidence and interpersonal skills necessary to make decisions, a search for identity and life work, intense group loyalty and identification, and many more. It is a turbulent, trying period of behavioral extravagance and excess. Small wonder that teenagers are often overloaded with personal concerns and do not always welcome an overture of clinical assistance. Empathy that flows from understanding is a powerful force in establishing a working relationship.

b. There is an intense desire to be like others, not to stand out from the group in any way that would suggest frailty. Hence, the adolescent may find it extremely difficult to reveal a speech impairment, even if help is desired. Often teenagers are simply sent for evaluation or treatment by parents. In some instances, the teenager with a chronic problem may have been in treatment for a long time and is weary of the idea of more therapy. Many will tend to cover up true feelings with a sullen bravado or a dense "it-doesn't-bother-me" shell. Denial is a particular forte. "Coolness" and image are very important. You can neither beat this down nor simply dismiss it with a shrug. Nor is silence a particularly effective tool in dealing with adolescent resistance. We advocate a straightforward approach; acknowledge the forces that are bearing on the individual; point up objectively the paths that others have taken; provide information about the economic and social penalties that accrue to the person with a communication disorder. The young client may need more time to become accustomed to the idea of therapy. Basically, try to demonstrate by your demeanor and what you say that you care about the client; a growing person needs lots of nourishment, and personal involvement and commitment are key factors.

c. Do not abandon your professional role for that of a teenager. Be yourself. As Will Rogers pointed out, if they don't like you the way you are, they are sure not going to like you the way you are trying to be.

d. Approach adolescents with tolerance and good humor. Do not be shocked or annoyed by their overstatements and superlatives; do not overreact to expressions of hostility or tempests of other emotions. Sometimes adolescents will, in order to uphold their protective armor, resort to all sorts of strategies to confuse, defeat or anger the clinician. The ability to laugh at yourself and to use humor in a gentle, needling manner is an asset. Remember, though, to always treat the adolescent with honesty and dignity—don't make fun of intense or idealistic views.

e. Explain the diagnostic process as much as possible by explaining what we are about, the reasons for the various tests and examinations, and how we will use the information. We encourage the adolescent to challenge and question what we are doing. Finally, we usually give the client an idea of the route we would follow when therapy commences, or we even do some trial treatment activities.

f. If the client is highly critical of parents or school officials, we must keep the person's confidences and not act in a judgmental manner. We do not enter into the criticism or side with the client against others, nor do we try to defend the institution or retreat to moralisms.

g. Discuss the results of the evaluation with the client before talking with the parents or school personnel. Be sure to let the client know exactly what you intend to tell parents and teachers and determine any feelings the client has about these suggestions.

These recommendations have been distilled from our clinical experience and are not presented as magical touchstones for all diagnosticians or all clients; nor do these recommendations represent the full range of possibilities for successful interaction with teenage clients. We present them here to encourage other workers to develop clinical generalizations on the basis of their experience (O'Connor and Eldredge 1981).

3. *The Elderly Client.* Older clients may present some rather special problems for the diagnostician, or they may need no particular special handling. Although the concept of "elderly" is relative, we refer here to persons in their sixties or older. A word of caution: Although there are certain generalizations that are useful for planning and conducting evaluations, elderly people are not any more "all alike" than are children or adolescents.

The clinician should be alert to fatigue, disorientation, failing eyesight, and hearing loss. With advanced age, the person may find it more difficult to focus attention on a task and generally may have trouble remembering directions because of possible short-term memory decline. Many of these potential problems are exacerbated when the person has experienced a neurological insult, as in a good number of elderly clients. We need, therefore, to explain each step of our clinical procedures at greater length and repeat instructions when necessary to ensure understanding. Our pace should be geared to the client's abilities if necessary to a slower level. Organize the testing sequence carefully to reduce distractions, noise, or interference. Older people are often more cautious and have a greater need to be certain before they respond, so adapt the tasks with this in mind; following standard procedure may not be as important as providing an environment in which the person is able to perform at an optimal level.

Since many older clients tend to feel useless and discarded in our youth oriented culture, and resentful that their bodies are betraying them, we may find it important to spend some time listening to their memories of past achievements. Older clients should always be treated with respect and not referred to by their first names. The clinician should also guard against using a louder vocal intensity and increased pitch range as if talking to a child. It is grossly offensive to infantalize an adult client. Many of our elderly clients will come to us with neurologically based disorders, serious vocal pathologies, and other medically related problems. There will be a tendency among many to talk about medical issues, since their problems have originated from this area. It is important for the diagnostician to be patient with these clients and listen to their concerns, while still not allowing conversation about medical issues to interfere with the testing.

In most cases, clinicians will find older clients to be interesting, socially adept individuals to be treated with courtesy and respect. The number of people over sixty composes a significant proportion of the population, and we cannot afford to perpetuate the stereotype that old people are expendable or that they should be relegated to demeaning idleness. As with children and adolescents, the diagnostician should know as much as possible about aging. Many references pertinent to communication disorders are readily available (Beasley and Davis 1981; Moore and Sherman 1981; Mueller and Peters 1981; National Council on Aging 1982; Shadden 1988).

Putting the Diagnosis to Work

Perhaps the most demanding of all diagnostic ventures is the ultimate synthesis of findings into a coherent statement of the nature of the problem. The skilled clinician draws the findings together by using the data available, past experience, knowledge, and intuition to formulate a total picture of the condition. At this point textbooks, research findings, and academic lectures fail to provide all of what is needed to succeed. Maturation of skills will only develop in an extensive practicum under the close supervision of a knowledgeable diagnostician. The essence of the synthesis process is a comparison of what is observed with what we expect to observe from our knowledge of the normal process. The incongruities between the observed and the normal provide the building blocks for completion of the picture. Figure 1.3 identifies a model of diagnosis as a synthesis of findings and shows a number of outcomes to which the synthesis might lead. This figure points out several important concepts.

First, the bedrock of the entire model is the clinician's knowledge and skill base. Without adequate training and experience the administration of tests and tasks becomes meaningless.

A second important point in the model is the series of six boxes that are immediately above the clinician's knowledge and skill base. These boxes highlight the diversity of information that the diagnostician should ideally obtain in order

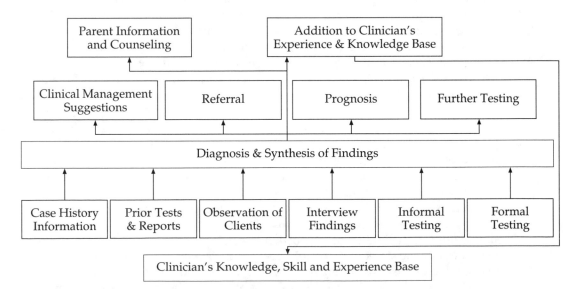

FIGURE 1.3   Components of an Effective Diagnosis/Evaluation

to make a principled judgment about a client's disorder (case history, prior reports, observation, interview, informal testing and formal testing). Interestingly, it is not unusual for prior reports and tests to be missing or unrequested, case history information to be returned by the client at the time of evaluation instead of prior to it, the case history forms to be incomplete or lost, and the interview cut to a ten-minute conversation because of time pressure. It is also not unusual for the clinician to spend the entire assessment time giving tests with little opportunity left for informal testing or observation of clients in relevant situations. While it is difficult to obtain information from all six boxes in the model, we must try to get as close to the ideal as possible. In many settings, the evaluation will not take place unless the client has submitted all pertinent information and unless reports from other agencies have been received. It is certainly that way in many other professions (medicine, psychology, etc.). We must ask ourselves about the quality of the diagnostic evaluation that is done with incomplete information. What is the efficacy of performing an evaluation if we do not have access to critical information and are not willing to spend the time to carry on a decent interview and do informal testing and client observation.

A third area in the center of the model is the synthesis of findings. This is where we begin to see overlaps in the data from case history, interview, reports, observations, and testing results. We should look for common threads among all of these information sources and tie them together in the synthesis and diagnosis. Often, this is where certain informational components begin to disagree with one another—which is also informative. For example, the parents indicate intense concern over their child's articulation in the case history and the interview. They also bring a host of prior reports that indicate the child has no clinically significant problem, and they look to you for guidance. If your own test results, informal task performance, and observations indicate that the child is performing within normal limits, the discrepancy between these components and the parents' perceptions is obvious. The prior reports also now gain significant importance in terms of counseling the parents and pointing out the disparity between their views and the perceptions of many professionals. Another example may point out the foibles associated with one or more of the sources of information. For instance, a child may not perform within normal limits on formal tests of language ability. Yet, that same child communicates well in informal tasks and observations of play interactions with caretakers and peers. The clinician must question the formal test results if the child's communication exceeds that which these measures suggest he or she is capable of.

A fourth series of five boxes in the model point out some important components important of a diagnostic evaluation that are present after the synthesis of information. As we mentioned earlier, a good diagnostician will make suggestions for treatment in terms of which goals may be logically selected for initial intervention. The parents need to be counseled about the results of the evaluation, and any problems or feelings they express must be dealt with. Often we are so zealous in performing the evaluation and in scheduling time for doing everything we feel is necessary that we give the client or parents short shrift in explaining our results.

In many cases, the results we report to parents or clients represent a significant affective burden. For example, even though parents usually know in their hearts that their child has a communication disorder, they often hold out the hope that their child really is not disordered and will grow out of a language or articulation difference. By telling parents that their child is indeed showing an impairment and is now officially in the ranks of the handicapped, it forces them to come to terms with this problem. Diagnosticians frequently experience parents or clients who cry at the culmination of the evaluation session when they are told something that confirms the idea of a disorder and/or commits them to an undetermined length of time spent in rehabilitation. Other emotions also emerge, such as anger and denial, which must sometimes be dealt with at the end of the diagnostic session. Emotions aside, it is enough of a challenge simply to communicate the complex evaluation results to parents of different educational levels and abilities. A skilled diagnostician has the ability to summarize assessment results and recommendations on the correct level of abstraction for different parents and spouses. Another aspect to deal with after synthesis is the possibility of referral. Many cases require a consultation by other professionals, such as audiologists, laryngologists, neurologists, special educators, psychologists, and others. Often the assessment raises more questions than it answers, and this is perfectly acceptable. We need to know the parameters of the patient's problem and many times this insight can only be gained from professionals who have expertise in areas with which we are not totally familiar.

Prognosis is another variable depicted in Figure 1.3. Prognosis may be defined as a prediction of the outcome of a proposed course of treatment for a given client: how effective treatment will be, how far we can expect the client to progress, and, perhaps, how long it will take. Inasmuch as diagnosis is a continuing process, prognosis should, like treatment planning, have both long-range and immediate facets. Immediate prognosis covers what the person can do now, what steps in therapy are possible, and what is the best route to take. Prognosis for specific communication disorders will be discussed in subsequent chapters; in this section we will present some generic purposes and a possible danger involved in predicting a client's response to treatment.

One basic purpose in making a prognosis is to economize our therapeutic efforts. There is only so much time and energy, and we must focus it on those clients who show the greatest promise of improvement. Patients and families also want to know what they may expect in terms of progress. Some general factors that the clinician must consider when making predictions are as follows:

1. *Age.* The chronological age of the client is a gross predictor of treatment success. In general, the younger the client, the better the treatment outcome. This can be seen in childhood disorders where the earlier the intervention is begun, the more progress can be made prior to school entrance. The earlier we involve children in treatment, the more likely we are to prevent the formation of secondary problems (Shine 1980; Starkweather, Gottwald, and Halfond 1990) such as social, psychological, and educational penalties. In adult cases, it is well known that patients who develop neurogenic disorders at younger ages (40–60) are generally given better prognoses than patients who develop these problems at later ages (70–90) (Rosenbeck, LaPointe, and Wertz 1989). This, of course, is due to a variety of reasons that include psychological, motivational, and physical factors. Thus, age is a macrovariable that in and of itself is not a potent variable, but it subsumes many factors that do have an influence on prognosis.

   2. *Length of Time Impairment Has Existed.* The length of time a client has had a disorder of communication may relate to prognosis. Obviously, if the impairment has a component of habitual activities (motor patterns, processing strategies, etc.) these are more difficult to alter in clients who have performed them for a lengthy period. In addition to the habit patterns developed over time, the client has also learned complex ancillary adjustment patterns to compensate for the communication impairment that may involve social, psychological, and motoric activities. These compensatory patterns eventually become part of the problem and often must be eliminated, as in the case of operant behaviors learned by stutterers (head jerks, timing devices, etc.).

   3. *Existence of Other Problems.* It is axiomatic that the more problems a client has, the more difficult it will be to deal with the disorder. A client with aphasia who is also hearing impaired will be more difficult than one with the language disorder alone. A child with a cleft palate and articulation problems will be more difficult than one with the articulation problem alone. A child who is language impaired and mentally retarded is different from one who presents only a language disorder.

   4. *Reactions of Significant Others.* A child with a communication disorder is going to make better progress in treatment if the parent takes an active role in the intervention. Many parents are interested in participating in treatment and will carry on home programs. On the other hand, if a child is brought to the clinic by a social worker and the parents do not appear interested in treatment, this child will probably take longer to succeed in remediation. If the spouse of a patient with aphasia is disinterested in facilitating communication, the client may make slower progress. The same can be said about the cooperation of teachers, aides, day-care providers, siblings, peers, and anyone else who comes in significant contact with the client and is in a position to help with treatment. Generally, the more assistance available from significant others, the better the prognosis.

   5. *Client Motivation.* While we have no reliable way to measure motivation in a client, most diagnosticians can recognize it when they see it. If the client appears enthusiastic, interested, and anxious to begin treatment, it is clearly a plus. If the client is an adult, was he or she self-referred? This may be a positive indication as opposed to a person referred by an employer or teacher or dragged to the evaluation by a domineering spouse. There may also be some positive prognostic value in cases where the client has something to gain from successful treatment (better social life, higher-paying job, etc.). Motivation is always difficult to quantify, but few would totally disregard the importance of this admittedly blurry construct.

   Accurate prognoses can help establish our credibility with other professions. The ability to predict with reasonable precision is perhaps the highest form of scientific achievement. Needless to say, however, these predictions should be based on something more than clinical intuition. Impressionistic conclusions, especially when made by experienced workers, can often be startlingly accurate, but they should always be labeled as impressionistic: A prognosis should be supported by a substantial amount of information. We never say that "the prognosis is favorable" without some documentation, both impressionistic and scientifically based. It is much better to say the following: "The prognosis is good because the child is stimulable for all error sounds, trial therapy has indicated good attention and a cooperative attitude, parents have committed to a home program, the client has stated he wants to change his speech, he has normal hearing, and language problems are not evident."

In what sense might a prognosis be dangerous? First, no one really knows the future. A client's prognostic variables might soon change with unforeseen circumstances (e.g., the uninterested parents become involved, the client develops motivation, the client makes a "breakthrough" in the ability to perform certain functions). This means that prognosis as a construct is dynamic, not static. A second danger is that the prognosis may well influence a client's performance and/or perceptions. If a clinician has certain expectations regarding the case's potential performance, this could be inadvertently communicated to the client or the family and could negatively affect the course of therapy. It could also influence the level of effort exhibited by the clinician. The old notion of a self-fulfilling prophecy is still alive and well. We must always be willing to alter prognostic judgments in light of new data; and perhaps more important, we must be willing to restrain from making prognostic statements in the first place if we do not know what we are talking about. It is better to say "I don't know how he will do in treatment; let's see what happens" than to jaundice the whole enterprise with a negative prognosis that has no real basis or that may disappoint all concerned with a positive prognosis that never was realized. This is *not* an exact science!

Precepts Regarding the Clinical Examination

In this chapter we have presented some suggestions for general conduct of the diagnostic session. We dislike diagnostic formulas, and our purpose has not been to give out recipes, but rather to describe some way of approaching various problems without going too far astray. By way of summary, we now present a list of interrelated and overlapping precepts regarding the clinical examination.

1. We examine persons, not speech defects or speech defectives. Our primary concern is with communicators, not just communication.
2. The clinical examination is conducted interpersonally; the catalyst of a diagnostic session is the person-to-person relationship between clinician and client.
3. There is an element of magic in every transaction between people. A diagnostic session can, in some instances, ameliorate a problem situation by engendering hope or be deeply disappointing to a client who hopes that a test or examination will resolve a difficulty.
4. A most important requisite for conducting a clinical examination is a thorough understanding of normalcy.

5. Diagnosis is the initial phase of treatment. The very first contact with a client—the manner in which he/she is treated during a clinical examination—is a crucial determining factor in response to therapy.
6. Diagnosis is not necessarily confined to a single session.
7. Treatment is often diagnostic; we often discover the nature of a client's problem in the initial stages of therapy.
8. The clinical examination is performed to provide a working image of the individual; it is accomplished by interviewing, examining, evaluating, and testing.
9. An important aspect in acquiring a working image of an individual is determining the person's self-perception and situation.
10. An individual makes certain adjustments to a problem (attempts to solve the difficulty) that may include a protective cover of defenses. These may be a part of the problem, but must not be confused with the problem.
11. Behavior is a function of the individual and the situation. We should be aware that our test results reflect not just the client's abilities but also performance in the diagnostic setting rather than the natural environment.
12. Our diagnostic activities should include an assessment of a client's larger social context (home, family, peers, job, school, etc.).
13. Tests are only tools to provide a systematic guide for our observations. They enable the clinician to scrutinize a client in a structured manner.
14. Although for the examiner the testing situation may be very familiar and routine, for the client it is a novel experience.
15. Examination and testing can be iatrogenic. It can suggest problems to the client that he or she had not previously considered.
16. Simply because a testing device is made up of a series of precisely defined tasks, administered and scored in a rigidly structured manner, this does not mean that a client's responses are similarly precise.
17. It is as important to observe *how* the client responds during a testing procedure as it is to obtain a score. Informal evaluation tasks are as important or more important than formal, standardized procedures.
18. The needs of the client, not the work setting in which the clinician labors, should determine the scope of diagnostic activities. A good diagnostic is over when sufficient information about a client is gathered and should not be short-circuited because of administrative red tape, arbitrary guidelines of a facility, or government regulations. A good clinician will find ways to obtain critical information even if the evaluation extends into the realm of treatment.

This chapter has served to generally introduce diagnosis and evaluation. The following chapters will focus more closely on important parameters of this interesting process with specific areas of communication disorders. We hope that students can see that this is an exciting enterprise that combines instruments with interpersonal relationships, testing with talking, and measurement with personal magnetism. The assessment process is the portal through which real people with real problems come to us for help. We must offer them the best of scientific as well as human resources.

Bibliography

American Heritage Dictionary (1985). Boston, MA: Houghton Mifflin.

Barker, R. (1953). *Adjustment to Physical Handicap and Illness: A Survey of the Social Psychology of Physique and Disability.* Bulletin 55. New York: Social Science Research Council.

Beasley, D., and Davis, G. eds. (1981). *Aging and Communication.* Baltimore, MD: University Park Press.

Buscaglia, L. (1982). *Living, Loving and Learning.* New York: Ballantine.

Cowley, M. (1980). *The View from 80.* New York: Viking.

Deutscher, M. (1983). *Subjecting and Objecting.* Oxford, Eng.: Basil Blackwell Publishers.

Ehren, B. (1993). "Eligibility, Evaluation and the Realities of Role Definition in the Schools," *American Journal of Speech Language Pathology* 2, no. 1:20–23.

Emerick, L. (1984). *Speaking for Ourselves: Self-Portraits of the Speech or Hearing Handicapped,* Danville, IL: Interstate.

Emerick, L., and Hood, S. (1975). *The Client-Clinician Relationship.* Springfield, IL: Charles C. Thomas.

Fuchs, D., Fuchs, L., Dailey, A., and Power, M. (1985). "The Effect of Examiner's Personal Familiarity and Professional Expertise on Handicapped Children's Test Performance," *Journal of Educational Research* 78:3–14.

Haynes, W., and Oratio, A. (1978). "A Study of Clients' Perceptions of Therapeutic Effectiveness," *Journal of Speech and Hearing Disorders* 43:21–33.

Hubbell, R. (1977). "On Facilitating Spontaneous Talking in Young Children," *Journal of Speech and Hearing Disorders* 42:216–231.

Johnson, D. (1972). *Reaching Out.* Englewood Cliffs, NJ: Prentice-Hall.

Lidz, C. (1991). *A Practitioner's Guide to Dynamic Assessment.* New York: Guilford Press.

Moore, J., and D. Sherman (1981). "Special Considerations with the Elderly Patient," *Journal of Communication Disorders* 14:299–309.

Mueller, R., and Peters, T. (1981). "Needs and Services in Geriatric Speech-Language Pathology and Audiology," *Journal of the American Speech and Hearing Association* 23:627–632.

National Council on Aging (1982). *Service Learning in Aging: Implications for Speech, Language and Hearing.* Washington, DC: National Council on Aging.

O'Connor, L., and Eldredge, P. (1981). *Communication Disorders in Adolescence.* Springfield, IL: Charles C. Thomas.

Olswang, L., Bain, B., Rosendahl, P., Oblak, S., and Smith, A. (1986). "Language Learning: Moving from a Context-Dependent to Independent State", *Child Language Teaching and Therapy* 2:180–210.

Oratio, A. (1977). *Supervision in Speech Pathology: A Handbook for Supervisors and Clinicians.* Baltimore, MD: University Park Press.

Paul, R. (1995). *Language Disorders from Infancy through Adolescence: Assessment and Intervention.* St. Louis, MO: Mosby.

Pena, E. (1996). "Dynamic Assessment: The Model and Its Language Applications." In *Assessment of Communication and Language,* ed. P. Cole, P. Dale, and D. Thal (Baltimore, MD: Brookes).

Ringel, R., Trachtman, L., and Prutting, C. (1984). "The Science in Human Communication Sciences," *Journal of the American Speech Language and Hearing Association* 26:33–36.

Rogers, C. (1942). *Counseling and Psychotherapy.* Boston, MA: Houghton-Mifflin.

Rosenbek, J., LaPointe, L., and Wertz, R. (1989). *Aphasia: A Clinical Approach.* Boston, MA: College-Hill.

Shadden, B. (1988). *Communication Behavior and Aging: A Sourcebook for Clinicians.* Baltimore, MD: Williams and Wilkins.

Shine, R. (1980). "Direct Management of the Beginning Stutterer," *Seminars in Speech, Language and Hearing* 1, no. 4:339–350.

Silverman, F. (1984). *Speech Language Pathology and Audiology.* Columbus, OH: Merrill.

Starkweather, C., Gottwald, S., and Halfond, M. (1990). *Stuttering Prevention: A Clinical Method.* Englewood Cliffs, NJ: Prentice-Hall.

Van Riper, C., and Emerick, L. (1984). *Speech Correction: An Introduction to Speech Pathology and Audiology,* Englewood Cliffs, NJ: Prentice-Hall.

Van Riper, C. (1972). *Speech Correction: Principles and Methods,* Englewood Cliffs, NJ: Prentice-Hall.

Vygotsky, L. (1978). *Mind in Society: The Development of Higher Psychological Processes.* Cambridge: Harvard University Press.

Wade, K., and Haynes, W. (1989). "Dynamic Assessment of Spontaneous Language and Cue Responses in Adult-Directed and Child-Directed Play: A Statistical and Descriptive Analysis," *Child Language Teaching and Therapy* 5:157–173.

Chapter *2*

Interviewing

The clinician sets in motion the process of recovery at the very first contact with a client. This is accomplished through the vehicle of the spoken word—in short, by means of the initial interview. Because the intake interview ushers the client into treatment, it is the key link in the evaluation process. In order to assess and treat persons with communication disorders, it is essential that we know how to talk with them in a manner that reflects our expertise and inspires confidence and trust.

The Importance of Interviewing

Although clinical evaluation obviously involves more than proficiency at conducting interviews, it is central to the role of the diagnostician. By means of verbal exchange, we gather data about the individual, transmit information, and establish and sustain a working relationship. The interview is also the means by which treatment is carried out and, as such, serves both as a tool and as a relationship (Figure 2.1). For the clinical speech-language pathologist, interviewing is an extremely important activity.

Although widely used, interviewing is often one of the least understood aspects of the worker's role. Prospective clinicians are expected to acquire an impressive array of knowledge, but often it is merely presumed that they know how to communicate effectively with clients. The mastery of interviewing is either taken for granted or expected to accrue somehow as an artifact of required course work and practicum experiences.

Some clinicians consider interviewing to be secondary; they use paper to replace personal interaction. An elaborate case history form containing a plethora of questions is mailed to the parents, and they are asked to fill it out and return it before the diagnostic appointment. The rationale for this procedure is that it saves the clinician time and alerts him/her to problem areas that can then be explored in the personal interview. Although the clinician certainly should get some idea of

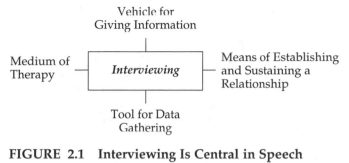

FIGURE 2.1   **Interviewing Is Central in Speech Pathology**

the problem before the diagnostic examination, there is no substitute for an in-depth interview. There are several reasons for disenchantment with an approach that only uses paper and pencil techniques. First, the questions on forms are often generic—they cover all possible respondents—and thus are ambiguous or not applicable to any particular clients; a parent may not understand the relationship between the questions posed and the child's speech problem. Face-to-face interviews permit greater flexibility in formulating precise and germane inquiries. Second, the queries may be threatening or may engender guilt, and the clinician is not present to observe the respondent's reactions or to support and assist the respondent as he searches for an answer. Does the mailed questionnaire allow time for the respondent to plan a defense? Is it more likely that we end up with a view of what the respondent wants us to see? More complete information can be obtained in an interview, where primary questions may be followed up with pertinent secondary inquiries. Third, the questions, if answered by the respondent in one particular way, may prevent the respondent from developing any other possible answers. Spoken language does tend to create a reality for the individual, but writing lends an air of permanence. During an interview, however, the clinician can determine not only what a client says but also how the respondent says it—for example, how does the respondent assign priority to items? associate items with one another? reveal attitudes by vocal quality or body language?

The Nature of Interviewing

An interview is essentially a process, not an entity—a process of verbal and non-verbal intercourse between a trained professional worker and a client who is seeking services. More specifically, an interview, in a clinical and diagnostic sense, is a *purposeful* exchange of meanings between two persons, a directed conversation that proceeds in an orderly fashion to obtain data, to convey certain information, and to provide counseling. The professional worker, by reason of his/her position and clinical expertise, is expected to (and usually does) provide the direction for the verbal exchange. Thus, an interview is not just an ordinary conversation in terms of a desultory exchange of opinions and ideas but rather a specialized pattern of verbal interaction directed toward a specific purpose and focused on specific content. The roles of interviewer and respondent are more highly specified in a professional interview than in a conversation. An interview differs from a social conversation in a number of other important respects. First, the time and location of an interview is specified formally. Second, the inquiries are generally unilateral—the clinician may ask about the parents' relationship with their child, for example, but it is not expected that the client will reciprocate with questions about the worker's children. Third, the clinician does not necessarily avoid unpleasant topics in the interest of social propriety.

In a good diagnostic interview, the clinician and client must become co-workers, multiplying their efforts by creating a mutual feeling of cooperation. It is futile to expect straightforward answers to simple questions. A good diagnostic interview always involves more than making queries and recording answers.

Interviewing is a unique kind of conversation. Perhaps for the first time, the respondent can talk freely without fear of criticism or admonishment. The *clinician* knows that an interview is a unique and distinct mode of verbal exchange. But does the *client* need to know? Probably not. Indeed, we typically advise students to refer to an interview as a "chat" or "a chance to share information" when they contact clients or parents to request an appointment time. An "interview" sounds rather ominous and frightening, perhaps even like a summons to account for one's failings.

In summary, a diagnostic interview is a directed conversation, carried out for specific purposes such as fact finding, informing, or altering attitudes and opinions. The clinician's efforts are directed toward the creation of mutual respect and team effort in the understanding and solution of the communication problem.

Common Interviewing Considerations

Several factors can prevent the establishment of effective communicative bonds between a speech clinician and those whom the clinician interviews. Although the list could obviously be expanded, we have picked several aspects that in our experience are the most-common interviewing barriers.

Multicultural Considerations in Interviewing

More than ever before in our history, the United States has become a multicultural society. Soon after the turn of the next century, the country will no longer have a majority of White, European residents. The populations of Hispanic, Asian, and Black individuals are the most rapidly growing segments of the society; and within the next few decades, most Americans will be from these groups. While multicultural issues affect all aspects of any profession, there are some important factors to consider in interviewing that relate to our burgeoning multicultural society. First, as mentioned previously, the clinical interview represents the meeting of two or more individuals who each contribute unique experiences, perceptions, views, values, and characteristics. When two people meet in a professional setting, the nature of the clinical relationship itself is sometimes problematic. That is, some people simply have trouble coming to a clinical situation, even if they are dealing with a clinician from the same culture as their own. When client and clinician represent differing cultural or racial backgrounds, there is an additional potential obstacle to overcome. Some clients may not feel as comfortable when they must reveal certain information to a stranger, and this discomfort may be intensified when the clinician represents a different race or culture. The solution for this is clearly not to make certain that clients and clinicians are culturally homogeneous. Given the diverse nature of our society, this homogeneousness would be impossible from a scheduling standpoint and unwise from a philosophical one. The best way to deal with cultural diversity in clinical situations is to make certain that clinicians have a sensitivity to cultural differences and a knowledge of multicultural issues in assessment and treatment. Recently, the American-Speech-Language-Hearing Association has mandated that every accredited training program in communication disorders infuse multicultural information into each area of academic preparation and clinical practicum. Hopefully, our students will have increased opportunity to deal with culturally different clients, parents, and children and to develop their interpersonal skills with and knowledge of these groups.

A second important implication of multicultural influence on interviewing concerns the specific information that is exchanged. We have indicated that much of the information exchanged in a clinical interview is of a highly personal nature and possibly charged with considerable affect. Many cultures (e.g., Native Americans and certain Asian groups) find it difficult to share personal information with unfamiliar people. Thus, in the interview it is extremely uncomfortable for them to reveal some types of data. The clinician must be sensitive to such cultural beliefs and should not press the client to provide information too soon. In some cases it will be necessary to conduct multiple interviews and to establish a strong relationship with the client before the client will give information or take advantage of clinician suggestions for treatment. This issue alone is a strong indictment of some rigid policies wherein an evaluation must be completed in an hour or two or IEP goals must be written in limited time frames. We must learn that different cultures may require alterations in our methods if we are to serve them optimally.

An obvious multicultural influence on interviewing is the possibility of dealing with the many children and adults from bilingual backgrounds. In some cases, the clinician must be bilingual, and in others the interviewer must make use of interpreters. The use of an interpreter, however, is a very specialized operation, and the clinician must be certain that the interpreter has adequate knowledge and experience to perform this specialized task. In some areas of the country, there is an increased likelihood that the SLP will encounter a bilingual population, and the SLP should reflect on how these clients will be served appropriately in assessment and treatment. It is not possible to provide adequate services to these populations without a knowledge of and sensitivity to multicultural issues. Lynch (1992) describes the ideal interpreter as someone who is

1. *proficient in the language (including specific dialect) of the family as well as that of the interventionist*
2. *trained and experienced in cross-cultural communication and the principles (and dynamics) of serving as an interpreter*
3. *trained in the appropriate professional field relevant to the specific family-interventionist interaction*
4. *able to understand and appreciate the respective cultures of both parties and to convey the more subtle nuances of each with tact and sensitivity. (52)*

Lynch (1992) cautions against the use of family members as interpreters because they rarely meet the above criteria and could inject significant bias and family difficulties into the clinical situation. Most authorities on the use of interpreters emphasize the importance of thorough preparation of the interpreter prior to the clinical encounter in terms of the goals/purposes of the evaluation, potentially sensitive clinical/family issues, the format of the interview, and any technical terms and/or paperwork to be used in the conference. It is helpful to provide proper introductions and clarify the goals and purposes of the interview so the family will know what to expect. Diligent clinicians may take the time to learn several social phrases in the language of the family so that greetings, thank yous, and leave taking can be done in a manner comfortable to the clients. This demonstrates respect for the family and shows that the clinician is making an attempt to understand and appreciate cultural differences. During the interview it is customary for the clinician to address remarks and questions to the family, not the interpreter. Also, while listening to the family, it is appropriate to look at the person who is speaking, not just at the interpreter. In this situation it is clearly beneficial to avoid technical jargon and figurative language that not only is difficult to translate but may be confusing to the clients. As the interview progresses, especially in the portion where information is provided to the clients, it is wise to periodically check the family's understanding of facts presented and of any recommendations given by the clinician. Finally, most experts on the use of interpreters recommend a debriefing session in which the clinician and interpreter can discuss the information collected, any difficulties encountered in the conference, any problems with the interpreting process, and any subtle impressions gleaned by the interpreter that go beyond the literal translation of the client's utterances (e.g., anger, hostility, fear). While such impressions are subjective on the part of the interpreter, they may represent important information about the family's acceptance of the problem, perceptions of the clinical situation, and possible compliance with a treatment program. Good interpreters are difficult to find and often "burn out" quickly because of the time commitment, requests to appear with little advance notice, and sometimes lack of adequate compensation for their work. As a result, the SLP must do everything possible to develop and cultivate mutually beneficial relationships with interpreters.

A final implication of multicultural issues on interviewing is the belief systems of the various cultural groups regarding disabilities. People from some cultures believe that a handicap is a condition about which nothing can or should be done, or they believe that this condition requires spiritual rather than clinical help (Cheng, 1989). If the clinician charges into the interview and makes a host of recommendations without addressing cultural attitudes toward remediation, these suggestions may fall on unsympathetic ears. The clients may also be offended and may not return for treatment. There is a growing literature in communication disorders concerning multicultural issues, and it is the ethical responsibility of every student and clinician to become familiar with this body of work. We cannot serve our clients well unless we take this cultural information into account.

Fears of the Clinician

There are two points in a student clinician's career when the anxiety rises to very high levels: the confrontation with his or her first therapy case and the first diagnostic interview. It is—and should be—an awesome responsibility to undertake the professional treatment of another human being. There is always an element of risk in offering help.

Perhaps the most-common fear expressed by the beginning clinician is that clients will not accept the clinician in a professional role because of the clinician's youth. The clinician doubts that he or she can bridge the age gap, especially when the clinician deals with parents: "Who am I to be asking questions and giving suggestions to them when they are older and more experienced?" The clinician sighs, "Won't they look down on me if I don't have children?" Most of this is pure projection on the clinician's part (Haynes and Oratio 1978). If the clinician indicates deep concern for the welfare of the child, then nearly every parent will respond in a positive manner, without scrutinizing the clinician for wrinkles, or grey hairs, or looking for photographs of children on the clinician's desk. The clinician, of course, should not communicate the uncertainty felt in the interview situation; otherwise, he/she will never establish competence or inspire confidence.

Another common fear among beginning clinicians—and one that is also largely projected—is that the client will become defensive or resentful during questioning. We have seen students omit a whole series of important questions when a client, especially a parent, responded curtly or showed mild annoyance. While it is not uncommon for parents to feel ashamed because they think of their child's communication disorder as an outward and visible sign of their own failure, in our experience few parents are resentful or defensive about the clinician's sincere efforts to determine the nature of the child's problem. The important point is, again, to make the clients and their families feel that they have done the best they could do, and now, with some assistance from the clinician, they can do better. The clinician should *always maintain a nonthreatened posture in the clinical transaction.*

Many beginning clinicians are leery of questions directed at them. "What do you do when the client starts asking *you* questions?" the beginning clinician frequently despairs. "Will I be able to explain to the client adequately what he or she needs to know? How will I know if I have communicated properly if the client just sits there and nods?" We shall return to this important topic of client questions in a later section of this chapter.

The Lack of Specific Purpose

Many beginning clinicians either have purposes that are too broad and general or interviewing goals that are too nebulous. It is important to write out carefully and rather explicitly the purposes for an interview before meeting with the client. We must know *why* we want the answers to the questions we ask. Specifying the purposes of an interview is also an effective way to reduce the interviewer's uncertainty and anxiety. Kadushin (1972) summarizes the importance of planning in this way: "To know is to be prepared; to be prepared is to experience reduced anxiety; to reduce anxiety is to increase the interviewer's freedom to be fully responsive to the interviewee"(2). The clinician should keep in mind, however, that thorough planning does not mean the application of an inflexible routine.

An Approach to Interviewing

We now present an interviewing approach, an eclectic product of our clinical experience together with an intensive study of relevant bibliographic materials. No doubt the reader will want to modify our approach in order to suit individual settings. It is desirable to do so, for only through critical self-evaluation and modification can any clinician acquire an interviewing procedure that is uniquely personal.

There are three basic goals in diagnostic interviews: to obtain information, to give information, and to provide counseling. For the purpose of discussion, each goal will be considered separately, a procedure rarely possible in an actual interview.

Goal One: Obtain Information

Although it may seem obvious, it is worth restating that as clinicians we must listen before we speak. There are essentially three reasons for this: (1) it gives clients an opportunity to talk out problems, to ventilate fears and feelings, thus enabling them to profit better from the direction and advice that the speech clinician will offer; (2) it gives the clinician an idea of the nature and scope of the information the client will need; and (3) it allows the clinician to formulate hypotheses concerning the individual's communication disorder.

Setting the Tone. The first important task of the clinician is to set the right tone for the interview, to get a structured conversation initiated and channeled in the proper direction. How does one go about that? Research by McQuire and Lorch (1968) has underscored the importance of proper structuring. Their findings indicate that the initial style of interaction may well determine the style of interaction for the entire interview (see Matarazzo and Wiens 1972). We find that defining the roles is an effective procedure for setting the tone:

Mrs. Seelos, I'm Miss Sullivan, Terry's speech clinician. I really appreciate the opportunity to chat with you about Terry and the things we are doing in speech. First, though, you can be of great help to me since you know Terry so much better than I do. There are several things about his early development and how his speech seems to be at home that I need to understand before planning a long-range therapy program. Before you came in today, I made some notes for myself so that we could best use this half hour before my next session.

It is helpful to think of the interview as a kind of role-playing situation. The clinician defines the roles for the client and indicates the rules and responsibilities that accrue to these roles. The clinician tells who he/she is, what he/she intends to do, and what he/she expects of the client. In other words, the interviewer structures the situation by explaining the purposes of the interview—why the information is needed and what will be done with it. Initially, of course, the client accepts the respondent role because of the nature of the situation and the official sanction of the interviewer's position. Then it is up to the clinician to demonstrate his/her empathy and clinical expertise in order to solicit further cooperation. Two problems sometimes arise here. First, some clients may be inhibited by such explicit role definitions; respondents from lower-middle or lower social classes have had little experience in holding directed conversations. In this case, a clinician can prolong the small-talk phase, emphasize the nature of the interview as chatting, and gently ease into the more-structured situation as the relationship develops. When two or more people get together, even for serious purposes, a certain amount of social and idle talk seems to foster positive attitudes toward continued interaction. Czikszentmihalyi (1975) describes this feature of group interaction as "flow."

The second, more-difficult problem concerns the site of the interview. Although it is generally best to conduct interviews in a clinical setting, sometimes this is not possible, and one has to seek out the client or parents at home. This is rarely satisfactory, not only because of the distractions inherent in the situation (children, pets, and neighbors) but also because the interview frequently becomes a social visit.

It is vital that the interviewer convey sincere interest in the situation as the client sees it. The SLP must demonstrate to the client that he/she is genuinely trying to comprehend what the problem is and what it means to the client personally. The clinician can show interest by carefully attending to the respondent: Assume a relaxed, natural posture; maintain eye contact; and offer minimal verbal encouragements that reveal you are listening ("Yes," "I see," etc.).

Rapport, of course, is not a separate substance that one pours into a session; it is mutual respect and trust, a feeling of confidence in the clinician, and a large measure of understanding. Empathy, warmth, and acceptance are crucial aspects; the worker must strive for the ability to understand sensitively and accurately the interviewee's situation. We should also try to be genuine, not contrived, with a professional-character armor that signals "clinician on duty." As a matter of fact, it is helpful to avoid interposing a desk—a symbol of authority—between the respondent and the interviewer. The interview is more effective without such a barrier. In addition to the words spoken, a number of forces shape the interview. Some things are conveyed by the setting and by the dress, manners, and expressions of the participants. If our office is located in a boiler room or a storage area, we have already conveyed something of our attitude toward the client and his/her problem by the very physical space that we use. In professional interviewing, the goal is to provide an atmosphere that fosters communication between client and clinician (Staples and Sloane 1976).

Asking the Questions. Preferably, the clinician should use an interview guide rather than one of the more-elaborate questionnaires—that is, instead of a formal set of questions written out to be read and answered, we should use a form that indicates areas to explore. Rather than read prepared questions, the speech clinician should word questions in keeping with his or her understanding of the individual's situation and thus conduct an interview that is much more spontaneous and meaningful. In most cases, formal questionnaires operate as another type of barrier or crutch for the insecure interviewer.

The specific content of the queries addressed to a respondent depend on, among other things, the age of the client, the nature of the problem, and the purposes of the interview. Most clinicians find that the younger the client being evaluated, the more important the parent interview. Because we intend to focus on style of interviewing in this chapter, we will not include lists of questions that pertain to particular disorders of communication. There are, however, seven general topics or areas of inquiry that are useful in any diagnostic session.

1. *What is the respondent's perception of the problem?* We seek here a global description of the communication disorder. In a parent interview, for example, we frequently open the session with an open-ended question: "Tell me why you brought Jamie to the speech clinic" or "What concerns do you have about Jamie?"

2. *When and under what conditions did the communication disorder arise?* The purpose of this question is to determine the history of the development and of the onset of the problem. An example of where this etiology would be especially important might be the development of a voice disorder (e.g., rapid versus gradual onset, occurrence of vocally abusive behaviors, changes in medication).

3. *In what ways has the communication disorder changed since its onset?* When interviewing the parents of a child who is exhibiting early signs of stuttering, for example, we are interested in how the speech disfluency has changed since it was first noticed.

4. *What are the consequences (the handicapping conditions) of the problem?* In what manner—socially, educationally, occupationally—does the communication disorder affect the person's life? In what ways has he/she adapted to the disorder?

5. *How has the client and family attempted to cope with the problem?* What lay remedies have been tried by the client and family? How has the client responded to them?

6. *What impact has the client's communication disorder had on the rest of the family?* When a child has a handicapping condition, it creates fertile ground for familial conflict (see Featherstone, 1980). In order to obtain a description of the child's ongoing behavior, and how he/she fits into the family regimen, ask the parents to describe a "typical" day, from the time the youngster gets up until he or she goes to bed.

7. *What are the client's (or parents') expectations regarding the diagnostic session?* The client often comes to a professional with an "agenda." The client may want the problem finally diagnosed after months of wondering about it. The parents may want a recommendation for treatment because they already know that their child has a communication problem. Sometimes parents have been agonizing over some hypothesis that has been advanced by a relative ("He's tongue-tied" or "He's mentally retarded") and their biggest concern is that the clinician address this issue. Whatever the client's expectations, the clinician must do his or her best to determine what those expectations are and to provide some sort of resolution if possible.

A good diagnostic interview is characterized by a shifting of styles: objective questions that ask for specifics, subjective queries that deal with feelings and attitudes, and finally the indeterminate questions, like "Tell me more," that keep the respondent going.

Classically, the interviewer should start with the least anxiety-provoking queries, mostly objective questions that have high specificity (Woolf 1971), and then proceed to more-subjective questions as the relationship develops. Quite often, however, we find it useful to employ a "funnel" sequence of inquiry during the course of a diagnostic interview—starting with broad, open-ended questions and then progressing to more-specific or closed questions (Stewart and Cash 1974). Here is an example of a funnel sequence from a parent interview:

- How does Jimmy function in the family setting?
- How does he get along with his brothers and sisters?
- How does his older sister "help" him communicate?
- Can you describe an instance in which she talked for him?

The "inverted funnel" approach, proceeding from specific to general, is also useful. It is best to avoid the checklist or long series of "tunnel" questions that call for information on one level of specificity, all of which are asked in a similar style (e.g., "Did your child have earaches, fevers, head injury?").

The Presenting Story. Most persons who anticipate visiting a clinic or discussing a speech problem with a public school speech clinician will have mentally rehearsed what they intend to say. Often the interviewer will have to contend with events that occurred prior to the session—the family car's failing to start, a burned breakfast, absence of a convenient parking place. A few words to reveal the interviewer's understanding of the distracting antecedents will generally assist the respondent in shifting to the topic of the interview. In some cases the client may even have a pseudoconversation with the clinician before the visit occurs. Think of the last time you visited your physician with a medical problem. While driving to the doctor's office, a person often rehearses how he/she will describe his/her symptoms. We must allow this story to be unraveled, or the respondent will be left with a sense of frustration and lack of closure. A question such as "What seems to be the problem?" will permit the flow of conversation to begin. The clinician should remember that the client's description is how the *client* perceives the problem—it is the client's unique way of looking at the situation. The client's description may be grossly inaccurate, but the interviewer should hear it out; nothing turns a respondent off more quickly than for the interviewer to suggest by word or action that the respondent's views are silly or misguided. Sometimes the presenting story will become a motif that recurs again and again during the course of the interview.

This is generally a crucial point in an interview. The interviewee may cautiously extend a portion of himself/herself verbally, carefully scan the interviewer's response, and then decide whether or not to tell the whole story. Sometimes a respondent may even set up a straw man to see how the interviewer deals with it.

This is not the proper time for the clinician to debate an issue with the client. The story can be accepted initially on the level of feeling, and later in the interview—when rapport is stronger—an issue can be discussed more fully. We feel very strongly that these initial stories, these primitive theories, should be respected as the best possible answer that clients have been able to come up with. It does not mean that the clinician agrees with a client's conclusions; it just means that the clinician accepts a client's judgment with understanding so that the clinician can form a basis for further communication.

Actually, the presenting information can be a very rich source of clinical hypotheses to be explored during the course of the interview. How do the client and parent present themselves (Goffman 1959)—as long suffering, anxious, diffident? How do they associate ideas or items of information sequentially? What priorities do they assign to issues they raise? Do they seem to be realistic in their expectations regarding the diagnostic session and treatment?

Nonverbal Messages. Respondents do not communicate by words alone, and the discerning clinician attends to body as well as oral language during an interview. As a matter of fact, some observers (Bosmajian 1971; Harrison 1974; Hinde 1972; Mehrabian 1972) suggest that a large portion of the total message—particularly messages involving strong feelings—is carried by nonverbal cues. However, the diagnostician should resist the urge to interpret a client's every twitch; each instance of nonverbal behavior should be related to the *content* of the oral message and to the *context* in which it occurs (Birdwhistle 1970; Feldman 1973; Knapp 1972):

> *If a parent leaves her coat on during an interview it may mean she feels vulnerable and the garment provides a bit of protective armor. It may also mean that she has a spot on her dress, or that all the hangers in the waiting room were taken again by forgetful students, or that the room is chilly. However, if she shifts her chair away from the clinician, sits with her arms and legs tightly crossed, avoids eye contact, and responds to questions with one-word answers, then it may be concluded that she is defensive and guarded in the clinical setting.*

The issue here is to avoid making one item of nonverbal behavior the sole basis for interpretation; the interviewer should be on the lookout for patterns (Weitz 1974).

Although research into the nonverbal facets of dyadic interviewing is still in its early stages, there are several useful questions that can assist the interviewer's scrutiny of body language (Egolf and Chester 1973), such as:

1. What clues are evident during the initial contact with the client? Does he/she enter the room hesitantly and wait to be seated? What can be discerned from clothing or personal grooming? Does he/she avoid eye contact and shake hands limply?

2. Is the respondent's facial expression congruent with the content of his oral message? Does the face flush or show other emotions when discussing different aspects of his or her speech problem? Does he/she reveal tension by constant bunching of his jaw muscles?

3. How does the respondent use eye gaze during the course of the interview? As a general rule, persons maintain less eye contact when talking than listening, particularly when responding to questions that provoke reflection and recall. The amount of mutual gaze between two individuals is increased markedly when they like each other and are involved in a joint concern. Keep in mind, however, that unwavering eye contact by the clinician, particularly when asking questions, may be interpreted as a threat signal or an attempt to dominate (Argyle and Cook 1976).

4. Attend to the client's body movements and postural shifts: What is the rate and extent of movement and the degree of tension shown? Does the respondent's postural shifting congruently mirror that of the interviewer?

5. How does the client speak with his/her hands? Are the hands tightly clasped? Does he/she wring them or play continually with a ring? Are a number of "adaptors" used such as adjusting clothing, scratching, or inspecting the fingernails (Knapp 1972)?

6. How does the respondent communicate by use of the available space? In which chair does a client choose to sit with respect to proximity with the interviewer?

7. What can be discerned by attending to nuances to the client's use of pitch, loudness, or vocal quality? Does the rate reflect apprehension, excitement, or depression? Is the respondent's recital of the presenting story punctuated by heavy sighs?

8. In what respect do the stigmata associated with various communication disorders (e.g., stuttering, cerebral palsy) interfere with or confound nonverbal messages (Eisenberg and Smith 1971; Goffman 1963)? How does body language vary with respect to the factors of sex, age, and culture (Morsbach 1973)?

The most important thing to look for may be lack of congruence between the respondent's verbal and nonverbal messages; in cases where the two conflict, body language is generally a more accurate indicator of how a person feels about an issue:

During a diagnostic session we opened the parent interview by asking the parent to describe the nature of his child's speech problem (the child was multiply handicapped). Before the parent responded verbally, he made a short, chopping gesture with his right hand, stamped his right foot, and wrinkled his face in a fleeting expression of disgust. However, he then proceeded to tell us calmly what a wonderful relationship he had with his son. The nonverbal message occurred so swiftly that later we were uncertain if we had really seen it; when we played back the videotape, however, the graphic body language was evident even to the father. This vivid self-confrontation seemed to release some long-repressed feelings, and the father then talked at length about how disappointed he was in his son, how much attention his wife devoted to the child—often, he felt, at his expense, and what a financial drain the various treatment programs had been. The consequence of the interview was a referral to a family service agency where both parents received the type of counseling they needed.

Although persons vary in terms of their skill at "reading" nonverbal cues, it is possible to improve with training (Rosenthal et al. 1974). Since body language is continuous—there is no way to turn it off, not even for the clinician—the interviewer will want to investigate the topic of nonverbal communication more fully (Duncan and Fiske 1977; Ekman 1980; Leathers 1976; Scheflen 1972; Spiegel and Machotka 1974).

Things to Avoid in the Interview. Beginning interviewers commit several common errors. The list that follows is not meant to be exhaustive, but it does cover the most glaring mistakes.

1. It is usually best to avoid questions that may be answered by a simple "Yes" or "No." Although open-ended questions do produce longer responses in general, it is interesting to note that respondents from lower socioeconomic groups, who have less education, become more anxious as the questions become less structured. We have interviewed several clients who are confirmed yes-men. No matter what the clinician asks, no matter what comments he/she makes, these respondents simply nod in passive agreement. Perhaps they are fearful of exposing their ignorance and feel that it is better to remain silent and be thought a fool than to say something and make it obvious.

We find that requesting the client to rate himself on a simple scale is more effective than "either-or" questions. We frequently ask the client to tell us not whether something is difficult or easy but to what degree. A simple rating procedure, with lower values (1 or 2) indicating relative ease and higher values (4 or 5) indicating relative difficulty, may be used.

2. Avoid phrasing questions in such a way that they inhibit freedom of response. Do not say, "You don't have any difficulty with ringing in your ears, do you?" or "You don't tell Billy to stop and start over again, do you?" Such leading questions are not effective interviewing. The beginning interviewer tends to be anxious about asking open-ended questions. The interviewer is afraid that silence will result and that this will damage his relationship with the client. So the interviewer will ask an open-ended question and then close it: for example, "How do you feel about David's stuttering? Does it bother you?" Leave it open! Although open-end questions consume more time and may produce some rambling and irrelevant responses, there are many advantages to recommend their use:

> *They let the respondent do the talking while the interviewer plays his role as listener and observer. The freedom to determine the nature and amount of information the respondent will give may communicate to him that you are interested in him, as well as his answers, and that you respect his ability to give accurate and relevant data.* (Stewart and Cash 1974, 28)

Try also to avoid abrupt shifts in your line of questioning. For example, if you are exploring the client's feelings or attitudes on a particular issue (subjective questions), don't suddenly ask an objective question. Inexperienced interviewers, fearful that they are too deep in an area, tend to jump around. Often they persist with objective queries; and once a pattern of response is established, the client finds it difficult to shift to more elaborate answers.

3. Avoid talking too much. This is perhaps the most-common mistake of the beginning interviewer. He/she feels that every pause must be filled with verbiage. It is much better to rephrase what the respondent has said or make some comment like "I see," "Tell me more," or "Anything else?" Sometimes a smile and an understanding nod are effective when it is felt that the client has more to say but needs some silent time to conjure it up. If there is a positive attitude—a good rapport—and if the client feels comfortable in the situation, then these encouragements increase the length of the response. If the topic or situation is neutral, these comments tend to expand the message. However, if the topic is negative or if the client feels uncomfortable, the "hmm, hmm" may be taken as a criticism—that is, if the client *cannot* respond at length, he/she will feel pressured to do so. Parents with little education are perhaps the most vulnerable to this kind of pressure.

Be careful not to fall into stereotyped verbal habits. One of our students used "Very good" as reinforcement so frequently with a severely aphasic patient that one day, after making a particularly effective response to a problem, the patient—who had said very little since his stroke—finished the clinician's "Very" with a resounding "good," surprising them both.

4. Avoid concentrating on the physical symptoms and the etiological factors to the exclusion of the client's feelings and attitudes. There is a little bit of physician in all of us; we yearn to play the role of omniscient healer. This is further compounded by instructors who dwell interminably on causation in their courses dealing with speech disorders. But it is possible to track each suspicious symptom with such zeal that we fail to obtain a basis for understanding the emotional and environmental complications of a speech or hearing disability. The interviewer should remember to distinguish between items of information that are simply interesting and background information that is really important.

5. Avoid providing information too soon. There will be plenty of time to clear up misconceptions later in the interview. The surest way to cut off the flow of information is to stop a parent, for instance, after he says, "I just tell Michael to stop, take a deep breath, and start all over again," and counsel him on the proper responses to nonfluency.

6. Avoid qualifying and hemming and hawing when asking questions. Ask them in a straightforward fashion and maintain eye contact. Rather than asking, "Did you find that, well, you know, when you were, uh, shall we say . . . with child, did you experience any untoward conditions?" say, "Did anything unusual happen during your pregnancy?" Instead of inquiring, "Did you discover, hmm, I mean, well, after your father, uh, passed away, did your stuttering problem increase?" say, "What impact did your father's death have on your speech?"

7. Avoid negativistic or moralistic responses, verbal or nonverbal, to the client's statements (avoid even the response "Good" since it implies a value judgment). The flow of information will stop rapidly and the relationship will be impaired severely if the individual senses that we find him or his behavior distasteful. We do not have to subscribe to a person's values or code of behavior for us to show compassion for and understanding of his/her situation. Use inquiries that begin with "Why . . . ?" very sparingly because beginning a question with the word *why* is often perceived as a challenge or threat; this way of questioning is too reminiscent of disciplinary sessions ("Why were you late for class?" "Why can't you behave properly?"). In a clinical setting we must not let our values obscure our perception of the client's frame of reference (Benjamin 1974). An interview is not the place to push the clinician's personal points of view. We had a student clinician who once wore a political button on her collar during a diagnostic interview. This can immediately alienate certain clients. Another student wore a button that said, "Jesus is the answer," which certainly would not have been the case for her Jewish clients.

8. When the client causes the interview to wander, avoid abrupt transitions to bring it back to the point. Most of those whom you will interview have had little experience in directed, orderly conversation. They tend to follow chance associations and wander far afield. The experienced interviewer has the ability to make smooth transitions. How does one go about getting the interview back on track? The best way is by building a bridge to the respondent's previous statements: for example, "That's interesting, Mrs. Davis, maybe we can come back to that in a little while. Now earlier you were mentioning that your child's loss of hearing occurred suddenly. . . ." The goal here is to use respondent antecedents—things that the person has said earlier in the interview. If we use only the interviewer's antecedents—questions that the interviewer has asked before—the client will not feel that he/she has been understood and will sense that what he/she has said was of little consequence. The inexperienced interviewer asks lots of questions either with no antecedents or with his/her own antecedents. This person is afraid of losing control of the interview and thus becomes preoccupied with formulating the next question.

9. Avoid allowing the interview to produce only superficial answers. We need ways to get deeper, more-significant responses from our clients. There are several interviewing devices, termed *probes*, that the clinician will find helpful.

Crosshatch, or *interlocking,* questions are useful when we need to elicit more detail about a topic that has been glossed over. Often there are discrepancies that must be resolved. Essentially, the way to go about this is to ask the same thing in different ways and at different points during the interview. For instance, the father of a young stutterer responded in a superficial manner to our query about his relationship with the child. He assured us that he had a "loving relationship" with his son and then complained at length about his working conditions. Later in the interview when we asked him to describe the sorts of things he did with the child, he was unable to mention a single one. We don't mean to imply that the clinician should attempt to catch the client lying and then demand an explanation. The clinician must examine discrepancies, however, in order to enhance understanding of the problem, since such discrepancies could have a significant effect on the mode of treatment.

Pauses can be very helpful. When there is a lull in the interview, it may mean simply that the client has exhausted his/her store of information, that a memory barrier has prevented further recall, or that he/she senses lack of understanding by the clinician. It can also mean, however, that a sensitive area has been touched upon. Do not feel that pauses harm the interview. Much significant information can be forthcoming if we keep quiet and indicate with a smile or a nod that we expect more.

Another aid is to encourage *time regression* and *association.* Memories are weak. In order to pinpoint some significant data, we may have to take the person back in time to find a memory peg, such as a wedding, or a natural calamity, that may call forth more information. One father, a long-time Air Force sergeant, cataloged everything in terms of the make and model of the car he was driving. Another client, an inveterate bird-watcher, remembered incidents by the times he had seen the marbled godwit or the prothonotary warbler.

The *summary probe* is one of the best ways to keep the interview moving smoothly. The clinician summarizes periodically what the client has said, ending perhaps with a request for clarification or further information. Incidentally, this procedure also demonstrates to the interviewee that the interviewer is indeed trying to understand the former's problem. We generally use "minisummary probes"—echo questions—all the way through an interview:

Respondent: After my husband's stroke, my whole world collapsed.

Interviewer: You were overwhelmed by the sudden change in your life.

Respondent: Yes, one day he was happily planning our trip to Sanibel Island . . . and then, in just a moment, he was paralyzed and couldn't talk. Now all our plans are up in the air . . . the new car, the checking account, he took care of all that.

The *stumbling probe* is a variation of the summary probe; we have found it helpful, especially with the reticent respondent. The interviewer rephrases a portion of the respondent's communication and then, attempting to interpret or comment upon it, the interviewer pretends to halt or stumble. For example, when interviewing the mother of a child allegedly beginning to stutter, the clinician might say: "Now, you were saying that Bruce first started to repeat and hesitate after he caught his finger in the car door. Under these conditions, it would be natural for you to . . . uh . . ." This really works. The respondent's need for closure will precipitate significant information and, perhaps more important, significant insights.

Finally, there is the *assuming probe*. If the client has avoided an important area, if he/she has left much unsaid regarding his/her speech or hearing problem and what it means to him/her, then it is up to the interviewer to bring this out. One adolescent boy who had been vehemently denying that his stuttering bothered him, unburdened himself when we said, "It bothers you so much that you don't want anybody to know, do you?"

10. Avoid letting the client reveal too much in one interview. You may have had similar experiences. A good friend encounters severe trouble and you come to his aid, helping him through the crisis. A curious thing often happens when your friend recovers his equilibrium. He feels obligated to you; he felt exposed to you as a raw human being during the crisis, and now he is embarrassed, somewhat resentful, and perhaps even hostile. It is as if you are now an outward and visible sign of his former debacle. Sometimes a beginning interviewer makes the mistake of trying to get everything in one sitting. The client, sensing perhaps that he is talking to the first person who really understands him/her, may want to pour out his/her whole sad tale of woe. Later, however, the individual will feel embarrassed and foolish, perhaps even exposed and guilty at revealing so much of himself/herself to this comparative stranger.

Bringing an interview to a graceful close can sometimes be more difficult than getting it started. In our experience, an interview is most effectively terminated by summarizing what has been discussed and reviewing the specific actions to be taken. It is probably best not to consider new material at this time when neither the interviewer nor the interviewee can devote sufficient attention to it. It is always important, however, to leave the door open for future contacts (see Stewart and Cash 1974, 197–201, and Kadushin 1972, 207–214, for more information on leave-taking).

11. Avoid trusting to memory. Record the information as the interview progresses. Tell the client that you will take some notes during the interview so that you can plan his/her treatment program more effectively and make recommendations for other services. Such note taking, or even recording devices, are rarely questioned. Indeed, we have found that clients expect you to write down some of the information they are giving you; they doubt that you would be able to remember all of their answers. You obviously would lose your relationship, however, if you scribbled furiously while the client was revealing some sensitive information. It is axiomatic that the respondent's confidence will be respected, but we have mixed feeling about mentioning this explicitly to the client. The clinician's manner should suggest that all information received is to be held strictly confidential.

Prepare a report of the interview as soon as possible. Commit your observations to paper while the encounter with the respondent is still fresh in your mind (see Chapter 9 for information on writing reports).

Goal Two: Give Information

No one likes uncertainty. Ironically, all too frequently the information, if not supplied by the professional worker, will come distorted from other sources. We can do an admirable job on our evaluation, but if we drop the ball on communicating the results to our client, we have not been successful. When not correctly informed, parents become misinformed, and this misinformation leads to confusion, misunderstanding, and further compounding on the problem. It is our responsibility, therefore, to provide accurate, unemotional, objective information of the status of the individual's speech and hearing problem. This forwarding of information is generally accomplished during the postdiagnostic conference (Martin 1977).

The clinician should summarize the findings of the clinical examination in simple, nontechnical language, using common terms compatible with the client's background. We prefer to commence, if possible, with results that show a client's area of normal functioning, to review findings that indicate what is good before describing deficiencies. Relate comments to normative values whenever possible. Clarify and help the respondent to ask questions by using examples and simple analogies. If the interviewer is in doubt concerning the client's understanding of the diagnostic material (clients will rarely ask if they don't understand), the interviewer should talk more slowly, employ longer descriptions, and use many examples and more redundant language (Longhurst and Siegel 1973).

The Questions Clients Ask. An interview is much more than a clinician's posing questions and recording the client's answers. It is an important forum for *exchange*—a reflexive, dynamic experience of sharing between the diagnostician and the informant. Indeed, we find that a client—especially a parent of a young child being evaluated—frequently is eager to probe the clinician's expertise. But often the questions the clinician asks may have a hidden meaning or purpose. The clinician must evaluate the informant's inquiries and determine, What is the person *really* asking? Is there an unstated concern behind the questions? Luterman (1979) divides the questions clients ask into three categories: *content, opinion,* and *affect.* We will describe and illustrate these three types of inquiries with excerpts from an initial interview with the mother of a three-year-old child brought to the speech clinic as a beginning stutterer.

1. *Questions dealing with information or content.* In this instance, the client seeks an informative or factual response from the clinician. The inquiry usually takes the form, "I want to know about something, and I hope you have the right information."

Mrs. Bell: The type of choppy speech [disfluency] Jesse has—is it common among children his age?

Clinician: It sure is. Most children between the ages of two-and-a-half and five do a lot of repeating and hesitating.

2. *Questions with predetermined opinions.* Here the client has an opinion regarding a particular subject and wants to determine if the clinician agrees with it. The clinician must be careful not to merely demolish the client's opinion until the clinician understands *why* and *how strongly* the client holds it.

Mrs. Bell: Um, on TV a couple of times, I've seen a demonstration of the airflow technique for stuttering. What do you think of it?

Clinician: Those demonstrations are very dramatic, aren't they? What's your impression of the technique as it applies to Jesse?

3. *Questions that are a "faint knocking on the door."* In this case, the client is not asking for information, or to determine the clinician's opinion, but rather for emotional support and reassurance. The question conceals a feeling that the client either is unaware of or is reluctant to reveal.

Mrs. Bell: Do you think my divorce and remarriage had anything to do with Jesse's speech problem?

Clinician: It's pretty easy for parents to feel guilty about something they might have done to cause their child to begin stuttering.

No doubt the reader has already detected a flaw in the triad: On the surface, each question posed by Mrs. Bell could be classified in any of the three categories. How does a clinician know *what* the client means? The clinician doesn't know in every case, but he/she tries to determine the purpose of a question by scrutinizing *how* a client asks it—by vocal inflection and body language—and by examining the context in which the inquiry appears. Interestingly, as long as the clinician is *trying to understand,* a client will not be alienated by an inaccurate interpretation (Chinn, Winn, and Walters 1978).

In our experience, speech clinicians, probably because the bulk of their training focuses on information, do a good job of responding to content questions. However, many beginning clinicians find it difficult to respond appropriately to a client's expression of emotion. Although Luterman (1979) is discussing clinical audiologists, his remarks pertain to many speech clinicians as well:

> *Professional training programs rarely provide any information or experience for the student in how to deal with parents. They concentrate instead on providing considerable information and practicum experience with the handicapped child. As a result of that imbalance in emphasis, the young therapist feels very insecure in dealing with parents, who may be older and more experienced in the care of children. So the therapist begins to adopt defensive strategies to "distance" the parents, the most common one being to impart information. The content-based relationship is completely controlled by the teacher and subtly puts the parents down by increasing their feelings of inadequacy. That one-sided way of dealing with parents becomes habitual with time, and older teachers rely on content strategy almost exclusively. In some circles that approach is considered very professional. It is only when professionals feel secure as people that they can allow more intimacy and more freedom in their relationship with parents. (48)*

Avoid superficial statements of reassurance. Most people can see through this sort of sham. The client's anxiety and uncertainty will be better relieved once he/she begins to understand his/her particular speech problem; the best antidote to fear and uncertainty is knowledge. Be sure, however, to avoid iatrogenic errors. Do not use terms or suggest consequences that will precipitate more stress for the client. One parent was told that his child's hearing problem was caused by atrophy of the hearing nerve. It is difficult enough to have a hard-of-hearing child without worry about mysterious nerves atrophying, something about which the parent can do very little. Do not communicate your negative expectations regarding the outcome of therapy to the client. We are convinced that the client will do what the clinician thinks the client can do. In other words, the client's behavior expands to fit the clinician's concept of the client's potential. Do we precondition our own therapeutic behavior when we make a prognosis? Is this communicated to the client and his/her relatives in some manner and on some level? We think it often is.

Below are six basic principles, addressed to the beginning clinician, for imparting information to clients that we have found useful:

1. Emotional confusion may, and often does, inhibit the client's ability to understand cognitively what you are trying to say. Just because you have once reviewed the steps of therapy is no reason to expect that its importance will be grasped.

2. Refrain from being didactic; do not lecture your clients. Focus on sharing options rather than giving advise.

3. Use simple language with many examples and illustrations. If you must err, err in the direction of being too simple rather than too complex. And repeat, repeat, repeat the important points—rephrasing each time.

4. Try to provide something that the client—especially a parent—can do. Action reduces the feelings of futility and anxiety. The activity should be direct and simple and should require some kind of reporting to the clinician.

5. Say what needs to be said pleasantly—but frankly. Do not avoid saying something that must be said on the assumption that the client cannot take it or that you will be rejected. People often display an amazing reserve of courage in difficult situations (Buscaglia 1975).

6. Remember, however, that the one who finally communicates what the client may have been dreading to hear is often hated and maligned. If you are the first to say the feared words, you may become the focus for all the hostile, negative feelings thus aroused. As a professional worker, you will have to be strong enough to be the lightning rod for these emotions.

Clients and their parents expect to receive help from the clinician but often will resist change. No matter how maladaptive a client's behavior may seem from an objective point of view, it represents the client's best solution. In fact, the client will often resist attempts to alter his/her equilibrium, precarious as it may appear to others. Change is stressful; diagnosis and treatment imply change; therefore, assessment and therapy are stressful.

According to Carkhuff and Berenson (1967) and others (Ginott 1965; Gordon 1970), the key feature of *creative listening* is the ability to scan a client's comments and respond in a way that fosters understanding and releases the potential for growth. Creative listening represents empathy in action: Before anyone can or will listen, he/she must first be listened to.

The particular kind of understanding we are referring to involves two facets: a *cognitive* aspect (the content) and an *affective* aspect (the feelings). In order for genuine understanding to take place, both aspects must be included in the interviewer's response to the client's statement. If the clinician is successful in crystallizing both aspects of his/her response, this provides an *interchangeable base* that allows the interview to move forward to levels of helping that involve direct action. Here are some examples taken from diagnostic interviews:

Client: (in response to a query regarding his marital status): No, I'm single. . . . Who would want to marry a clod who stutters like me?

Clinician: You feel rejected because of your speech problem, is that right?

Parent: We tried to be good parents, we really did . . . but somehow we messed up in helping Peter learn to talk.

Clinician: You feel a sense of failure, perhaps even guilt, that your child has a speech problem.

Client: I stutter so badly that life is worthless. . . . I can't get a job. . . . The business of living just doesn't seem to meet expenses.

Clinician: You feel thwarted and frustrated by your speech problem. Sometimes you wonder if you can go on.

Note the clinician's responses carefully. The clinician does not simply repeat the client's comment but attempts to restate it in clarified form. Observe that the interviewer used the second-person singular "you" in referring to the client's affect. Feelings are commonly stated first, since they are more important than content. We sometimes add a tag question ("Is that right?") to check on the client's intake of our responses.

Goal Three: Provide Release and Support

The clinician does not, of course, wait until the end of the interview to provide release for the frustrations and fears of the client. Most of the parts of the interview already discussed will serve this purpose. By helping the client talk out his/her problems, the clinician is providing an excellent escape for pent-up feelings. We maintain that our purpose is not just to remove discomfort but also to promote a state of comfort and well-being.

More than advice is needed during interviews for the purpose of helping a client take some specific action or move in a particular direction. The client needs help in sorting out confusing choices. To support a respondent's real strengths, we need to make it clear that we understand what the situation means to him/her and that we uncritically sympathize with his/her feelings and attitudes. We can restore the client's self-esteem and ability to function more appropriately if we convey our interest in him/her as a person and our solid acceptance of the client's importance. If the client feels appreciated and understood, he/she can sometimes drop his/her self-protective behavior and see how the experience will eventually be of benefit.

There is an unfortunate tradition of "sweetness and light" in client counseling. A person has a problem. The person is sad and depressed, and we try to cheer him or her up. Sometimes this degenerates into a debate, with the interviewer's attempting to persuade the person that he/she should not feel miserable. When a person feels depressed, anxious, and fearful, he/she does not want to count his/her blessings. That person wants you to feel miserable, too. He/she wants you to share and identify with him/her on his/her own level. Thus, the interviewer is given a basis for communication with the person. We start where he/she is, accept it as the proper place to start, and agree that it is a sad state of affairs that would make anyone sad and depressed. Then, using this bond of identification, which becomes a basis for communication, we can assist in solving the problem. The main ingredient is *empathy*, the capacity to identify oneself with another's feelings and actions. The best way to demonstrate our attempt to understand a client's point of view is by listening creatively. In our judgment, of all the skills inherent in effective interviewing, the most important is the ability to listen carefully and empathically. This skill can be learned, although beginning clinicians find it difficult to employ remarks that facilitate a client's expression of feelings (Volz et al. 1978).

How does one handle emotional scenes? They are bound to arise at some point in your interviewing experience. Some clinicians excuse themselves from the room and allow the respondent to recover his/her dignity alone. Others try to change the subject to something less emotional. Both of these approaches may, with certain clients, give the impression that the clinician is rejecting their feelings. It is more effective to indicate one's understanding of the feelings that are being expressed and accept them as natural human reactions: for example, "That's okay to let it come out, Mrs. Moody. You have been holding it back too long. Sometimes it helps to get it out in the open."

Not all clients seen by the speech clinician will need or even want extensive supportive interviewing. In some cases, the procedures discussed here would be grossly inappropriate. Visualize an interview as ranging along a continuum from affective concern, such as feelings and attitudes, to objective matters, such as goals and advice. Some respondents simply need objective information so that they can take over and modify their behavior. The clinician's role in some interviews may consist of simply listening to and supporting a client. We quite agree that love alone is not enough in a helping transaction; a good relationship is a *necessary* but not a *sufficient* condition for good interviewing. Although it may sound trite, it is true that the secret of care *of* a client is caring *for* the client. The sense of being understood by a helping professional is a powerful stimulant to the client's growth (Llewelyn and Hume 1979; Sherman and Fields 1982).

Improving Interviewing Skills

We hope the material in this chapter will be useful to students majoring in clinical speech pathology and to our colleagues working in various settings. However, no one ever became proficient in interviewing solely by reading about it. Nor, it seems, are interviewing skills enhanced by increasing knowledge about communication disorders (Janz 1982; Wolraich et al. 1982). It took us many years of constant searching and experimenting to evolve the interviewing approach presented here. And, with the indulgence of our clients and many long-suffering parents, we continue to explore for better ways.

We have included below a series of activities and projects for your own practice. Let them serve as the beginning steps in a continual learning effort toward improved interviewing. You will find that the time devoted to such training exercises is well spent. Now, consider these steps on how to improve your interviewing skills:

1. Read widely from a variety of sources. We have included a list of selected references to get you started. Find out what people are like by reading in sociology, psychology, anthropology, and philosophy. This is, of course, a lifetime project, which we feel is delightful since there is always a new frontier, an open horizon toward which we can set our sails. Our profession has arisen so abruptly, has grown so rapidly, and has been so concerned with the urgent scientific and clinical issues that it has ignored the important issue—the development of a philosophical basis for our work. A speech-and-hearing clinician without a rationale is like a ship without a rudder. The fundamental and mandatory basis for sound, purposeful therapy is an overall point of view, a workable theory that does not necessarily include the specific activities that will be used to carry it out. Nothing is so pathetic as the clinician who, in a willy-nilly manner, empties a bag of therapeutic homilies on the client's lap, hoping somehow that one of them will work. Only a sequential system of logically interrelated theorems will enable us to evaluate our clinical effectiveness.

2. Listen to all sorts of people, to their dreams, their rationalizations, their insights—or lack of them—and their gripes. Get acquainted with the way common people think and talk, by following the example of Caldwell (1976) and others (Coleman 1974; Least-Heat-Moon 1982; Morris 1972; Steinbeck 1961; Terkel 1980; Walters 1970).

3. Form small heterogeneous groups of students majoring in speech pathology and audiology. Conduct some sensitivity and values clarification training, particularly as it relates to your self-concept, your assets and liabilities, your responses to people, and your relationship with your own parents and other older adults (Kaplan and Dreyer 1974). In order to provide assistance to others, we must know our own foibles and potential blind spots and have them under reasonable control. Remember, too, that the way in which our academic preparation teaches us to explain a situation will tend to determine the way in which we perceive it.

4. Role-playing is still one of the best methods to prepare for interviewing (Finn and Rose 1982; White 1982). Set up several typical interview situations in front of a class and play, for example, the roles of the reluctant parent, the spouse of an aphasic patient, or the hostile father. Discuss the interaction and replay the situations with others assuming the roles. Write out interview purposes prior to the role-playing and determine, or have the class determine, how effectively the interviewer accomplished avowed purposes. Whenever the viewers feel that the interview went wrong or the responses were ineffective, see how many different ways the interview could have been handled. This builds up the beginning interviewer's repertoire of adaptive responses. You can do a surprising amount of intrapersonal role-playing in your spare time. While we are waiting for a class to begin, for a light to change, or for our father-in-law to cease talking, we frequently imagine ourselves in various interviewing situations and then explore alternate statements, probes, and so forth.

5. Make recordings of your first few interviews, then analyze them carefully with your clinical supervisor or a colleague (Adler and Enelow 1966; Cannell, Lawson, and Hausser 1975; Irwin 1975). We believe that multiple interviewers simply do not work (although seeing multiple interviewees—such as a mother and father at the same time—can be useful and productive); hence, we would suggest that your supervisor not observe your performance in the same room, especially for your first ventures. In a dyadic interview there are only two possible directions for communication ($1 \times 2 = 2$). When a third party is added it increases the potential interaction to six ($1 \times 2 \times 3 = 6$). Add yet another person, and the possibilities for communicative exchange reach unwieldy proportions ($1 \times 2 \times 3 \times 4 = 24$). We have found that when the supervisor stays in the room, the student has a tendency to seduce him/her into taking over as interviewer; and if the supervisor refuses to assume the mantle, he/she can only sit there looking at the clients as if they were bugs in an insect collection. We have no role sanction in our social structure for the silent scrutinizer, and this presence can seriously impair the effectiveness of the interview.

Play back your interview again and again, revising statements, underscoring errors, and scanning for the good parts. Have typed protocols prepared from some of these tapes—the errors really leap out at you from the printed page—and discuss them with your instructors, fellow students, or colleagues.

Stewart and Cash (1974) have devised a set of questions that you can use as a guideline for evaluating your performance. Explore also the methods prepared by Iwata et al. (1982) and Molyneaux and Lane (1982) for the assessment and training of clinical interviewing skills. Finally, we suggest you evaluate your diagnostic interviews by using the Checklist of Interviewing Competencies (Figure 2.2). Obviously, no beginning clinician will remember, let alone exhibit, all the skills delineated in the checklist; practice only a few at a time, and provide constructive feedback for each other.

We would like to end this chapter with a challenge to the reader. We challenge you to utilize the interviewing approach delineated above, find the errors, the

FIGURE 2.2   Checklist of Interviewing Competencies

Interviewer: _____   Date: _____

Client/Respondent: _____

   I. *Orienting the Respondent*
      A. Attends to comfort (coats, seating, and so on)
      B. Engages in appropriate "flow" talk
      C. Explains purposes, procedures
      D. Structures roles

  II. *Engendering Communication*
      A. Attending behaviors (demonstration receptiveness)
         1. Relaxed, natural posture
         2. Appropriate eye contact
         3. Responses that follow the client's comments (restating, overlapping the client's message)
      B. Open invitation to share (open-ended questions)
      C. Nondistracting encouragement to continue talking
         1. Verbal ("Yes," "I see," and the like)
         2. Nonverbal (nodding, shifting posture toward client)
      D. Obtains an overview of the presenting problem

 III. *Use of Questions and Recording*
      A. Orderly, sequential questions
      B. Nondistracting note taking

  IV. *Active Listening*
      A. Reflects feelings (empathic statements)
         1. Matches affect
         2. Matches content
      B. Periodic summarizing of affect and content message

   V. *Monitoring Nonverbal Clues*
      A. The diagnostician's
      B. The respondent's

  VI. *Skills in Presenting Information*
      A. Transmission of information
         1. Content
         2. Style and language
      B. Responds to questions appropriately
      C. Appropriate use of humor, "flow" talk

 VII. *Closing the Interview*
      A. Summary, review of findings
      B. Recommendations
      C. Supportive comments

VIII. *Analysis of Information*
      A. Major themes in the client's presentation, association of ideas, inconsistencies and omissions
      B. Descriptive report

Note: This checklist is designed to help monitor the performance of beginning interviewers. It can be used as a self-rating device or a format for supervisory feedback. (See also Enlow and Swisher 1972; and Maier 1976.)

things that just don't work for you, and then develop your own methods. We have given you the foundation blocks. Can you use them to make stepping-stones?

Bibliography

Adler, L., and Enelow, A. (1966). "An Instrument to Measure Skill in Diagnostic Interviewing: A Teaching and Evaluation Tool." *Journal of Medical Education* 41:281–288.

Argyle, M., and Cook, M. (1976). *Gaze and Mutual Gaze.* London: Cambridge University Press.

Benjamin, A. (1974). *The Helping Interview.* 2nd ed. Boston: Houghton Mifflin.

Birdwhistle, R. (1970). *Kinesics and Context.* Philadelphia: University of Pennsylvania Press.

Bosmajian, H., ed. (1971). *The Rhetoric of Nonverbal Communication.* Glenview, IL: Scott, Foresman.

Buscaglia, L. (1975). *The Disabled and Their Parents: A Counseling Challenge.* Thorofare, NJ: Charles B. Slack.

Caldwell, E. (1976). *Afternoons in Mid-America.* New York: Dodd, Mead.

Cannell, C., Lawson, S., and Hausser, D. (1975). *A Technique for Evaluating Interviewer Performance.* Ann Arbor, MI: Institute for Social Research.

Carkhuff, R., and Berenson, B. (1967). *Beyond Counseling and Therapy.* New York: Holt, Rinehart, and Winston.

Cheng, L. (1989). "Service Delivery to Asian/Pacific LEP Children: A Cross-Cultural Framework." *Topics in Language Disorders* 9:1–14.

Chinn, P., Winn, J., and Walters, R. (1978). *Two-Way Talking with Parents of Special Children.* St. Louis: Mosby.

Coleman, R. (1974). *Blue-Collar Journal: A College President's Sabbatical.* New York: Lippincott.

Czikszentmihalyi, M. (1975). *Beyond Boredom and Anxiety.* San Francisco: Jossey-Bass.

Duncan, S., and Fiske, D. (1977). *Face-to-Face Interaction: Research, Methods and Theory.* Hillsdale, NJ: Lawrence Erlbaum Associates.

Egolf, D., and Chester, S. (1973). "Nonverbal Communication and the Disorders of Speech and Language." *Journal of American Speech and Hearing Association* 15:511–518.

Eisenberg, A., and Smith, R. (1971). *Nonverbal Communication.* New York: Bobbs-Merrill.

Ekman, P. (1980). *The Faces of Man.* New York: Garland Press.

Featherstone, H. (1980). *A Difference in the Family: Life with a Disabled Child.* New York: Basic Books.

Feldman, S. (1973). *Mannerisms of Speech and Gesture in Everyday Life.* New York: International Universities Press.

Finn, J., and Rose, S. (1982). "Development and Validation of the Interview Skills Role-Playing Test." *Social Work Research Abstracts* 18:21–27.

Garrett, A. (1972). *Interviewing: Its Principles and Methods.* 2nd ed. New York: Family Service Association.

Ginott, H. (1965). *Between Parent and Child.* New York: Macmillan.

Goffman, E. (1959). *The Presentation of Self in Everyday Life.* Garden City, NY: Doubleday.

Goffman, E. (1963). *Stigma: Notes on the Management of Spoiled Identity.* Englewood Cliffs, NJ: Prentice-Hall.

Gordon, T. (1970). *Parent Effectiveness in Training.* New York: Peter H. Wyden.

Harrison, R. (1974). *Beyond Words: An Introduction to Nonverbal Communication.* Englewood Cliffs, NJ: Prentice-Hall.

Haynes, W., and Oratio, A. (1978). "A Study of Client's Perceptions of Therapeutic Effectiveness." *Journal of Speech and Hearing Disorders* 43:21–33.

Hinde, R., (1972). *Nonverbal Communication.* New York: Cambridge University Press.

Hodges, K., et al. (1982). "The Development of a Child Assessment Interview for Research and Clinical Use." *Journal of Abnormal Child Psychology* 10:173–189.

Irwin, R. B. (1975). "Micro-Counseling Interviewing Skill of Supervisors of Speech Clinicians." *Human Communication* 4:5–9.

Iwata, B., et al. (1982). "Assessment and Training of Clinical Interviewing Skills: Analogue Analysis and Field Replication." *Journal of Applied Behavior Analysis* 15:191–203.

Janz, T. (1982). "Initial Comparisons of Patterned-Behavior Description Interviews vs. Unstructured Interviews." *Journal of Applied Psychology* 67:577–588.

Kadushin, A. (1972). *The Social Work Interview.* New York: Columbia University Press.

Kaplan, N., and Dreyer, D. (1974). "The Effect of Self-Awareness Training on Student Speech Pathologist-Client Relationships." *Journal of Communication Disorders* 7:329–342.

Knapp, M. (1972). *Nonverbal Communication in Human Interaction.* New York: Holt, Rinehart, and Winston.

Least-Heat-Moon, W. (1982). *Blue Highways: A Journey into America.* Boston: Atlantic–Little, Brown.

Leathers, D. (1976). *Nonverbal Communication Systems.* Boston: Allyn and Bacon.

Llewelyn, S., and Hume, W. (1979). "The Patient's View of Therapy." *British Journal of Medical Psychology* 52:29–35.

Longhurst, T., and Siegel, G. (1973). "Effects of Communication Failure on Speaker and Listener Behavior." *Journal of Speech and Hearing Research* 16:128–140.

Luterman, D. (1979). *Counseling Parents of Hearing-Impaired Children.* Boston: Little, Brown.

Lynch, E. (1992). "Developing Cross-Cultural Competence." In *Developing Cross-Cultural Competence,* ed. E. Lynch, and M. Hanson, (Baltimore, MD: Brookes).

Mcquire, M., and Lorch, S. (1968). "A Model for the Study of Dyadic Communication." *Journal of Nervous and Mental Diseases* 146:221–229.

Maier, N. (1976). *Appraising Performance: An Interview Skills Course.* La Jolla, CA: University Associates.

Marshall, N., and Goldstein, S. (1969). "Imparting Diagnostic Information to Mothers: A Comparison of Methodologies." *Journal of Speech and Hearing Research* 12:65–72.

Martin, A. (1977). "Post-Diagnostic Parent Counseling by a Speech Pathologist and a Social Worker." *Journal of American Speech and Hearing Association* 19:67–68.

Matarazzo, J., and Wiens, A. (1972). *The Interview: Research on Its Anatomy and Structure.* Chicago: Aldine-Atherton.

Mehrabian, A. (1972). *Nonverbal Communication.* Chicago: Aldine-Aterton.

Molyneaux, D., and Lane, V. (1982). *Effective Interviewing: Techniques and Analysis.* Boston: Allyn and Bacon.

Morgan, H., and Cogger, J. (1973). *The Interviewer's Manual.* New York: Psychological Corporation.

Morris, T. (1972). *The Walk of the Conscious Ants.* New York: Knopf.

Morsbach, H. (1973). "Aspect of Nonverbal Communication in Japan." *Journal of Nervous and Mental Disorders* 157:262–277.

Nideffer, R. (1976). *The Inner Athlete.* New York: Crowell.

Pratt, L., Seligman, A., and Reader, G. (1958). "Physicians' Views on the Medical Information Among Patients." In *Patients, Physicians, and Illness.* New York: Free Press.

Richardson, S., Dohrenwend, B., and Klein, D. (1965). *Interviewing: Its Forms and Functions.* New York: Basic Books.

Rosenthal, R., et al. (1974). "Body Talk and the Tone of Voice: The Language Without Words." *Psychology Today* 8:64–68.

Scheflen, A. (1972). *Body Language and Social Order.* Englewood Cliffs, NJ: Prentice-Hall.

Sherman, J., and Fields, S. (1982). *Guide to Patient Evaluation.* 4th ed. Garden City, NY: Medical Examination Publishing Company.

Sigelman, C. (1982). "Evaluating Alternative Techniques of Questioning Mentally Retarded Persons." *American Journal of Mental Deficiency* 86:511–518.

Spiegel, J., and Machotka, P. (1974). *Messages of the Body.* New York: Free Press.

Staples, F., and Sloane, R. (1976). "Truax Factors, Speech Characteristics and Therapy Outcome." *Journal of Nervous and Mental Disorders* 163:135–140.

Steinbeck, J. (1961). *Travels with Charley.* New York: Viking.

Stewart, C. and Cash, W. (1974). *Interviewing: Principles and Practices.* Dubuque, IA: W. C. Brown.

Terkel, S. (1980). *American Dreams: Lost and Found.* New York: Pantheon.

Volz, H., Klevans, D., Norson, S., and Putens, D. (1978). "Interpersonal Communication Skills of Speech-Language Pathology Undergraduates: The Effects of Training." *Journal of Speech and Hearing Disorders* 43:524–542.

Walters, B. (1970). *How to Talk with Practically Anybody about Practically Anything.* Garden City, NY: Doubleday.

Weitz, S. (1974). *Nonverbal Communication: Readings with Commentary.* New York: Oxford University Press.

White, R. (1982). "Observer's Presence and Self-Focused Attention in Role-Rehearsal Activities." *Perceptual and Motor Skills* 54:839–842.

Wolraich, M., et al. (1982). "Factors Affecting Physician Communication and Parent-Physician Dialogues. *Journal of Medical Education* 57:621–625.

Woolf, G. (1971). "Information Specificity: A Correlate of Verbal Output in Diagnostic Interview." *Journal of Speech and Hearing Disorders* 36:518–526.

Chapter 3

Psychometric Considerations in Diagnosis and Evaluation

Let us interest you in purchasing a standardized test to use in assessing communication disorders. It has the following characteristics:

1. Test administrators have trouble agreeing on whether a response on the test is correct or not.
2. Clients seem to perform differently on the test each time they take it.
3. The test really does not focus on the aspects of communication that are relevant to treatment or diagnostic decision making.
4. The test manual is vague about how to administer the instrument and how to interpret the results.
5. The test does not really examine the true process that you are attempting to assess.
6. The test was normed on 200 normal, White children from Idaho.
7. The test does not adequately discriminate between those clients with disorders from those who are normal.

No one in their right mind would buy the instrument described above because it would provide little valid and reliable information to use in assessment. Do tests in communication disorders ever have this many shortcomings? Unfortunately, *many* formal tests in our field suffer from the problems listed above (McCauley and Swisher 1984a, 1984b; Muma 1983, 1984, 1986; Muma, Lubinski, and Pierce 1982; Plante and Vance 1994)! This, however, is not likely to happen. The authors of these tests no doubt begin with the notion of designing a useful instrument; however, when conceptual and psychometric limitations manifest themselves, the test designer is typically reluctant to scrap the whole enterprise. Usually, the test is submitted, warts and all, to a publisher because, even though it suffers from inadequacies, it represents a significant amount of work in its development. It is therefore up to the consumer to carefully evaluate any instrument in terms of psychometric adequacy before purchasing it. We must become educated in evaluating any instruments that we buy, not only because purchasing an inadequate test is a waste of our money but, more important, is a waste of our time. We have just mentioned the effects of buying and using inadequate tests on the clinician, but it also affects our clients since they must spend money paying for the administration of these tests and also must invest their time to take the tests. In addition, a client can be misdiagnosed, mislabeled, and mistreated on the basis of testing with psychometrically poor instruments. One can readily see that psychometric adequacy of standardized tests is a significant issue and one that we must deal with in a textbook on diagnosis and evaluation.

It is important to note that it is not only standardized instruments that require some measure of psychometric adequacy. While many authorities apply psychometric principles only to standardized, norm-referenced tests, it is the feeling of the present authors that most of the informal or descriptive measures that we use in communication disorders are also susceptible to considerable error. Just because we are not using a standardized test does not relieve us of the responsibility of checking our validity and reliability. The same psychometric rigor applied to standardized examinations could easily be applied to our informal evaluation procedures (Hegde 1987). Informal measures can clearly vary in the degree to which they are valid and reliable. Validity is the degree to which a procedure actually measures what it purports to measure. Validity can be compromised in both formal or informal procedures. For instance, we can ask a person with velopharyngeal incompetency to blow a pinwheel and we can time how long it spins to get an indication of velopharyngeal closure. This measure may have good reliability in that two clinicians could time the pinwheel with a stopwatch and agree on how long the wheel spins. Perhaps the client could even be reliable in terms of blowing the wheel in a similar fashion over several trials and making the wheel spin a fairly consistent length of time each trial. The problem, however, is validity. We know that blowing a pinwheel may not relate at all to the ability to maintain velopharyngeal closure during speech production. Reliability is useless if the measure being taken is not valid.

There are many potential problems with reliability as well with the use of informal measures. For instance, many behaviors that we observe, count, or time are often not clearly defined, and this imprecision contributes to a lack of reliability. In order to have good agreement, two examiners would have to be looking for the same behavior and coding it in a similar manner. The difficult aspect of informal assessment is that many behaviors that we examine are transient (phonemes, disfluencies, facial grimaces, laryngeal tension, slight head jerks, etc.) while others may be ill defined and subjective (pitch changes, topic changes, cohesive adequacy, voice quality changes, stress alterations, intelligibility, severity, etc.). In research reports, it is incumbent on the investigator to provide evidence that behaviors studied are both valid and reliable. Clinicians must devote the same attention to these issues if they use informal measures so that these measures can be replicated over time as indications of treatment progress. Without validity and reliability, informal measures are nothing more than the "artsy," subjective judgments of one person that may tell us little about client performance.

Common Types of Tests

Most textbooks on psychometric issues focus on norm-referenced tests. Norm-referenced tests also are called standardized tests or formal tests, depending on the designer's preference. Just because a test is standardized, however, does not mean that it is norm-referenced. Standardization can only imply that the procedures for test administration are standard while no norms may be provided with the instrument. In developing norm-referenced tests, the designers have created some tasks they feel are relevant (valid) and have administered the instrument to large groups of subjects who hopefully represent the population on whom the test is to be used. From these large-scale administrations, the designers are able to calculate normative data that reflect the performance of the large sample. When an individual is given the test, his/her score is compared to the performance of the normative sample and it is determined how this person performed similarly relative to the large group. The purpose of norm-referenced tests is to determine if an individual obtains a score similar to the group average or, if not, how far away from average the score is. Generally, if the individual scored within 1.5 to 2 standard deviations above or below the mean, he/she is said to reflect performance within "normal limits." If the score was more than 2 standard deviations above or below the mean, the performance is said to be exceptional, since only about 5% of the normative population scored in a similar manner. Thus, norm-referenced tests have the major purpose of determining if there is a problem, or a significant enough difference from standard performance to warrant concern with regard to normalcy. We will have more to say in a later section regarding some qualifications that must be taken into account when considering this purpose of standardized tests.

The other type of test typically mentioned in psychometric texts is the criterion-referenced instrument. Salvia and Ysseldyke (1981) describe such tests as follows:

> *Rather than indicating a person's relative standing in skill development, criterion-referenced tests measure a person's development of particular skills in terms of absolute levels of mastery. . . . Items on criterion-referenced tests are often linked directly to specific instructional objectives and therefore facilitate the writing of objectives. Test items sample sequential skills, enabling a teacher not only to know the specific point at which to begin instruction but also to plan those instructional aspects that follow directly in the curricular sequence.* (30)

The criterion-referenced test, then, serves a different purpose compared to a norm-referenced instrument. It is clearly more related to defining specific skills in assessment and treatment and emphasizes individual performance, while the norm-referenced tests focus on group similarity (Muma 1973). McCauley (1996) provides guidelines for the evaluation, selection, and development of informal criterion-referenced measures in communication disorders. Unfortunately, there are precious few criterion-referenced measures in our field. Most of our formal instruments are norm-referenced, so the focus of the rest of the chapter will be on these types of tests.

Validity: The Foundation of the Test or Measure

As we mentioned above, a test can be reliable but may lack validity. Validity basically refers to the extent to which a test measures what it sets out to measure. Validity is highly related to the purpose for which the test is used, and a particular test can be valid for one purpose and invalid for another (Plante 1996). If we say we are going to measure a child's language comprehension, we hopefully select a test that can accomplish this goal. If the test is measuring something other than the child's language comprehension, then the test is invalid. So many of the behaviors we assess in communication disorders are extremely complex and involve multiple systems. Language, for example, has many areas (semantics, syntax, morphology, phonology, pragmatics), and it is influenced by other systems (cognitive, social, psychological, neurolinguistic, etc.). If we develop a test of "language ability" that can be administered and scored in twenty minutes, and this test has the child imitate, name pictures, and point to photographs, we have not really looked at language ability completely. We have taken a few tasks and we are willing to make judgments about a very complex linguistic system based on the child's ability to perform these operations, which are totally unnatural and unrelated to normal language use. This is tantamount to a cardiologist's making a clinical judgment about a significant heart condition only by feeling the patient's pulse. Such a judgment is just not valid, especially when we have the technology available to do a thorough evaluation of heart function by using EKG and other measures. The major point here is that without validity we are fooling ourselves as we look at complex behaviors. Even if we can demonstrate that the items on the test are reliable, it does not matter. We have only developed a reliable way of looking at "garbage." This point is made painfully clear by several authors who raise ethical concerns about the administration of tests that lack validity (Messick 1980; Muma 1984). If we use such tests, we not only waste time and money, but we can arrive at erroneous judgments about our clients, resulting in incorrect goal selection, or worse, placement in inappropriate programs.

Classically, discussions of validity focus on three types: construct, content, and criterion-related validity. Construct validity is "the degree to which a test measures the theoretical construct it is intended to measure" (Anastasi 1976, 151). To obtain this type of validity "the test author must rely on indirect evidence and inference" (Salvia and Ysseldyke 1981, 108). Thus, a test in any area of communication disorders must ideally reflect the underlying construct it is attempting to assess. A second type of validity is content validity. Typically, content validity is derived by: "a careful examination of the content of a test. Such an examination is judgmental in nature and requires a clear definition of what the content should be. Content validity is established by examining three factors: the appropriateness of the types of items included, the completeness of the item sample, and the way in which the items assess the content" (Salvia and Ysseldyke 1981, 102). Typically, expert judges are included to examine the content of the test in order to make the determination of content validity.

A final type of validity is criterion-related. There are two types of criterion-related validity. First, concurrent validity is a measure of how an individual's current score on one instrument can be used to make an estimate of his/her current score on some other criterion measure, typically another test in a related area. Predictive validity is a measure of how an individual's current score on one instrument can estimate scoring on a criterion measure taken at a later time. A critical variable, however, is the validity and reliability of the criterion measure selected for use in criterion-related validity. The instrument you design must be valid, and so must the criterion measure.

The three types of validity mentioned above would ideally be used in concert to determine the overall validity of a test instrument. There is, however, a tendency among some test designers to believe that only one or two types of validity are required to validate an instrument and that perhaps the three types of validity are equally powerful and thus interchangeable. This is *not* the case. The most potent type of validity is construct validity. Construct validity is viewed by most authorities as the *keystone* of test development (Messick 1975, 1980; Muma 1985). We have separated this section on validity from the rest of the psychometric background in this chapter and discuss it first because it is probably the most important issue in psychometric adequacy. It does not matter how popular a test is, how easy it is to administer, or how much statistical hocus-pocus is found in the examiner's manual. If the test lacks validity, it is nothing more than a wasteful, empty exercise.

Reliability

The notion of reliability is critical to formal as well as informal measures. If one were to develop a valid norm-referenced test or informal measure, it would be useless if the test developer could not demonstrate that different examiners could use it with similar facility and that clients performed consistently from one occasion to another. Several types of reliability are classically discussed.

1. *Interjudge Reliability.* This term refers to the agreement of two independent judges on the occurrence and type of responses performed by a client. Almost every clinician has had the experience of asking another SLP to take a look at a difficult case. We question our abilities to judge aberrant vocal qualities and pitches. We often want another opinion on a child's intelligibility or pragmatic abilities. Clients who stutter often present many complex avoidances and timing devices that we ask our peers to scrutinize, just to make sure we are on the right track. Sometimes, even in standardized tests, we ask the opinions of others to check some arbitrary scoring convention that we have used because the manual did not tell us what to do in enough detail. All of these factors have to do with interjudge reliability.

The types of responses that we ask children and adults to perform in diagnosis and evaluation tasks are many and varied. Some responses are relatively straightforward and easily agreed upon by two independent judges. For example, if we ask a client to point to one of four pictures in response to an auditory model (e.g., "Point to 'running'") most judges would agree on the correctness of the client's response. Other types of responding may not be quite as clear to judges. For instance, judges may not be able to agree on the occurrence of a distorted /s/ or /r/ phoneme.

Judges may have difficulty determining whether a response was correct if the client initially makes the wrong response and then self-corrects it. Does the test provide guidelines for examiners in terms of accepting a self-corrected response as "correct"? In informal tasks, it is often difficult for judges to agree on certain behaviors, such as the amount of time spent in symbolic play. An adequate operational definition of symbolic play would be necessary and criteria for when such play begins and ends would be required if two judges are to agree on time sampling of behavior. Thus, we can see that the behaviors that judges must agree upon vary in terms of their observability, definition, and subjectivity. If judges cannot agree on what they are observing, then the test or procedure is unreliable. There are some obvious contributing factors that decrease interjudge reliability:

a. *Incomplete or Ambiguous Definitions.* If a behavior is to be counted, timed, observed, or interpreted, there must be an adequate definition of the behavior so that independent judges can agree on behavioral occurrences. For example, if one goal of treatment is to reduce behavior problems in a client with language impairment, the measurement of this construct (behavior problem) must be guided by a specific definition. Do behavior problems include only tantrums, or do actions such as pushing the materials away, whining, repetitive vocalizations, and refusal to participate in tasks also constitute behavior problems? One can readily see that two examiners could experience major disagreement on this measure unless the definition was quite precise. The two judges need to know what to count or time and what behaviors to exclude from the concept of behavior problems. Sometimes the operational definition selected by an examiner may not be universally agreed upon, and this may affect the *validity* of the measure. Even if the definition is somewhat incomplete, however, reliability can be increased by limiting the behaviors under scrutiny so that everyone can agree when they occur. Regardless of whether the measure is a formal, standardized test or an informal evaluation measure, interjudge reliability is critical to psychometric adequacy of the test. Formal tests should include data on interjudge reliability. Test manuals should include detailed definitions of the behaviors to be scored and as many guidelines as possible about potential response modes that may be difficult for the examiner to interpret as a correct or incorrect response. Some tests (Porch 1967) have multidimensional scoring systems in which the client's response is not merely judged for correctness but also for the way the response occurred and for levels of acceptability. If the scoring system is complex enough, the test developer may even recommend taking a training course in test administration. This training is routinely done for tests of intelligence that require many judgment calls about client responses and some consistency in these decisions.

b. *Training.* For any procedure to be reliable, the judges need to receive similar training in the observation, coding, and interpretation of the data. Most researchers put reliability judges through training periods, sometimes lasting several hours, prior to actual computation of the reliability scores. It makes good sense that prior to using any procedure a clinician will have adequate exposure to the methods and some practice using them.

c. *Practice.* Reliability is a function of practice. Both formal tests and informal evaluation measures require practice to efficiently administer and score. If one judge has much experience with a particular test or measurement and another judge has had none, lack of reliability can be expected. The more we perform procedures, the more systematic and consistent our decision-making becomes.

d. *Response Complexity.* Generally, the more complex the response, the greater the lack of reliability. If the system you are using to examine teacher-child interactions has a host of teacher and child variables, it will be more difficult to use than one with fewer aspects to examine. Another common example is the poor reliability associated with narrow phonetic transcription. The more molecular we become in what we do, the more difficult it is to obtain adequate reliability. In this age of writing generative phonologies from children's spontaneous samples, you can imagine how many specific disagreements could occur between two clinicians. First, there is error in just transcribing the sample, and there is the opportunity for many disagreements. Second, there is error in detecting the specific errors within the transcript. Third, there is further error in trying to arrive at a list of phonological processes or idiosyncratic rules that account for the child's sample. Finally, there is error in determining the frequency or percent of occurrence of each rule derived from the sample. The result could be a catalog of chaos. The more guidelines these clinicians have in making decisions, the better the reliability; in addition, the less complex the decisions, the better the reliability. This is why some authors have developed specific guidelines and definitions to use in phonological analyses (Ingram 1981; Shriberg and Kwiatkowski 1980).

e. *Live Scoring Versus Tape Analysis.* Scoring behaviors "on-line" is always more difficult than being able to replay video- or audiotapes for second and third opportunities to examine a behavior. Probably, videotape scoring would tend to be more reliable simply because it is difficult to accurately observe behaviors in rapid sequence and to take the time to note their occurrence on an observation form (which further takes away from one's ability to observe).

There are several ways to compute reliability. One method involves statistical procedures known as reliability coefficients or correlation coefficients (Hegde 1987; Salvia and Ysseldyke 1981). Typically, formal tests compute such correlations on judges to determine if the scores they derive are in general agreement as far as moving up and down together is concerned. It is preferable for standardized tests to have interjudge reliability coefficients of .90 or above to show good agreement among examiners. For example, if Judge A scored a series of tests as 89, 62, 53, and 36 and if Judge B scored the same tests as 90, 60, 50, and 35, there would be general agreement and a possible correlation of .99. The closer a coefficient of reliability is to 1.0, the more reliable the scoring. Some reliability coefficients take into account variance in the examiner's judgments (e.g., intraclass correlation, Winer's Coefficient of Reliability). Other test developers have used a simple correlation coefficient (e.g., Pearson Product Moment), which is far less effective in evaluating reliability (Bartko 1976). In the example above, the judges did not agree exactly on any of the test scores, but there was a general trend for the two judge's scores to go up and down together. There was also a tendency for the scores to be rather close (within 3 points of each other). This type of reliability may be acceptable for general responses, but if we want to gain insight into more specific behaviors, the correlation coefficient is too general a measure.

For instance, if we wanted to count specific articulatory errors, it would be important to agree on the type of error produced. It also would be important for the judges to be counting the *same* errors. The following scenario is possible. A child is asked to produce ten words for two judges who are going to count misarticulations. Both judges come up with five misarticulations. If the two judges made these kinds of responses over many subjects, they would appear to represent perfect agreement (1.0 in a correlation). Further analysis, however, reveals that Judge A found errors in the first five words and Judge B found errors in the last five words. In essence, they did not agree on *any* of the misarticulations, but came up with the same total number.

This example points out the importance of a different type of reliability measure called *point by point* or *percent exact agreement*. In this type of reliability, a formula such as the following is used:

$$\frac{\text{Agreements}}{\text{Agreements} + \text{Disagreements}} \times 100 =$$

Thus, one takes the total number of specific agreements and divides this number by the total number of agreements plus the disagreements and arrives at a percentage of exact agreement. In this way, we get a good idea of the behaviors that judges rate in exactly the same way. Any clinician can compute such a simple formula and determine interjudge reliability for almost any clinically relevant behavior in a diagnostic or treatment context. Often it is good to check our perceptions every once in awhile to see if we are fooling ourselves with regard to the occurrence of client behaviors. This type of reliability is especially important in behaviors that lend themselves to error because of subjectivity. Unfortunately, this includes many of the relevant measures in communication disorders.

2. *Test-Retest Reliability.* Some behaviors are highly stable over time. We would hope that most of the responses we assess to gain insight into various processes underlying communication are of this variety. If we are attempting to examine language comprehension, we assume that client performance on one day will be similar to that on another day. Vocal differences found one week would hopefully be observed the next week. If it were not for these behavioral consistencies, we really would have difficulty justifying treatment. A person's voice is either disordered, or it is not. Clearly, there are behavioral fluctuations in some disorders (e.g., stuttering, voice problems that vary with fatigue, etc.), but in others one can expect a fairly consistent occurrence (e.g., articulation errors, language errors). Tests are supposed to be designed to probe a particular error in such a way as to show consistent problems with a client's communication. If a patient with aphasia showed drastically different performances from week to week, it would be impossible to formulate a treatment program since the targets would always be changing. If a person's IQ was not relatively stable from week to week, it would be impossible to diagnose mental deficits. If a laboratory test for cancer varied from day to day in its diagnosis of tissue samples, it would be unusable. It is easy to see that test-retest reliability has much to do with the behavior being evaluated, and also with the test items chosen to reveal the skill you are testing. Reliability coefficients, as described above, also are used to examine test-retest reliability, and those coefficients close to 1.0 indicate stability in performance on a particular task. One could also use the point-by-point procedure to determine if the errors made on one day are similar to those made at a later time. It depends on how molecular the clinician wants to be in examining client performance.

3. *Split-Half Reliability.* Many formal test developers want to evaluate the internal consistency of the items on their instrument. In essence, they want to determine if both halves of the test tend to be reliable or agree in terms of scores obtained.

Some Quantitative Background for Test Interpretation

There are some basic concepts in measurement that are necessary in order to appreciate most standardized tests. Many traditional quantitative aspects will not be covered, since they rarely are found on tests we use (e.g., mode, median, semiquartile range, types of curves, kurtosis, and skewedness). While we are omitting these, we are certainly not suggesting they are of diminished value. We simply want to discuss aspects that are useful for interpreting most tests in communication disorders. For more detailed accounts of these concepts, the reader is referred to other sources that provide more in-depth coverage (Anastasi 1976; Messick 1980; Salvia and Ysseldyke 1981).

Central Tendency, Variation, and the Normal Curve

Whenever someone takes a test they earn one or more scores. Part of test interpretation involves placing the score(s) of an individual in the context of others who also have been administered the instrument.

The most often encountered measure of central tendency in formal tests is the mean or arithmetic average of the normative sample. This is computed simply by adding up all the scores of the standardization sample and dividing by the total number of scores. As a clinician, you will probably not have to compute many mean scores on clients you test. You will see means in formal tests that have been used to examine differing age groups on a particular skill, and you will use this information as a reference point to compare the score of a specific child or adult you have tested. For example, if we have tested a four-year-old on a vocabulary test, we are interested in how his or her score compares to the normative sample of four-year-olds who took the same test as part of the standardization procedure. While some tests report data on other measures of central tendency (e.g., mode, median), the most frequently reported scores are means, and they are perhaps the most meaningful to a clinician.

The other important score we must deal with in order to make sense of normative data is some measure of variability (variance) in the standardization sample. The *variance* is "a numerical index describing the dispersion of a set of scores around the mean of the distribution" (Salvia and Ysseldyke 1981, 50). In computing the variance, the statistician first derives the amount by which each person's score deviates from the sample mean (e.g., if the score is 70 and the test mean is 60, the deviation is 10). After this is done for each subject in the sample, the deviation scores are all squared. Then, these squared scores are added up and divided by the total number of subjects minus one. This results in the variance. One can easily see that we are essentially obtaining a very gross measure of the average amount of variation from the mean (squared) by computing the variance. The variance is not particularly meaningful in test interpretation so its square root, the *standard deviation*, is used because it is a more interpretable measure of variation. Thus, if the variance is 25, the square root of this is 5, which is the standard deviation. This measurement is more interpretable since it is in the same units as the mean instead of squared values as in the variance. If the mean on a test is 50 points and the standard deviation is 5 points, one can actually use these numbers together to gain a picture of variability. If we used a mean of 50 points and the variance of 25, we are no longer talking about the same types of numbers (points) since the variance is the average number of points of deviation squared.

In most cases, whenever researchers gather data on a particular skill from a large sample of people, the scores tend to form what statisticians call a *normal curve*. This means that there will be a tendency for most of the scores to fall around an average value, while some scores will be scattered toward very high and very low values. If researchers weighed a random sample of two thousand adults between the ages of twenty and forty, they would probably find an average weight, with most people clustered around this value, and a much smaller number of people who were very fat and very thin who deviated markedly from this value. This is where means and standard deviations are helpful in describing the performance of a given population of subjects.

Figure 3.1 shows a normal bell-shaped curve that could theoretically depict the performance of a sample of people on any variable. For our purposes, let us say that the curve represents scores on a vocabulary test. Several things are important to note. First, the line in the center of the normal curve at the score of 45 represents the mean performance or the average score in the distribution. Notice that it is the tallest line in the curve because height represents the largest number of people (9) who earned this score. The lines on either side of the mean are shorter and represent smaller numbers of subjects (8) who earned these scores (e.g., 40 and 50). As the lines become shorter it indicates that fewer subjects earned the scores as they moved progressively higher and lower than the mean of 45. The two subjects scoring 10 and the two subjects scoring 80 are in the tails of the normal curve and are called "outliers."

Look again at Figure 3.1 that depicted vocabulary scores. Previously, we said that the mean was 45. If we said that the standard deviation was 10, this would mean that +1 standard deviation would be located at 55 and –1 standard deviation would be located at 35. Taking the example further, +2 standard deviations would be at the score of 65, and –2 standard deviations would be at 25. Now look at Figure 3.2 that depicts the percentage of cases under portions of the normal curve and the standard deviations at the bottom. We can see that about 68% of cases in the sample would probably score within –1 and +1 standard deviations from the mean. This means that on the vocabulary test, about 68% of the subjects would earn scores somewhere between 35 and 55. If we considered the cases scor-

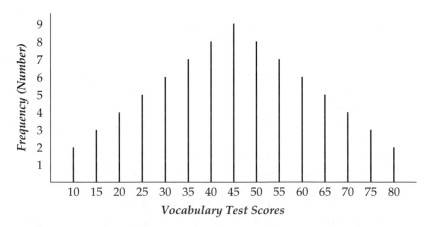

FIGURE 3.1   Example of Normally Distributed Data

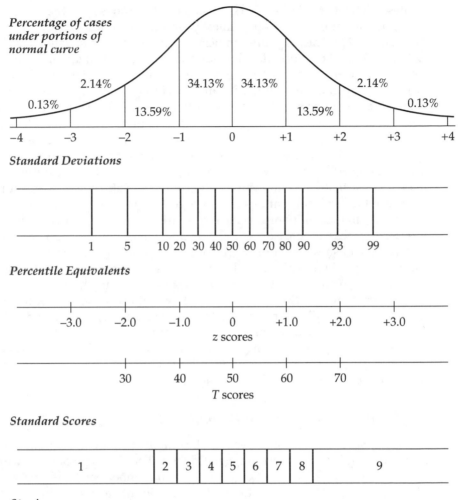

*Percentage of cases
under portions of
normal curve*

0.13%   2.14%   13.59%   34.13%   34.13%   13.59%   2.14%   0.13%

−4   −3   −2   −1   0   +1   +2   +3   +4

Standard Deviations

1   5   10 20 30 40 50 60 70 80 90   93   99

Percentile Equivalents

−3.0   −2.0   −1.0   0   +1.0   +2.0   +3.0

z scores

30   40   50   60   70

T scores

Standard Scores

1   2   3   4   5   6   7   8   9

Stanines

**FIGURE 3.2   Relationship of Various Types of Derived Scores to the
Normal Curve**

From: Carrow-Woolfolk, E. (1985) *Test for Auditory Comprehension-Revised*, DLM Teaching
Resources, Allen, TX. Used with permission.

ing between −2 and +2 standard deviations, about 96% of the subjects would earn
scores in this area somewhere between 25 and 65. Finally, if we looked at cases
scoring between −3 and +3 standard deviations, around 99% of the cases would
earn scores of between 15 and 75.

Thus, the use of means and standard deviations helps researchers and test developers to determine scoring patterns that are characteristic of the majority of a
particular population. It often has been stated in the assessment literature that

scores falling at or below –1.5 to -2.0 standard deviations from the mean are thought to be abnormal enough to be clinically significant (Ludlow 1983; McCauley and Swisher 1984b). This, of course, indicates that the score in question was lower than some 95% of the population included in the standardization sample. Thus, it should be clear that we use the means and standard deviations of the normative sample as a context for comparing an individual client's score on a standardized test. If the client's score falls below a particular standard deviation level (e.g., –2.0), we may decide to make a judgment about lack of normality in performance. This is why it is important to understand some basic facts about means and standard deviations. While many authorities advocate the use of cutoff scores as mentioned above, others (Plante and Vance 1995) dispute the use of such arbitrary guidelines and suggest that clinicians empirically derive specific cutoff scores for each test they use on local populations. This suggestion is based on research that shows variability in the ability of specific tests to discriminate normally developing children from those with disorders (Plante and Vance 1995). If tests are going to be used to establish whether or not a child has a problem, they should have demonstrated discriminant validity. All distributions, however, are not normal. Some are skewed positively (many low scores) or negatively (many high scores); others have much variation (platykurtic) or very little variation (leptokurtic). It is significant that most standardization samples tend to be normally distributed, which is important for the statistical analyses that are applied to them. There are many special problems in dealing with abnormally distributed data that are beyond the scope of the present text. It is enough if we are clear about normally distributed data and about the ways of describing these distributions.

Types of Scores Found on Formal Tests

There are several kinds of scores that the diagnostician will encounter when dealing with standardized, norm-referenced tests. The first type of score we will mention is the *raw score*. The raw score is the actual number you arrive at when grading the client's test. Many times the raw score amounts to the number of correct responses that the client gave to the test items. So, if the test has 75 items on it and the client got 50 of them correct, the raw score might be 50. On some tests the raw score is not simply the number correct but is some other number (e.g., maybe each test item is worth 2 points). At any rate, you score the test and arrive at some number that the test manual typically refers to as the raw score.

Most standardized, norm-referenced examinations include a manual to be used by the diagnostician in scoring and interpreting the test results. These test manuals typically contain a series of tables that are designed to convert raw scores into more interpretable numbers. Raw scores by themselves are not readily meaningful. For instance, the raw score of 50 out of 75 does not tell us anything about how our client's score compares to the performance of the normative sample. Perhaps this is normal performance for the client's age group and perhaps it is not. Thus, we must convert the client's raw score into a more meaningful type of number to allow comparison with the normative sample. Another reason to convert the raw scores to some other type of derived score is that one cannot compare the results of two different tests by using raw scores. For instance, if a child obtains a raw score of 50 out of 75 on a vocabulary test and then earns a raw score of 125 out of 200 on a metalinguistics test, it would be difficult to compare these results. If, however, the raw scores were converted to some derived score, we could generally compare the performances on the two measures.

One type of converted score is called the *percentile rank*. Percentile ranks reflect the percentage of subjects or scores that fall at or below a particular raw score. For example, if a child scored in the 20th percentile, this means he/she scored as well or better than 20% of the children of the same age in the normative sample. Likewise, if a child was in the 90th percentile, the score was as good or better than 90% of the children taking the test. Another way to look at it is that only 10% of the normative population scored higher than a child who performed in the 90th percentile. If you look at Figure 3.2, you will see that percentile ranks are arranged under the normal curve. It can be seen that the 50th percentile rank basically represents the middle or median performance of the normative sample. A percentile rank of 10 is slightly more than –1 standard deviation below the mean. Remember from the prior discussion that some authorities view performance below –1.5 or –2.0 standard deviations to constitute clinical significance or abnormality. Some authorities suggest that consistent performance below the 10th percentile is cause for clinical concern (Lee 1974) because this is between –1 and –2 standard deviations. One can see that conversion of the raw score into a percentile rank allows the clinician to put an individual client's performance into the context of the normative sample. It is meaningless to say that the client got a raw score of 90, but it is much more valuable to be able to say that a client scored in the 90th percentile.

Another way to derive more interpretable data from a client's raw score is to convert it into a *standard score*. There are a number of types of standard scores that the diagnostician will encounter on formal tests; however, we will discuss only the two most common types: *z-scores* and *T-scores*. Standard scores transform the raw scores into sets of scores that have the same mean and standard deviation. A z-score has a mean of 0 and a standard deviation of 1. One can see from Figure 3.2 that the z-scores are exactly equivalent to the standard deviations in the normal curve. Thus, a z-score of –1.0 is in the same place on the curve as a standard deviation of –1.0. A raw score can be converted to a z-score by subtracting the raw score from the mean of the normative sample and dividing the resulting number by the standard deviation of the normative sample. Test manuals typically include tables for the conversion of raw scores into z-scores so that the clinician will not have to perform the mathematical operation mentioned above. It is easy to see that when a client's raw score is converted to a z-score, it is much more interpretable. For instance, it is meaningless to that say a client had a raw score of 59 on a test because it does not relate to the normative sample. If, however, the client has a z-score of –2.0, we can look at Figure 3.2 and see that this is equivalent to performing at –2.0 standard deviations, which is a clinically significant abnormality according to the criteria mentioned earlier.

Another standard score is the T-score. This operates basically the same way as the z-score, except that the mean is 50 and the standard deviation is 10. Thus, the performance of a client with a t-score of 30 would be equivalent to –2.0 standard deviations.

A final type of standard score depicted in Figure 3.2 is the *stanine*. Tables for conversion of raw scores to stanines are not found as often in standardized tests. As stated by Salvia and Ysseldyke (1981),

> *Stanines are standard score bands that divide a distribution into nine parts. The first stanine includes all scores that are 1.75 standard deviations or more below the mean, and the ninth stanine includes all scores 1.75 or more standard deviations above the mean. The second through eighth stanines are each .5 standard deviation in width and the fifth stanine ranging from .25 standard deviation below the mean to .25 standard deviation above the mean.* (73)

It can be seen from the above discussion that standardized, norm-referenced tests provide the diagnostician with a variety of possible scores to use in the interpretation of a particular client's performance. We must remember, however, that while standard scores are useful to the diagnostician, they are valid only if the score distribution in the normative sample is normal. Percentiles do not require a distribution to be normal and can be computed on any distribution shape; thus, they have fewer requirements than standard scores for accurate use and interpretation.

The Age and Grade Score Trap

Many formal tests include tables for converting raw scores into age-equivalent and/or grade-equivalent scores. Thus, a nine-year-old child who earns a raw score of 50 might be said to have an age-equivalent score of 7.5 (seven years, five months). A fourth-grader might earn a grade-equivalent score of 2.2 (second grade, second month). It is easy to be seduced into using these types of scores because they appear to relate to development. On the surface, these age and grade equivalents seem to place the child in a developmental context with peers who took the test. It is tempting to say that the nine-year-old mentioned above is really at the seven-and-a-half-year-old level, or the fourth grader is performing at the second-grade level. All of these assumptions could be wrong. Most authorities who focus on psychometric interpretation indicate that age-equivalent and grade-equivalent scores are the *least* useful and *most dangerous* scores to be obtained from standardized tests because they lead to gross misinterpretations of a client's performance (Lawrence 1992; McCauley and Swisher 1984b; Salvia and Ysseldyke 1981). Basically, age-equivalent scores indicate that the client's raw score approximated the average performance for a particular age group. In the example above, the nine-year-old earned a raw score that was the average of the children in the seven-year-old group of the normative sample. A similar relationship holds for grade-equivalent scores.

There are several commonly discussed problems with age- and grade-equivalent scores. McCauley and Swisher (1984b) discuss these problems:

For most tests, as age increases, similar differences in age-equivalent scores are the result of smaller and smaller differences in raw scores. Therefore, an age equivalent score that is 6 months behind an individual's chronological age may indicate a larger difference in actual test performance for younger test takers than for older ones. . . . The 1-year delay . . . reported for Paul, who is 4 years old, may have resulted from 12 missed items; whereas a 1 year delay for a 10 year old child taking the test might be due to only one or two missed items. This causes the reliability of age-equivalent scores to be poorer for developmentally more advanced test takers. A second psychometric problem with age-equivalent scores is that they are not necessarily based directly on evidence collected for children of that chronological age. . . . Instead, a given age-equivalent score is often calculated indirectly either by interpolating between two ages for which data are available or by extrapolating from ages for which data are available to older or younger ages, for which data were not gathered. For example, Paul's raw score . . . probably fell between the average scores of the 3-year-olds and 4-year-olds in the normative sample, and he was assigned the age-equivalent of 3:2 by interpolation although no children of age 3:2 were sampled in the normative studies. (340)

The psychometric problems above lead to a number of misinterpretations of age-equivalent scores. First, as Salvia and Ysseldyke (1981) indicate, it leads to "typological thinking." As they say, "The average 12-0 child does not exist. The child is a composite of all 12.0 children. Average 12-0 children represent a range of performances" (68).

A second misinterpretation is that laymen and some professionals may believe that a nine-year-old child who earns an age-equivalent score of 7-0 is *performing like a seven-year-old*. This is probably not true. While the nine-year-old may have earned the score obtained by the average seven-year-old, the test items that were correct and missed may be totally different in the client and the normative sample of seven-year-olds. As McCauley and Swisher (1984b) state: "Similarly, a 60-year-old suffering from aphasia might receive an age-equivalent score of 10 years on the vocabulary test. It is unlikely, however, that such a client would make the same kind of errors as the 10-year-old or that he would exhibit similar communication skills" (341).

A final danger in using age-equivalent scores is their use in attempting to define impairment in a client. Often, the assumption is made that a child exhibits a disorder if his/her age-equivalent score is lower than his/her chronological age (e.g., a four-year-old earning an age-equivalent score of 3.0). It is important to understand that these age-equivalent scores do not take into account the variation in performance expected in a particular age group. If a child performs below the average score for his/her age group, it may be within the range of normal variation for that group and not an indicator of impairment at all. McCauley and Swisher (1984b) provide a graphic example shown in Figure 3.3:

Paul—and all of those 4-year-olds whose scores fall in the shaded area of the curve—would be said to have received an age equivalent score of 3 years or less. However, when the variability shown by the 4-year-olds as a group is taken into account using z scores, the same score may not be found to be sufficiently different

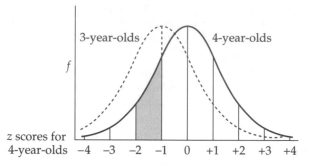

FIGURE 3.3   Hypothetical Distributions of Scores Received by Two Groups of Children. The Shaded Area of the Distribution for 4-Year-Olds Includes Scores That Would Yield Age-Equivalent Scores of 3 Years or Less but z Scores of −2 or Better.

From McCauley, R. and Swisher L. (1984). Use and Misuse of Norm-Referenced Tests in Clinical Assessment: A Hypothetical Case. *Journal of Speech and Hearing Disorders*, 49, 338–348. Used with permission.

from the average obtained by this group to suggest impairment. Certainly, if a z score better than −2.0 were considered within the normal range, almost all of the scores falling in the shaded area on the figure would be considered normal, despite their correspondence to age-equivalent delays of up to a year or more. Thus, age-equivalent delays do not necessarily indicate delay or impairment. (341)

It is almost universally agreed that the least useful and most perilous types of scores are the age-equivalent or grade-equivalent scores mentioned above. They tend to distort a client's performance and lead to misinterpretations by laymen and professionals alike. Yet, many state departments of education mandate use of age-equivalent scores for purposes of determining eligibility for services (Lawrence 1992). Most authorities advocate the use of percentile ranks and standard scores for test interpretation since these do not suffer from the problems mentioned in relation to developmental scores. Perhaps the percentile rank is the easier of the scores to use in communicating with parents and spouses since most people can understand this concept readily. Clinicians who are consumers of formal, standardized, norm-referenced tests would be wise to refuse to purchase examinations that offer only age-equivalent scores and that omit standard scores and percentile ranks.

Standard Error of Measurement and Confidence Intervals

Two final concepts that we will deal with regarding standardized tests are the notions of *standard error of measurement* and *confidence intervals*. When used with the concepts previously discussed (mean, standard deviation, standard scores), these measurements give the diagnostician some very powerful quantitative tools to use in evaluating test performance.

Even though a standardized test may be developed very carefully, a client's responses to test items may not really reflect the underlying ability that the examination is attempting to tap. Statisticians realize that *any* measure is susceptible to error. Error is ubiquitous—it is in everything we measure, and especially in evaluating human performance. Thus, we know that no test is perfectly reliable (1.0) and that some distortion is present in any measurement device. Some statisticians use the terms *observed score* and *true score* to refer to the actual raw score that the test taker earns and to the "ideal" score that the person would have earned if there were no error in the measuring instrument. The true score, then, does not really exist; it is only hypothesized. We would ideally like the observed score to be highly similar to the true score, and this is the case in using tests that have high reliability. As the reliability of a test decreases, the disparity between true and observed scores increases.

A statistic called the standard error of measurement (SEM) has been developed to increase our precision in determining whether the observed score of a client is reasonably close to his/her possible true score. While one could calculate the SEM and associated confidence intervals from one of several statistical formulas, many tests provide tables from which to arrive at this information. Basically, the calculation of SEM involves three things (McCauley and Swisher 1984b): "(a) an estimate of the test's reliability, (b) the mean and standard deviation of scores obtained by the normative sample to which the test taker's score is to be compared, and (c) the test taker's observed score" (339). We should be able to look up the SEM in a test manual and find a table that indicates the confidence intervals around the client's true score for at least a 95% level of confidence. Thus, if a subject had an observed score of 50 on a test and we calculated the true score and it was 53, there would be a pretty good correspondence between the observed and true scores. If we look up the 95% confidence interval in a table included in the test manual, we might find that the confidence interval is 5. Next, we subtract 5 from the subject's true score and arrive at 48 and add 5 to the true score and get 58. Thus, we have a range from 48 to 58, with the subject's true score in the middle. We can have confidence that the subject's true score would fall in this range 95 times out of 100 test administrations.

McCauley and Swisher (1984b) point out the importance of using confidence intervals, especially when attempting to determine cutoffs for abnormality (340). Figure 3.4 shows a normal curve with an observed and true score for a particular subject expressed in z-scores. If one were to use the traditional cutoff of –2.0 standard deviations as an indication of abnormality, the observed score would clearly fall below this point, and the client would be considered impaired. The 95% confidence interval, however, straddles the –2.0 standard deviation cutoff. We see that the client's observed score is below the cutoff and that the calculated true score is above the cutoff. If this were the case in making a clinical decision, it would be difficult to say that the client is exhibiting impairment just because of the observed

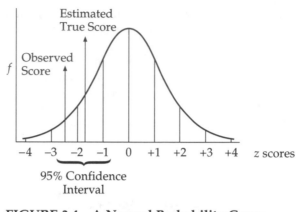

FIGURE 3.4   **A Normal Probability Curve
Showing the 95% Confidence
Interval and Estimated True Score
(•) for an Observed Score (○)**

From McCauley, R. and Swisher, L. (1984). Use and Misuse of
Norm-Referenced Tests in Clinical Assessment: A Hypotheti-
cal Case. *Journal of Speech and Hearing Disorders, 49, 338–348.*
Used with permission.

score. There is enough error in the test to suggest that the client's true score might
be above the cutoff, and this assessment suggests normal performance. This type
of decision would be clear only in a case where the true score and its associated
confidence interval does not overlap an arbitrary cutoff. This problem becomes especially important in cases where psychometrists are attempting to determine if a
child is mentally retarded. If an IQ below 70 is indicative of mental retardation, it
would be important for the client's true score *and* confidence interval to be well
below 70 to make a judgment. If the confidence interval overlaps the cutoff, it is
possible that the true score could lie in the area above the cutoff even though the
observed score is below it. Important decisions should not be dealt with lightly,
and clients should be given the benefit of the doubt, especially where program
placements are concerned.

Criteria for Evaluating Standardized Tests

We would be remiss if we did not report the most-common considerations in evaluating formal tests. These criteria have been reported by many authors, but basically flow from the *Standards for Educational and Psychological Tests* compiled by the
American Psychological Association. We will paraphrase these considerations
here, but the reader should know that the actual standards go into much more detail. Hutchinson (1996) offers a very useful and practical guide for clinicians to use
in interpreting the technical manuals of standardized tests. The criteria should be

used by a consumer of formal tests in communication disorders to make principled decisions about selection and purchasing of instruments:

1. The test should be accompanied by a comprehensive manual that provides detailed information on (a) the rationale behind the test, (b) a detailed description of the development of the test, (c) the specific purposes for which the test is to be used and not used, (d) qualifications of the test administrator, and (e) specific instructions for administering, scoring, and interpreting the test.

2. The test manual should also provide information on construct-, content-, and criterion-related validity. The emphasis should be on construct validity, and reporting of other types without this emphasis is unacceptable.

3. The test manual should include a section that reports interjudge, test-retest, and internal consistency types of reliability.

4. Descriptive statistics, including means and standard deviations for all groups studied in the normative sample, should be included along with tables to use in converting raw scores into standard scores and percentile ranks. Information on the standard error of measurement and computation of confidence intervals also should be included.

5. The sizes of the normative sample should be reported; and most authorities suggest that if the test has subgroups, the number of subjects in each group should not be less than 100.

6. The normative sample should be fully described in terms of race, socioeconomic level, geographic residence, and normality on relevant variables (e.g., IQ, hearing, medical). If any subjects are included in the sample to represent disordered groups, these individuals should be described in detail in terms of relevant variables.

We could go into much detail on any of the above points or subpoints, but it should be clear that selection of a standardized, norm-referenced test should not be just an arbitrary decision on the part of a diagnostician. Every month we are inundated with flyers and catalogs attempting to sell tests. The choice of whether to purchase one of these instruments is significant in terms of cost and, more important, in terms of serving our clients well. Try to examine these tests at conferences and conventions, read reviews in professional journals, and/or examine the *Buros Mental Measurements Yearbook* (Conoley and Impara 1995) for critical reviews. The test brochures and catalogs may not tell us enough to make an accurate judgment. If possible, order a test "on approval," and pay for it only if you are satisfied with its psychometric adequacy and what it will actually tell you about a client. Most reputable publishers allow a customer to return an instrument that he/she is not satisfied with.

Common Errors in the Use of Norm-Referenced Tests

With very few exceptions, norm-referenced tests are designed to help the clinician determine if a client is performing within normal limits on a particular behavior.

We compare an individual's score to the normative data and decide if our client is impaired or not. Muma (1973) has said that the purpose of formal tests is to solve the "problem/no problem" issue. Often, the clinician could do this just by observation alone, but many institutions (e.g., school systems) may require some formal test score to include in a client's record instead of relying solely on clinical judgment. Public Law 94-142 requires that more than one standardized test be used in assessment. At any rate, solving the problem/no problem issue is a rather narrow payoff for taking the time to administer and score a standardized test. As a result, some clinicians try to make more of the test results than they should. Formal tests are only designed to go so far; and if we make other judgments about our clients based on these data, we are violating the assumptions of the tests. The following are some of the common ways in which clinicians misuse standardized tests:

1. *Measuring Treatment Progress with Norm-Referenced Tests.* We mentioned earlier that the purpose of norm-referenced tests is to determine if a client is performing in a way that is similar to a large standardization sample. The tests were not designed for the purpose of measuring progress in treatment. If the clinician administers a formal test at the beginning of treatment and readministers the test (or even an alternate form of the test) after a period of treatment, the resulting scores can lead to gross misinterpretations. First of all, the formal test samples a broad range of behaviors and may sample the behavior trained in therapy only in a few trials. Thus, much of the time spent in test administration would be devoted to assessing behavior that is unrelated to therapy. It would be much more logical to examine the trained behavior in detail by using an informal format that focused more fully on the particular behavior of interest. Second, a subject who scores abnormally low on an initial administration of an instrument will tend to score higher on a subsequent administration of the same test. This is a well-known phenomenon called *statistical regression*, which states that subjects earning extreme scores (either high or low) will tend to regress toward the mean of the sample population on subsequent administrations. Thus, a client may receive a higher score, not because of treatment effects but because of statistical regression. Third, clinicians may unconsciously "teach to the test" and prepare the client to do well on a second administration by practicing items in a format similar to the formal test. Fourth, all tests include elements of unreliability. It could very well be that an increase in an overall score on a formal test is simply the result of chance. We urge clinicians to never use standardized, norm-referenced tests as measures of progress. Criterion-referenced tests and informal probe tasks are the best way to gauge treatment progress.

2. *Analyzing Individual Test Items for Treatment Target Selection.* After administering a norm-referenced test, it is always tempting to examine the client's responses to particular test items and to try to determine some kind of pattern of impairment. For example, on a receptive vocabulary test one might find that particular prepositions are in error. A natural tendency would be to include the understanding of prepositions in a treatment program based on the analysis of the formal test performance. There are several problems with this. To begin with, clients cannot be expected to take tests that are of an inordinate length. As a result, a formal test must be relatively brief in order to be practical. On the other hand, most formal tests are fairly broad based in that they cover a number of areas (e.g., syntax, morphology, vocabulary) or one area that has several facets to it (e.g., assessment of all relevant, bound morphemes). This characteristic creates a dilemma for the person who is developing a test instrument. In order to cover all of the areas of interest, or even all aspects of one area, the test developer must be very selective in deciding how many items to include and how many times a particular behavior will be sampled. In assessing bound morphemes, for instance, the test developer must determine how many times each morpheme of interest will be sampled and in what contexts. Often, a particular form will only be sampled two or three times in order to make the length of the test manageable. Herein lies the tradeoff: Making a test of reasonable length necessitates the use of small samples of each behavior of interest. Thus, it would be difficult to make a judgment about a particular grammatical morpheme (e.g., plurals) based on only two or three occurrences. This observation is especially true when client responses on formal tests can be due to a variety of reasons. As much as test developers would like to believe that an incorrect response indicates lack of ability on a particular item or that a correct response suggests mastery of an item, it is well known that test takers are human. Clients make lucky guesses, are distracted during test administration, do not fully understand instructions, experience a variety of internal states (fatigue, boredom, pain, need to use the bathroom, etc.) that could all affect test performance. Be wary of selecting treatment objectives from any norm-referenced test.

3. *Forgetting That Formal Tests Almost Always Distort What They Are Designed to Examine.* Almost every construct one might desire to measure in communication disorders is highly complex. Whenever we deal with human behavior and try to translate a complex activity into a single score, there is a considerable amount of information lost in the process. Is it valid to say the child's vocabulary is a 74 because he/she earned this score on a test? Does this tell us how many words are in the lexicon, or are understood? Does it tell us how words are retrieved? Does it tell us if the child's internal definition of the word is equivalent to an adult's? Do we know how the word is used for communication? Do we know how the word will be used in sentences or written language? We could continue to ask questions about how deeply we have examined the child's vocabulary by obtaining a formal test score, but you probably have the idea by now that such a score is quite superficial. In designing a test, developers have competing goals that make it almost impossible to create the perfect instrument. Figure 3.5 illustrates this dilemma. As the test becomes more specific and controlled, it becomes more unnatural. As we move toward a naturalistic task, we lose control over stimuli, tasks, and responses. Standardized tests have a number of ways in which they tend to distort the constructs that we wish to examine.

First, almost all tests that are standardized imply a circumscribed method of administration. The testing must be done in a particular setting, specific instructions

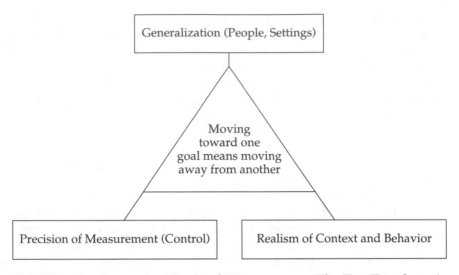

FIGURE 3.5   Competing Goals of Measurement: The Test Developer's Dilemma

Adapted from Sabers (1992)

must be given, and items must be administered in a particular order. In addition, the client's responses must be graded as pass or fail, based on the criteria set forth by the test developer (some tests do not classify client responses as pass/fail, but these are few in number). The vast majority of formal test scenarios involve a highly artificial, regimented way of assessing performance.

A second reason for distortion is that most of these tests designed to assess communication rarely examine *real* communicative efforts. The interactions are typically artificial. The client has no real communicative intent, communications are often about trivial topics (e.g., telling the examiner what is going on in a picture while both client and clinician look at it), and the topic of each task is constantly changing as the clinician flips the test plates. Thus, we must *always* remember that we have not examined real communication until we have analyzed the client's communicating in a natural situation.

A third source of distortion is the fragmentation of integrated systems often seen in formal testing. As Muma (1973) points out, many systems interact with one another in communication and to single out a particular area to analyze is in many cases ludicrous. For instance, how can one separate semantics from cognition, syntax from semantics, syntax from morphology, phonology from syntax, motor speech skills from language, intonation from meaning, or structural language from pragmatics? While this can be done on the formal test level, it certainly cannot be done on a construct validity level. We cannot evaluate a system or subsystem independent of the context in which it typically operates. If we do, we have not really evaluated the system of interest. Always be aware that when we use an artificial task as found on most formal tests, we are always a dimension or more away from looking at the reality of communication.

4. *Ignoring Possible Cultural Differences in Normative Data.* It is axiomatic in the psychometric literature that norms are not valid if the standardization sample differs significantly from the local population tested. Figure 3.6 shows selected tests in communication disorders and the percentages of certain cultural groups included in the standardization samples according to the test manuals. While many test instruments that are currently used have included children of different cultural groups in their norming samples, the percentage of these children may not be reflective of the proportion of such children in many local areas. For example, the general population of the United States is composed of approximately 12% African Americans; however, the concentration of this cultural group in many cities and states may be several times this proportion. As an illustration, let us look through the microscope at selected states in the country (Figure 3.7) and their percentage of cultural makeup mainly for African American and Hispanic residents (the "other" category includes Native American, Pacific Islander, and Asian individuals). It is clear from this figure that many states have significantly more than the national average of African Americans, for example. If we turn to a more powerful lens and focus on cities in the United States (Figure 3.8), you can see that the percentages of the various cultures change drastically. The 1990 census statistics show that over half of the United States population lives in the thirty-nine largest metropolitan areas. It is questionable, at best, to use a test that had included only 9% African American children in its standardization sample if one is working in a community where over 60% of the children represent this cultural group.

FIGURE 3.6   Selected Frequently Used Language Tests and Their Standardization Samples

Test	African-American	Hispanic	Other	White
AAPS	10	3	3	84
ALPHA	12	6	0	82
BRACKEN	15	9	3	73
BTBC	0	0	23	77
CELF-R	16	0	0	79
CAS	15	6	2	84
ELM	0	0	20	80
GFTA	15	12	1	73
M-Y	0	0	0	100
PPVT-R	10	3	1	85
SICD	0	0	0	100
TELD	8	0	2	90
TLC	16	16	0	69
TACL-R	7	0	0	84
TOLD2-P	11	0	5	84

FIGURE 3.7   Selected States and Their Cultural Makeup in Percentages

State	African-American	Other	Hispanic
Alabama	25.3	1	.6
Arkansas	15.9	1.3	.8
Arizona	3	16.2	18.8
California	7.4	23.6	25.8
Colorado	4	7.6	12.9
Florida	13.6	3.3	12.2
Georgia	27	2.1	1.7
Hawaii	2.5	63.4	7.3
Illinois	14.8	6.9	7.9
Louisiana	30.8	1.9	2.2
Maryland	24.9	4.1	2.6
Michigan	13.9	2.6	2.2
Mississippi	35.6	.9	.6
New York	15.9	9.7	12.3
North Carolina	22	2.5	1.2
South Carolina	29.8	1.1	.9
Texas	11.9	12.9	25.5

FIGURE 3.8   Selected Cities and their Cultural Makeup in Percentages

City	African-American	Other	Hispanic
Albuquerque	3	4.7	34.5
Atlanta	67.1	1	1.9
Baltimore	59.2	1.4	1
Boston	25.6	5.6	10.8
Charlotte	31.8	2.2	1.4
Chicago	39.1	4	19.6
Cincinnati	37.9	1.3	.7
Cleveland	46.6	1.3	4.6
Dallas	29.5	2.7	20.9
Denver	12.8	3.6	23
Detroit	75.7	1.2	2.8
El Paso	3.4	1.6	69
Fresno	8.3	13.6	29.9
Houston	28.1	4.4	27.6
Los Angeles	14	10.3	39.9
Memphis	54.8	1	.7
Miami	27.4	.8	62.5
New Orleans	61.9	2.1	3.5
New York	28.7	1.1	24.4
Philadelphia	39.9	2.9	5.6
San Francisco	10.9	29.6	13.9
Tucson	4.3	3.8	29.3
Washington, DC	65.8	2	5.4

A second problem with the standardization samples in their reflection of cultural differences may surface in a lack of specific description of the groups in the norming sample. For instance, saying that 120 African American children were included in the norming sample does not provide any information on their socioeconomic level or whether or not they spoke Black English. If the children were not dialectal speakers, then their scores may have no relevance for evaluators who want to compensate for language bias on the test or to compare these scores to a population in the inner city where dialectal usage is a prominent feature.

The concept of *local norms* has been discussed for years in the psychometric literature (Adler 1990; Evard and Sabers 1979; Hamayan and Damico 1991; Omark 1981; Owens 1995; Popham 1981; Seymour 1992). Owens (1995) states:

> *Often the norming sample does not represent the population with which the speech-language pathologist is using the assessment procedure. In this situation, the norms are inappropriate and should not be used. This situation occurs most frequently with minority or rural children or with children from lower socioeconomic groups. In these cases, local norms should be prepared by following the norming procedure described in the test manual. Some tests, such as the Test of Language Development-Intermediate (TOLD-I) and the CELF, explain this process in detail. (72)*

Some formal tests such as the TACL-R have developed software that the practitioner can use in generating local normative data (Swank 1987). The use of local norms does not mean ignoring national norms in evaluating a client. It is useful, however, to obtain both national and local perspectives in order to discover test biases and the most discriminating types of norms for identifying disorder versus cultural difference in performance.

Conclusion

Some students and clinicians feel frustrated when confronted with the type of information presented in the present chapter. This is especially true if the clinician has emphasized formal tests in his/her approach to diagnosis and evaluation. Others also may feel a bit guilty if they have misused norm-referenced tests or have used instruments and techniques uncritically without insuring the validity and reliability of those instruments or techniques. These practices, however, are probably the rule rather than the exception. Others might feel lost if all of their traditional tools are suddenly taken away from them and they may ask, "What are we supposed to do without our tests?" There is no simple answer. One obvious response would be that we can still use tests for the purposes they are intended to serve, but we need to tighten up our criteria for test selection, use, and interpretation. The other response would be that we need to develop and use more-informal methods for diagnosis and evaluation that will give us insight into the nature of a client's problem and the means for treating it. In many areas of communication disorders, we are beyond the basic question of the "problem/no problem" issue. We need ways to describe client performance and gain insight into individual differences, dynamism, ecological relevance, processes, and patterns of behavior (Bates, Bretherton, and Snyder 1988; Bronfenbrenner 1979; Chafe 1970; Donaldson 1978; Muma 1978, 1981, 1983, 1984). The field of communication disorders is moving more toward descriptive and criterion-referenced measures rather than toward norm-referenced tests. This trend, however, does not absolve each of us from the ultimate responsibility of incorporating sound scientific principles into our measurements. An informal probe or task used to describe client behavior is just as susceptible as a norm-referenced test to psychometric and examiner error. Students, professors, and working clinicians should adhere to high standards of measurement and should refuse to use inadequate test instruments or descriptive procedures that cannot be effectively replicated.

Bibliography

Adler, S. (1990). "Multicultural Clients: Implications for the SLP." *Language, Speech and Hearing Services in Schools* 21:135–139.

Anastasi, A. (1976). *Psychological Testing.* New York: Macmillan.

Bartko, J. (1976). "On Various Intraclass Correlation Reliability Coefficients." *Psychological Bulletin* 83, no. 5:762–765.

Bates, E., Bretherton, I., and Snyder, L. (1988). *From First Words to Grammar.* Cambridge, MA: Cambridge University Press.

Bronfenbrenner, U. (1979). *The Ecology of Human Development.* Cambridge: Harvard University Press.

Chafe, W. (1970). *Meaning and the Structure of Language.* Chicago, IL: University of Chicago Press.

Conoley, J., and Impara, J. (1995). *The Twelfth Mental Measurements Yearbook.* Lincoln: University of Nebraska Press.

Donaldson, M. (1978). *Children's Minds.* London: Fontana.

Evard, B., and Sabers, D. (1979). "Speech and Language Testing with Distinct Ethnic-Racial Groups: A Survey for Improving Test Validity." *Journal of Speech and Hearing Disorders* 44:271–281.

Hamayan, E., and Damico, J. (1991). *Limiting Bias in the Assessment of Bilingual Students.* Austin, TX: Pro-Ed.

Hegde, M. (1987). *Clinical Research in Communication Disorders.* Boston, MA: Little, Brown.

Hutchinson, T. (1996). "What to Look for in the Technical Manual: Twenty Questions for Users." *Language, Speech and Hearing Services in Schools* 27:109–121.

Ingram, D. (1981). *Procedures for the Phonological Analysis of Children's Language.* Baltimore, MD: University Park Press.

Lawrence, C. (1992). "Assessing the Use of Age-Equivalent Scores in Clinical Management." *Language, Speech and Hearing Services in Schools* 23:6–8.

Lee, L. (1974). *Developmental Sentence Analysis.* Evanston, IL: Northwestern University Press.

Ludlow, C. (1983). "Identification and Assessment of Aphasic Patients for Language Intervention." In *Contemporary Issues in Language Intervention,* ed. J. Miller, D. Yoder, and R. Schiefelbusch (Rockville, MD: American Speech-Language-Hearing Association).

McCauley, R. (1996). "Familiar Strangers: Criterion Referenced Measures in Communication Disorders." *Language, Speech and Hearing Services in Schools* 27:122–131.

McCauley, R., and Swisher, L. (1984a). "Psychometric Review of Language and Articulation Tests for Preschool Children." *Journal of Speech and Hearing Disorders* 49:34–42.

McCauley, R., and Swisher, L. (1984b). "Use and Misuse of Norm-referenced Tests in Clinical Assessment: A Hypothetical Case." *Journal of Speech and Hearing Disorders* 49:338–348.

Messick, S. (1975). "The Standard Problem: Meaning and Values in Measurement and Evaluation." *American Psychologist* 30:955–966.

Messick, S. (1980). "Test Validity and the Ethics of Assessment." *American Psychologist* 35:1012–1027.

Muma, J. (1973). "Language Assessment: Some Underlying Assumptions." *Journal of the American Speech and Hearing Association* 15:331–338.

Muma, J. (1978). *Language Handbook: Concepts, Assessment, Intervention.* Englewood Cliffs, NJ: Prentice-Hall.

Muma, J. (1981). *Language Primer.* Lubbock, TX: Natural Child Publisher.

Muma, J. (1983). *Language Assessment: How Valid is the Process?* Double miniseminar presented at the Annual Convention of the American Speech-Language-Hearing Association, Cincinnati, OH.

Muma, J. (1984). "Semel and Wiig's CELF: Construct Validity?" *Journal of Speech and Hearing Disorders* 49:101–104.

Muma, J. (1985). "No News Is Bad News: A Response to McCauley and Swisher." *Journal of Speech and Hearing Disorders* 50:290–293.

Muma, J. (1986). *Language Acquisition: A Functionalistic Perspective.* Austin, TX: Pro-Ed.

Muma, J. Lubinski, R., and Pierce, S. (1982). "A New Era in Language Assessment: Data or Evidence." In *Speech and Language,* Vol. 7, ed. N. Lass (New York: Academic Press).

Omark, A. (1981). *Communication Assessment of the Bilingual, Bicultural Child: Issues and Guidelines.* Baltimore, MD: Pro-Ed.

Owens, R. (1995). *Language Development: An Introduction.* Needham Heights, MA: Allyn and Bacon.

Plante, E. (1996). "Observing and Interpreting Behaviors: An Introduction to the Clinical Forum." *Language, Speech and Hearing Services in Schools* 27:99–101.

Plante, E., and Vance, R. (1994). "Selection of Preschool Language Tests: A Data-Based Approach." *Language, Speech and Hearing Services in Schools* 25:15–24.

Plante, E., and Vance, R. (1995). "Diagnostic Accuracy of Two Tests of Preschool Language." *American Journal of Speech-Language Pathology* 4:70–76.

Popham, J. (1981). *Modern Educational Measurement.* Englewood Cliffs, NJ: Prentice-Hall

Porch, B. (1967). *Porch Index of Communicative Ability.* Palo Alto, CA: Consulting Psychologists Press.

Salvia, J., and Ysseldyke, J. (1981). *Assessment in Special and Remedial Education.* Boston, MA: Houghton-Mifflin.

Seymour, H. (1992). "The Invisible Children: A Reply to Lahey's Perspective." *Journal of Speech and Hearing Research* 15:640–641.

Shriberg, L., and Kwiatkowski, J. (1980). *Natural Process Analysis.* New York: John Wiley.

Swank, P. (1987). *Compuscore for the Test for Auditory Comprehension of Language-Revised.* Allen, TX: DLM Teaching Resources.

$$Chapter\ \ 4$$

Assessment of Children with Limited Language

Our discussion of evaluation of child language disorders will be divided into two chapters. The present chapter deals with clients whose language does not exceed simple multiword combinations. Since most clients with limited language are children, we will refer to them as such in this chapter. Chapter 5 will focus on children who are using longer sentences and are typically school age or older.

The Process of Becoming a Communicator: Getting the "Big Picture"

MacDonald and Carroll (1992) have presented a useful conception of the developmental progression children must follow on their way to becoming effective communicators. The steps are deceptively simple, yet elegant. The following steps should be easy to remember, and they are important to consider in development, assessment, and treatment:

- **Play Partners (Implication: Cognitive Assessment).** Does the child play with objects appropriately? A child's play tells us about his/her conceptions of objects, events, and relationships in the world. A child who exhibits primitive play strategies with objects (e.g., mouthing, banging, sensorimotor exploration) is likely to have quite different cognitive abilities than a child who engages in functional object use and symbolic play. A child who does not know how to play with objects in productive ways is unlikely to learn to communicate about objects and events in an appropriate manner.
- **Turntaking Partners (Implication: Social Assessment).** After children learn some appropriate play strategies with objects, they begin to involve adults in

their play interactions. This social development is a critical prerequisite for communication. The development of reciprocity is important because communication involves social turntaking between partners.

- **Communication Partners (Implication: Assessment of Communicative Intent and Gesture System).** The initial communications of children are gestural in nature. They point, pull, push, and reach while looking at adults and objects. These initial nonverbal communications precede the use of words to regulate adult action and attention.
- **Language Partners (Implication: Language Model Analysis and Language Structure Analysis).** After the "flow" of communication is established through the use of gestures, children begin to approximate word productions that are modeled by their caregivers.
- **Conversational Partners (Implication: Pragmatic Analysis).** When the use of language is firmly established, the child gradually learns the pragmatic rules for taking into account listener perspective, topic manipulation, and appreciation of social context in participating in dialogue.

One can easily see that the five areas mentioned above build upon one another, and in assessment we can locate a child on this continuum. Each step implies a different evaluation focus and different treatment implications.

Focusing on the Child's Language Level: Nonverbal, Single-Word and Early Multiword Communicators

In talking about children with language disorders, it is not uncommon for authorities to refer to children's presenting linguistic-development level (Carrow-Woolfolk and Lynch 1982; Mclean and Snyder-Mclean 1978). Often, training programs in speech-language pathology offer one course that deals with language disorders in infants/toddlers and another course that focuses on language disorders of school-age children and adolescents. It is not the chronological age per se that is important here because a client with limited language can be from any age group (e.g., there are nonverbal teenagers and adults with mental retardation). Thus, it is unlikely that a single assessment procedure would be appropriate for *every* four-year-old because some of these children could be using advanced syntax while others could be using nonverbal communication. It is much more meaningful to discuss techniques that would be useful for a client who is communicating at the single or early multiword level regardless of his/her chronological age.

For purposes of assessment it is useful to consider children with limited language in three general categories. First, there are children, who are largely nonverbal. They use vocalizations and perhaps gestures, but their caretakers report no real use of language to control the latter's environment. Obviously, in dealing with a nonverbal child, a "test of language ability" would be too advanced. Faced with the virtual elimination of an entire shelf of standardized tests, the clinician must focus on more-informal assessment procedures. The following areas are especially important to consider in evaluation of nonverbal communicators:

- General developmental level/adaptive behavior
- Biological prerequisites (audiometry, neurological, medical)
- Case history (preevaluation questionnaire, detailed interview)
- Caretaker-child interaction analysis
- Communicative intent inventory (types, frequency, level)
- Vocalization analysis (use of phonetically consistent forms, syllable shape, phonetic inventory)
- Cognitive analysis (play analysis, screening tasks, formal scales)
- Lexical comprehension (parent reports, scales, tasks)

We will discuss each of the procedures mentioned above in more detail later in this chapter.

A second group of children consists of those who speak largely at the single-word level. The single-word stage has been reported in the developmental literature (Nelson 1973); and according to some authorities, the child may accrue a lexicon of about fifty words before starting the use of word combinations for generative language. Clearly, the assessment of a "single-word child" is both similar to and different from dealing with a child who is nonverbal. In terms of similarities, we are still interested in general developmental levels, biological prerequisites, case history, caretaker-child interaction, communicative intent, the phonetic inventory, cognitive development, and understanding of semantic elements. At the single-word level, however, we can add the following assessment areas to the ones listed above:

- Length measures from spontaneous sample (e.g., mean length of utterance, or MLU)
- Form/function analysis of single-word productions (What functions do the child's single word utterances serve?)
- Analysis of presyntactic devices (transitional elements related to development of multiword utterances)
- Analysis of lexical production (grammatical types of words, number of words in lexicon)
- Phonological-process analysis

The measures listed above will be discussed more specifically in later sections.

A third type of child is one who is using early multiword combinations. For this type of child, it is clear that some basic cognitive capacity for using a symbol system exists because the child is, in fact, using one. In studying an early multiword child, it is more important to focus on the types of word combinations used and the functions for which the child uses the utterances. The phonetic inventory and phonological-process analysis also become important for this type of case, because a child's oral language can only be functional if it is intelligible to listeners.

Thus, for the child who uses early multiword utterances, we must examine the language, but not necessarily in the same way as we would a language sample of a child who has a longer length of utterance. Thus, we would add the following to the prior measures:

- Analysis of semantic relations (types, frequency, productivity)
- Specific language development test
- Comprehension of simple commands

We have seen that there are at least three categories into which we can place children with limited language. The clinician's first step is to determine in which category the client is placed based on preponderant communication behaviors. The next step involves considering the high-probability diagnostic areas associated with the category. Finally, the clinician can use some of the specific procedures referred to later in this chapter which will allow evaluation of the pertinent areas. Implied in the categories are different assessment targets, most of which cannot be evaluated by using formal test instruments (Wetherby and Prizant 1992). Mc-Cathren, Warren, and Yoder (1996) identify four proven predictors of later language development in prelinguistic children: (1) use of babbling, (2) development of pragmatic functions, (3) vocabulary comprehension, and (4) the development of combinatorial/symbolic play skills. Unfortunately, most available formal assessment instruments do not measure these variables adequately. Notable exceptions are the *Communication and Symbolic Behavior Scales* (Wetherby and Prizant 1993) and *Assessing Prelinguistic and Early Linguistic Behaviors in Developmentally Young Children* (ALB) (Olswang et al. 1987). Crais and Roberts (1991) provide a useful conceptual framework for the clinician in the form of "decision trees" to help generate assessment questions, select procedures, and link these procedures to intervention recommendations.

Considering "Etiology"

Although we have characterized children with language disorders by their general linguistic development level, some students may be tempted to describe those disorders by using etiology (e.g., mental retardation or hearing impairment). We agree with those who suggest that classification of language disorder by etiology does not relate productively to assessment (Aram and Nation 1975; Lahey 1988; Newhoff and Leonard 1983; Paul 1995). The various etiological groups themselves are highly heterogeneous, and thus to refer to a child who is "mentally retarded" really means little in terms of predicting what one might be like. In addition, the language disorders manifested by these various groups may not be significantly different. Therefore, the language samples gathered from children who are hearing impaired, mentally retarded, learning disabled, autistic, and language delayed but with normal intelligence may be highly similar. Diagnostic grouping, then, does not necessarily provide the clinician with valid guidelines for assessment of language skills.

Why Is Early Language Assessment So Difficult?

Language assessment in children is one of the most difficult and challenging tasks faced by the SLP, and many clinicians are insecure about their diagnostic ability in this area.

1. *Heterogeneity of the population.* One complicating factor for the diagnostician is that the population that exhibits a language disorder is extremely heterogeneous (Aram and Nation 1975; Wolfus, Moscovitch, and Kinsbourne 1980). In addition, children from a wide spectrum of etiological groups manifest language impairment, and the practitioner is faced with youngsters who are mentally retarded, autistic, hearing impaired, learning disabled, or who exhibit a variety of other organically based conditions. This heterogeneity appears to make diagnosis quite difficult, especially for the clinician who knows only one approach to language assessment.

2. *Highly Varied Severity Levels.* A second variable that makes language diagnosis difficult is the difference in the degree of severity found in the language-impaired population. The children range from those who are nonverbal with a lack of social and cognitive bases for language, on the one hand, to youngsters who inconsistently misuse grammatical morphemes or exhibit subtle pragmatic problems on the other. Thus, for each evaluation the clinician must be prepared to assess the broad representation of linguistic and prelinguistic behaviors.

3. *Language Is a Complex Phenomenon.* A third variable that makes language assessment confusing is the complex nature of language itself. Most introductory courses discuss language as an area that is comprised of various domains. In fact, many textbooks are organized with reference to such language areas as semantics, syntax, morphology, phonology, and, more recently, pragmatics. Any or all of these areas can be affected in a language disorder. Most theorists agree that these domains are not isolated from one another but have complex interactions that proceed from "top-down" and "bottom-up" in models of language processing. Complicating the problem further is the fact that authorities in the area of psycholinguistics are not in total agreement regarding exactly how these domains of language interact with each other in spontaneous communication.

4. *A Multitude of Assessment Instruments/Procedures.* Another variable that makes it difficult to know what to do in language evaluation is the proliferation of assessment devices and procedures available on the market. We are inundated with flyers and catalogs, many reputed to offer "the best language assessment device." How does one select a test? Is one test really enough? The fact that people have designed tests of language for children with oftentimes very inclusive titles suggests that it is possible to find out all one needs to know from a single test. Unfortunately, the disclaimers that some authors place in their test manuals regarding the shortcomings of the instruments are forgotten, and the perhaps over ambitious title remains in the mind of clinicians and parents. Tests, also, are based on different theoretical points of view or models. The differing theoretical underpinnings result in dramatically different types of tasks and areas of emphasis on tests. The plethora of tests, then, is a source of confusion to many clinicians.

5. *Language Is Profoundly Affected by Multiple Processes and Domains.* It is also difficult to know what to do in language assessment because language development and disorders encompass so much more than just linguistic ability. In the literature on language acquisition, for instance, one routinely reads about cognitive development, neurolinguistics, linguistic theory, adaptive behavior, play development, social development, self-help skills, phonology, motor ability, caretaker-child interaction, and other areas that may not appear to be directly related to linguistic symbols but are critical to language development. Since language itself has many domains (semantics, syntax, phonology, morphology, pragmatics, etc.) and the related areas mentioned above are numerous, language assessment may take on quite different guises, depending on the focus of the evaluation. This complexity is clearly a source of confusion for clinicians and requires a very broad base of skill and knowledge.

The difficulties mentioned above probably contribute to many clinician's uncertainties in the area of language assessment. Models, as we indicate in the following section, are sometimes helpful in reducing the difficulties in understanding an area and in assisting diagnosticians in developing workable clinical procedures.

Models to Consider in Language Assessment

If we were to travel around the country and eavesdrop as SLPs evaluate children, we would find a confusing conglomeration of activities performed under the aegis of linguistic assessment:

A clinician has a child repeat sentences.

A child plays silently while the clinician takes notes.

A child is trying to obtain a toy, and the clinician resists.

A clinician is asking a child to point to one of three pictures.

A clinician is instructing a child to act out a scene with dolls.

A child is trying to get a piece of candy by pulling a string tied to the candy, and the clinician is scribbling on a clipboard.

A clinician is watching a child and the parents play.

A clinician with a child is pushing a car back and forth and suddenly pushes a horse on wheels instead of the car back to the child.

A child is trying to complete open-ended sentences presented by the clinician.

A child is describing pictures for a clinician behind a cardboard barrier.

What does it all mean? Are all these clinicians really performing language assessments? How does a clinician know which thing to do with a particular child? If one thing is clear today, it is that more than ever language assessment requires that the clinician possess more varied skills and diversity of educational background than before.

The clinician in a language evaluation must have some framework upon which to gather and organize the data. For years, authorities have been "model building." Many people, however, tend to think that the models that are built in paneled dens across the country are exclusively the stuff of intellectualization and idle theorizing. There is a point, however, where some models begin to have clinical relevance. When a clinician has some sort of guiding principle to use in assessment and treatment, the model appears as a relevant clinical concept. As Nation and Aram (1977) indicate, you cannot operate effectively unless you have some organization of your database. Models, then, are "organizing principles" that help to make the clinician more operational. The way in which the clinician conceptualizes language and communication will largely dictate how language disorders are assessed and treated. For instance, a strict behavioral model of language and communication would not necessarily consider cognitive or social prerequisites. It does not deal with intent or other unobservable phenomena. If a clinician subscribed exclusively to this model, there may be no evaluation of the areas mentioned above. Models that emphasize modalities of input and output, such as Kirk and Kirk's (1971), do not particularly focus on linguistic aspects such as syntax, morphology, and pragmatics. Prerequisite areas (cognitive, social, biological) also are ignored. These are just two examples of how the model of language that is adopted by a clinician can constrain thinking and clinical behavior. Thus, all models are not equally useful to a clinician, and certain important aspects of the language process can be missed.

There are some cautions. First, general semanticists have said for decades that the "map is not the territory". So it is with models. They are not the knowledge or behavior they represent. Clinicians should never forget that it is what they know that is important, far beyond any model. Models are perspectives and guides for organizing clinical information, nothing more. If the clinician is confronted with a real child that is performing at odds with a model's prediction, the validity of the child's behavior is not questionable, but the applicability of the model in this case is certainly a bit dubious. Do not, as they say, let the tail wag the dog. A second caution is that at the present time no one knows for certain all the details of exactly how language is developed, processed, or most efficiently assessed. Thus, any model is likely to be inaccurate or at least, incomplete. Clinicians, like theorists, must be open to change in their conceptualizations and evaluations of language and its evaluation.

Theoretical Considerations in Language Assessment

Following the lead of Muma (1973, 1978, 1983) we would like to echo some basic diagnostic precepts that we feel should underpin language assessment. First, the best language assessment device, as Siegel (1975) stated, is a well-trained clinician who keeps up with current developments. There is no "best" language test, just as there is no ideal language treatment program.

Second, language is a multidimensional process that has many facets of structure and use. There are also the prerequisite areas discussed earlier to consider in evaluation. The existence of the multidimensional process makes it unrealistic to separate structure and function or syntax from semantics or pragmatics. The most ecologically valid methods of analyzing the process are preferable. Whenever we fractionalize the communicative process, we are no longer really looking at it.

Third, Muma (1978) has reminded us that whatever we do in assessment must apply to treatment of the language disorder. If we administer tests and then do not consider these results in planning our treatment, the time spent in assessment is wasted. Our assessment and treatment procedures also should be based on similar assumptions about the communication process.

A fourth important concept also was articulated by Muma. He stated that the diagnostic paradigm seems to have two levels or issues associated with it. The most basic issue is the "problem/no problem" issue. Standardized tests help to solve the problem/no problem issue by comparing a child's test performance to that of other children. This type of testing emphasizes group similarity and minimizes individual variability. The "nature of the problem" issue, however, must be addressed through description of the individual child's communicative performance. This assessment is best accomplished through nonstandardized, descriptive techniques that are more ecologically valid. Fortunately, the problem/no problem issue is solved by many parents when they have referred their children for evaluation. These parents typically know that something is wrong when they compare the communication of their children with their children's peers. A standardized test can confirm this, but it rarely can be prescriptive in terms of specifying treatment targets (Millen and Prutting 1979).

A fifth important notion has to do with sampling. All we ever do in a diagnostic evaluation is obtain a sample of communicative behavior. There are several important implications that stem from the sampling idea. First, the samples we obtain should be "representative" of the child's communicative performance. The notion of representativeness has been with us for a long while, and we must not forget that a sample we obtain may or may not represent a child's typical or "best" performance. Secondly, speech pathologists have subscribed for years to the idea that an evaluation can and must take place within a one- or two-hour block of time. This kind of thinking can result in frustrated clinicians when they do not obtain the data they need in the allotted time, or if the child is uncooperative. Evaluation is ongoing, and there should be no pressure to find out all there is to know in a limited time frame. The medical profession does not feel compelled to diagnose in a limited time with short, abbreviated procedures. Physicians order examinations that they feel are appropriate, and the diagnostic process takes place over as much time as is necessary. This is not to say that we should emulate the lengthy testing procedures of the medical profession; but on the other hand, we should not become like purveyors of fast food. Third, whenever possible, the clinician should attempt to obtain multiple samples. Many children behave differently in the clinical setting than they do at home or in the preschool. There have not been many comparisons of language in preschool settings with clinical environments, but we suspect that there are important differences.

Case Example. *Tyrone had said nothing during the two-hour evaluation session. He was brought to the clinic by a caseworker from the state pensions and securities office as a foster child. The caseworker said that Tyrone did talk and could not explain why he was so taciturn upon meeting us. He seemed shy and reluctant to participate even in play with the clinicians. We decided to make an observation the next week at Tyrone's day-care center. We sat unobtrusively in a corner and watched Tyrone carom off the walls like a buzz saw going awry, pulling pigtails and spewing broken crayons. He yelled at his classmates, and when the teacher asked who wanted to play ball, Tyrone was one of the first to initiate his loud request. Lucas (1980) has observed that some preschoolers take on the role in the classroom of "starter of the rules." They tell other children "You can't do that," "The paper has to be over here," etc. (We often wonder what types of people these children develop into when they become adults. Know any?) Tyrone frequently made rule statements to the other children. We half felt that we had seen a "medicated" Tyrone at our clinic. Our goals for treatment would have been far different had we not observed Tyrone in more than one setting. It may have been appropriate, based on our first impression, to begin work on increasing child-initiated language.*

What we have described above is not an isolated case. We have often made the recommendation to clinicians in the field to observe children in other settings before deciding on treatment goals. In many cases the feedback from these professionals has been, "I thought he was a different child when I saw him in the classroom."

A sixth basic premise of language assessment is that for every technique or test that the clinician uses, he/she must realize that certain assumptions are implied about child language. To use an instrument, you should "buy the assumptions" that underlie it. Whenever we receive the myriad flyers and announcements of new language assessment instruments, we should remember that each is based on assumptions. We should ask ourselves, "What do I have to believe about language to use this instrument?"

Finally, we feel compelled to say that the quality of the information obtained is proportional to the amount of time the well-trained clinician spends in evaluation. In short, there is no free lunch. A twenty-minute screening test that is easily administered and scored will simply not yield as much information as various analyses of a twenty-minute spontaneous interaction.

The above suggestions should not be taken to mean that we are opposed to the use of standardized tests. We do, in fact, recommend the use of such instruments for the purpose they are most able to accomplish, namely, to determine if a child is performing similarly to other children of his/her age group. Standardized tests, however, cannot make a principled clinical judgment; clinicians make decisions. Assessment has aspects of both art and science (Allen, Bliss, and Timmons 1981). We advocate the use of a combination of standard measures coupled with nonstandardized tasks and more naturalistic sampling of communicative behavior (Lund and Duchan 1988; Paul 1995). We believe that reliance on exclusively either type of procedure will not provide as complete a picture of a child's performance as the use of both types. Additionally, school systems and other institutions often require some form of standardized testing.

Specific Assessment Areas: Procedures, Considerations and Directions for Further Study

In the sections that follow, we will discuss specific techniques for assessing important areas related to the communication of a child with limited language. We try to provide guidelines and references for the clinician to use in learning about these various aspects of language assessment. In cases where we cannot adequately summarize a procedure (which is most of the time), we refer the reader to a primary source with the hope that he/she will critically evaluate and perhaps learn techniques that will be clinically useful.

At the beginning of most sections, we will provide a brief sketch of some important developmental trends reported in the existing research. It is imperative that the clinician appreciate that each assessment technique mentioned is basically grounded in the research on communication development. While it is beyond the scope of this chapter to present an adequate view of any aspect of language acquisition, we would be remiss if we did not touch upon some "highlights" of the process that are related to language assessment. Many fine textbooks are available that summarize research in language acquisition, and the reader should become familiar with this information prior to engaging in any language assessment (Bloom 1974; Brown 1973; Carrow-Woolfolk and Lynch 1982; Devilliers and Devilliers 1978; Hubbell 1981; Ingram 1989; Lahey 1988; Owens 1995).

Preassessment and Pertinent Historical Information

Preassessment

In most clinical settings, prospective clients are required to complete some sort of case history information prior to being seen by the speech-language pathologist and/or other professionals. It is especially unnerving to meet a client for the first time, prior to receiving the completed case history information, because the clinician has little idea about how to prepare for the evaluation. Especially in the area of language disorders, the client could be at levels ranging from totally nonverbal to a syntax level with only subtle language problems. Thus, it is crucial for SLPs in any work setting to avoid performing an evaluation without access to important historical information. Prior knowledge of historical information can allow the clinician to plan the evaluation in such a way as to maximize the use of time and resources during the initial contact with the child and parents.

Gallagher (1983) suggested a preassessment procedure for use with language cases and outlined the advantages of such a process for the clinician in planning and conducting evaluations. Preassessment is more than the typical process of having the parents merely fill out a case history form. The notion of preassessment includes finding out some clinically useful data that could affect the way in which the initial evaluation is conducted. In our university setting, we use a preassessment form that contains components from a variety of research projects (Gallagher 1983). Clients are asked to complete the form and return it prior to the scheduling of the evaluation appointment. In some cases where the parents cannot read or have difficulty completing the form, an interview session is scheduled in which the parents are questioned about each item on the preassessment prior to our seeing the child. The important thing is that the clinician has a fairly good picture of the child's cognitive, social, play, and communicative behavior before the evaluation session. Typically, to provide additional information on noncommunicative behaviors that relate to cognitive, social, and language development, we also include a short adaptive-behavior scale that focuses on motor skills, self-help skills, and personal/social abilities. Gallagher (1983) gives a concrete example of the value of preassessment information:

> One child who was particularly sensitive to the communicative partner had an MLU value of 1.6 in the clinician-child sample and an MLU of 3.96 when she talked with her brother. One boy produced his most structurally complex utterances while he was playing with water toys in a plastic pan filled with water, an activity his mother had indicated "he would talk most about." One boy's most structurally complex language performance was obtained when he played with a younger friend who was his neighbor. For one child, it was talking about pictures in a family album. (14)

None of these language-facilitating situations would have been known to the clinician if the appropriate questions had not been asked on a preassessment instrument. The clinician can plan ahead and ask family members to bring specific stimulus items, toys, or interactants that would provide the best sample of a client's communication abilities.

The Parent Interview

Many questions will be raised by parent responses on the preassessment packet. The interview is a good place to clarify any missing information or inconsistencies in a parent's responses. The information obtained from caretakers of limited-language children is highly important. First of all, many of these children may not have the linguistic means or cognitive development to express themselves well, and the parent or guardian must be relied upon to provide pertinent background details and estimations of present skill levels. Second, recent research has suggested that expressive language disorders tend to run in families (Lahey and Edwards 1995), and information regarding symptoms, treatments, and outcomes related to disorders in other family members is most easily obtained in the interview format that allows for examples and follow-up questions.

As mentioned in Chapter 2, we do not recommend that the diagnostician write down specific questions prior to the evaluation. Appendix A contains an interview protocol for assessment of the limited-language child. The protocol is divided into broad areas covering the prerequisites to language as well as the beginnings of linguistic development. Much of the specific information can be filled in from responses to the preassessment packet, and the interview can simply follow up areas of interest to the clinician. The interviewer should ask questions in the broad areas, obtaining information in each subarea. The exact wording of questions is not provided owing to the pragmatics of the interview situation. Parents represent differing levels of education, intelligence, socioeconomic status, and experience, and we have found it more feasible to tailor interview questions for each individual case. The protocol was designed only to "jog the mind" of the clinician, who, it is hoped, will ask questions in specific topic areas. When remarkable information is reported in any area, the interviewer should formulate appropriate follow-up questions to clearly illuminate the area of interest. The major interview areas represent biological, social, and cognitive prerequisites to language as well as linguistic level and were gleaned from a variety of child-language-acquisition and language-impairment sources. The interviewer should especially focus the interview on the most applicable portions of the protocol and not ask unnecessary questions. For instance, if a child is using a wide variety of multiword utterances and is communicating effectively in the environment, it would be inappropriate for the interviewer to spend inordinate time on cognitive and social attainments.

One of the most revealing questions about the child's home environment is the item that asks a parent to describe a typical day in the life of his/her child. It is often surprising how many inconsistencies can be uncovered in the answer to this question. For instance, a parent may report that his/her child spends many hours watching television, or playing alone outside, or engaging in self-stimulatory activities—activities that have been allowed to continue despite their lack of productivity. Often, a pattern emerges that shows that the child spends little time in meaningful social interactions. Another pattern that reveals much about a child's problem is lack of a schedule or rules in the household. One mother reported that her nonverbal three-year-old child typically went to bed at 11:30 P.M. after a late night talk show and liked to sleep until 9:30 A.M. The child also ate all his meals while walking around inside the house, refused to wear pajamas, threw frequent tantrums, and was prone to writing on the walls. This scenario suggests that the parents and child may be in some need of counseling regarding behavior management. Much of this information would not have been gleaned from the preassessment packet or a formal test, but the information would be quite important when it comes to making recommendations for treatment. If, for example, we wanted these parents to begin to withhold desired items from this child in order to create communicative opportunity, they would have extreme difficulty with this procedure since there appear to be few existing rules in the home. Tantrums would inevitably increase, and the treatment plan would have a high probability of being aborted by the family.

The protocol in Appendix A is designed for the well-informed child-language clinician. The question areas will mean nothing to the interviewer who does not know the relevance, rationale, and research that underpins each major area and subheading. Finally, no single item on the protocol is significant in its own right. We are looking for patterns among the major areas. It should be remembered that the areas are divided upon the protocol only for convenience and that in reality the domains are interrelated. In obtaining the information the interviewer should do the following:

1. Tape record the interview and take notes after obtaining permission.
2. Frame questions on the correct level of abstraction for the parent.

3. Use many examples when asking questions, and do not use frequent yes/no questions. For instance, ask questions such as, "How does Randy let you know he wants something?" "What does he like to do when he plays?" "What kinds of sentences have you heard him say?" "Under what circumstances does he try to communicate with you?" If the parent is not providing enough specific information, the clinician can ask some specific questions, such as, "Does he seem to use objects for the purpose they were intended? For instance, does he use a comb to comb his hair?"
4. Ask the parent to give you *examples* of behaviors and language you are interested in.
5. Space is provided on the protocol for the interviewer to make a brief note as to remarkable findings in any area.

Assessment of Social Prerequisites and Caretaker-Child Interaction

Language development takes place in a social context. From the moment of birth, a child interacts with his/her caretakers and is bombarded with visual, auditory, and tactile stimuli that occur in this relationship. Current legislation (PL 99-457) also mandates the involvement of the family in both assessment and treatment. It is especially important in cases of nonverbal, single-word and early-multiword-level children to observe them as they interact with their caretaker. There are two reasons for this.

First, we want to observe the child with someone whom he/she is familiar with and feels comfortable being around. It is often the case that the best sample of the child's communication is obtained in this portion of the evaluation. When unfamiliar clinicians attempt to establish rapport with a child in strange surroundings, it may be quite difficult to observe natural communication, especially in a limited time period. Occasionally, we have seen children who refused to interact with us in an evaluation. In these cases the caretaker-child interaction provides the only data base available. In the early years of our field, we were frequently told that the initial step in an evaluation was to separate the child from his mother. Often, this resulted in a catastrophic reaction on the part of the child, and little information was gained from the evaluation (other than the fact that the child did not "separate well from the mother"). We must not lose sight of our goal, namely, it is to observe the child's communicative and prelinguistic skills through talking and play. If the caretaker can provide a more-effective demonstration of certain skills than the clinician can, then we must take advantage of this opportunity and not feel that we have failed as clinicians. Rather, we have succeeded in getting the data we were after as the result of making a sound clinical judgment. Establishing a relationship with a child can always be accomplished in the initial treatment sessions where we are not under as severe time constraints. Thus, the caretaker-child interaction can provide a rich sampling of the child's communication. As we will soon indicate, it also can give the clinician a meager, constrained, and repetitive sample.

A second goal of the caretaker-child interaction is to observe the quality of the language model provided by the parent. Research has shown that caretakers alter many aspects of their communicative behavior. Suprasegmentally, they raise their vocal fundamental frequency, increase their pitch range, speak more slowly, and use double primary-stress patterns (Garnica 1974). The caretaker is less disfluent when talking to an infant and pauses at major linguistic constituent boundaries. Linguistically, the mean length of utterance is reduced, and the vocabulary and syntactic complexity are simplified (Snow 1972). Developing children, in addition to being exposed to a simpler language model, are given an introduction to the reciprocity of communicative interchange. Snow (1977) has shown that with neonates as young as three months of age, mothers engage in turn-taking, reciprocal, behavior. Early on, the child's "turn" is a biologically programmed nonverbal action, such as smiling, sneezing, or burping. The mother simply responds to this with some sort of language response and oftentimes takes the child's turn for him/her linguistically. As the child develops, the caretaker demands that the youngster's turn more closely resemble the adult correct model.

As important as the model itself are the circumstances under which it is delivered. The youngster benefits cognitively from interacting with the caretaker. Mothers and fathers typically show the child "how the world works" by demonstrating the functional use of objects and body parts, the attributes of objects, and many other conceptual aspects of the environment. Children have been shown to follow a caretaker's line of visual regard (to look at an object a parent is focused on) very early in development (Mclean and Snyder-Mclean 1978). Adults also show the child how to play with a variety of objects and even stimulate symbolic play. We see then, that caretakers demonstrate language structure, language use, concepts, and the reciprocity of communication. Children are highly sensitive to their social environment, and they learn that language is a tool to be used for a variety of social and nonsocial purposes (Dore 1975; Halliday 1975). With young children, it is clear that their early exposure to language and their early use of it is highly social.

The clinician needs to answer many questions about the caretaker-child interaction. Does the caretaker talk about the "here and now" (Holland 1975) or about things removed in time and space? What kind of joint referencing takes place in the interaction? Does the caretaker talk about and participate in things that the child appears to be interested in? Does the caretaker direct the child's play to things that the former feels are significant and disregard the child's preferences? Is there a balance between when the parent joint references with the child and when the child joint references with the parent? Regarding the uses of language, does the parent force the child into limited or respondent modes of communicative function? It is not unusual to observe parents of early language-disordered children who ask incessant questions (e.g., "What's this?" "What color is this?") or who ask the child to constantly imitate (e.g., "Say 'ball' "). We are not intimating that the parent's interactive style is in any way causally related to the child's language disorder. In fact, a parent's way of talking to a child could be a result of the disorder rather than a cause. Whatever the relationship, the caretaker's model as it presently exists, may not be conducive to language development and should be changed. The only way to determine the quality of this relationship is through the observation of caretaker-child interaction. Evaluating and working with caretaker-child interaction is especially important when dealing with infants and toddlers who are "high risk" for language disorder. Providing the best-quality stimulation for these children will go a long way toward preventing, or at least reducing, the severity of potential language disorders.

It is also important to examine specific aspects of the child's social behavior in the caretaker-child interaction. Socially, the child's eye contact and willingness to participate in reciprocal nonverbal activities should be observed. A child who does not tolerate or seek out the participation of another person may not have any need for a communication system. Perhaps this child might need to work on some prelinguistic social skills prior to the development of language. Recall that Macdonald and Carroll (1992) said that a child must first become a play partner and a turn-taking partner before a communication partnership develops. Language is, after all, a social tool, and a child who is not "social" has little need of a code to use around people with whom he does not even communicate nonverbally.

> Case Example. *Natalie entered the examination playroom, and her attention settled on the juice. She ran to the table and tried to remove the top of the glass container. When she could not, she proceeded from item to item, pausing only a few seconds on each. When the clinician called her name loudly, she did not respond. Small noises in the hallway occurred several times, and she paused, transfixed on the door, with her head cocked to one side like a dog listening to a distant sound. The clinician physically caught her and tried to engage in reciprocal play with a car. Natalie would not look the clinician in the eye, and the car was thrown across the room behind her. Throughout the two hour session, the child never maintained eye contact longer than two seconds and never participated cooperatively with the clinician. More important, even when it was clear she wanted something out of reach, she never sought out help from the other human being in the room. The mother reported that Natalie plays alone most of the time and with animals outside in the rural farmyard. It is doubtful that this child has much need for social interaction, let alone a use for a communication system.*

Table 4.1 provides an example of a checklist that the clinician could use in examining caretaker behaviors during interaction in the evaluation session. Note that the "score" is not important; however, the clinician's impressions of the caretaker modifications could lead to treatment recommendations involving work with interaction patterns.

Cross-cultural studies of caretaker-child interaction have demonstrated cultural differences in interaction style, play, speech register, use of objects in joint referencing, parenting, family values/beliefs, and general opportunities for interaction (Bornstein, Tal, and Tamis-Lemonda 1991a; Bornstein et al. 1991b; Fogel, Toda, and Kawai 1988; Heath 1983, 1989; Saville-Troike 1986; Schieffelin 1985; Watson-Gegeo and Gegeo 1986). Anderson-Yockel and Haynes (1994) found differences in parental questioning behaviors during joint book reading between lower-socioeconomic-level African American and Caucasian mother-toddler dyads. These potential cultural differences in caregiver-child interaction must be taken into account as the clinician examines parents and children in clinical settings. Social interactions and selection of activities for joint referencing may be very different in the home envi-

TABLE 4.1   Caretaker-Child Interaction Attributes

Child: _____   Date: _____   Age: _____

Nature of interaction in terms of toys, room, and interactants:

General Parameters	No				Yes
1. Encourages communication by looking expectantly	1	2	3	4	5
2. Responds to communication by reinforcing it with action or utterance	1	2	3	4	5
3. Joint references with child	1	2	3	4	5
4. Alternates adult/child direction in joint referencing	1	2	3	4	5
5. Talks about present context (here and now)	1	2	3	4	5
6. Model is timed to coincide with joint referencing	1	2	3	4	5
7. Talks at child's eye level	1	2	3	4	5
8. Successful attempts at interpretation of child's utterances and communicative intents	1	2	3	4	5
9. Creates communicative opportunities by using sabotage or pause time	1	2	3	4	5
10. Does not anticipate child's needs ahead of time thus reducing communicative attempts	1	2	3	4	5

Language Model Parameters					
1. Reduces sentence length	1	2	3	4	5
2. Reduces sentence complexity	1	2	3	4	5
3. Repeats utterances frequently (redundancy)	1	2	3	4	5
4. Paraphrases utterances ("throw the ball; throw it")	1	2	3	4	5
5. Uses exaggerated intonation patterns	1	2	3	4	5
6. Places stress on important words	1	2	3	4	5
7. Uses concrete, high frequency vocabulary	1	2	3	4	5
8. Does not talk too much and dominate conversation	1	2	3	4	5
9. Does not use excessive questions and commands	1	2	3	4	5
10. Uses slower speech rate	1	2	3	4	5

Use of Teaching Techniques					
1. Self-talk	1	2	3	4	5
2. Parallel talk	1	2	3	4	5
3. Expansion	1	2	3	4	5
4. Expatiation (enlargement)	1	2	3	4	5
5. Buildup/breakdown sequences	1	2	3	4	5
6. Recast sentences	1	2	3	4	5

Average Score = _____

ronment, and we should not expect everyone to interact in the same way when using "mainstream" toys and objects provided in clinical settings. Clinicians must endeavor to learn more about child rearing and interaction in different cultures and should not impose ethnocentric views on the families we serve.

Adaptive Behavior Scales
Adaptive behavior scales typically rate a child's development of motor skills, social behavior, self-help skills, and language ability. Children are given tasks to

perform, or the parents are asked to respond to items on the interview protocol. The advantage of such scales is that their use helps to broaden the perspective of the SLP beyond exclusively examining language ability. Although we will assess social cognitive development as it relates to language, much of a child's adaptive behavior depends on cognitive and social attainments. We can obtain a better over-all picture of the child's level of functioning, and this information, when coupled with our other assessment data, can be valuable. In addition, many conditions (e.g., mental retardation) may show that a child is of generally low functioning in most areas and that language is only part of the problem. Knowledge of adaptive behavior also will be important to the clinician in making referrals. Language-treatment activities also can be designed to incorporate motor, social, and self-help areas so that the child is learning a variety of needed skills as well as the language associated with them. Several adaptive behavior scales are available (Balthazar 1973; Lambert et al. 1981; Project RHISE 1979; Sparrow, Balla, and Cicchetti 1984). In most work settings, including public schools and many medical settings, SLPs are part of a transdisciplinary or multidisciplinary team. Other professionals such as psychologists, psychometrists, occupational therapists, physical therapists, special-education teachers, and medical personnel can provide valuable interpre-tations of the noncommunication domains included on such behavior scales as self-help, motor skills, and social adjustment. The advantage of such a team ap-proach is not only in the interpretation of assessment findings but also in the pro-gramming of goals for multiple domains across the treatment regimen.

Assessment of Cognitive Attainments Associated with Communication

Conceptual holdings are thought to be important to linguistic acquisition for sev-eral reasons. First, language is a representational act. It represents reality or stands for objects and relationships in the world. Second, language is an abstract symbol system. In order to appreciate abstract symbols, we must be able to represent them mentally. Third, language is a tool that we use in social interactions. Tool use im-plies certain conceptual underpinnings such as the apprehension of relationships like means-end. Fourth, language use involves talking about objects, events, and relationships in the world. It is necessary that one knows the properties of these objects and relationships before talking about them coherently. As Nelson (1974) said, we use words as "tags" for the concepts that we have.

Perhaps the most well-known researcher in the area of children's cognitive de-velopment has been Jean Piaget. A most significant period in language development occurs between birth and two years. By the age of two, a child is typically beginning to use multiword utterances and has clearly demonstrated the symbolic capacity for dealing with language. Piaget calls the period between birth and age two the sensorimotor stage of cognitive development because most learning takes place through active sensorimotor exploration of a child's environment. There are many sources available that describe this period of cognitive growth in detail (Flavell 1977; Ginsburg and Opper 1969; Morehead and Morehead 1974). We hope to present a feeling for some of the developmental landmarks that a child is thought to pass on the way to becoming representational. The implication for the diagnostician is that these landmarks may be assessment targets for severely language-disordered children. It should be emphasized that not all of these cognitive attainments have been shown to directly or strongly correlate with language acquisition. However, many authorities have advocated the administration of Piagetian assessment batteries that examine cognitive attainments in the sensorimotor period (Mclean and Snyder-Mclean 1978; Newhoff and Leonard 1983; Ruder and Smith 1974). Some skills examined on these scales seem to be "logically related" to language development, and others have been shown to have a statistical relationship to linguistic acquisition. There is, however, a difference between correlation and causation. Actually, some authorities feel that the relationship between specific cognitive developments and specific language acquisitions has not been clearly shown (Leonard 1978). Others support the notion of relating more-specific cognitive skills to linguistic acquisition (Gopnik and Meltzoff 1987; Lifter and Bloom 1989). In reviewing the cognitive-development literature, however, there seem to be certain skills that are included on cognitive-assessment scales and often referred to by authorities as being potentially language related.

One cognitive skill that is logically related to language development is that of object permanence. At a certain point in development, an infant will not appear to be able to represent an object mentally when it is not in physical view. The infant seems to "forget" about the object, even if it is one that the infant desires. If you cover an object with a cloth, a child of a certain age and cognitive level may stop searching for the object. Some studies, however, have not shown a strong relationship between language development and object permanence (Bates 1979; Leonard 1978), although it is included in many scales that are often administered to language-developing children (Merhabian and Williams 1971; Uzgiris and Hunt 1975).

Another cognitive skill thought to be related to the acquisition of language is the ability to appreciate the means-end relationship (Bates 1979; Morehead 1974). The idea that a particular process is a means to accomplishing an end is similar to the use of language in affecting the environment of the language user. Language is, in fact, a means to accomplishing a variety of ends, such as regulating the environment, obtaining information, sharing information, and so forth. (Halliday 1975). If the child does not have the basic means-end concept, it is doubtful that language will be used as a means for accomplishing any purpose.

Functional object use has also been related to the development of communication (Steckol and Leonard 1981). Using an object for its intended purpose (e.g., combing hair with a comb), requires the mental representation of both the object and its use. In addition, when a child begins to talk about basic relations in the environment, utterances typically concern objects, their functions, and all the relationships an object enters into (Nelson 1974). Steckol and Leonard (1981) found that training in the functional use of objects resulted in an increase of protoimperative responses (using adults nonverbally to accomplish a task or manipulate objects) in nonverbal children.

Imitation and deferred (delayed) imitation also have been related to the development of language (Bates et al. 1979). Imitation requires mental representation of an act for a short time period, and deferred imitation requires holding onto an event for a longer duration. Both suggest at least being able to represent reality for a length of time and not having to depend on immediate stimulus support.

Finally, symbolic play (pretend behavior) is frequently regarded as evidence of a child's general symbolic capacity. One can think of symbolic play on a continuum from playing with exemplars of an object that are physically similar to the real object (e.g., a box representing a car), to playing with exemplars that are dissimilar to the real object (e.g., a comb for a car), and finally to playing with no object at all (pantomime) (Elder and Pederson 1978). The use of one object to "stand for" another is similar to the way in which words represent objects in the real world. A basic symbolic capacity must be present in order to use a symbolic play routine, and these routines should be noted in a child's behavior as a positive sign of increased symbolic capacity.

Thus far, the cognitive attainments of object permanence, the means-end relationship, the functional use of objects, imitation, deferred imitation, and symbolic play have been suggested as possibly important to the development of language. Of course, no one really knows how much each of these capacities or activities contributes, or whether any of them does contribute for certain, to the acquisition of language. They may only be correlated with language development (Newhoff and Leonard 1983).

Piaget has divided his sensorimotor period of cognitive development into six substages. Several investigators report that a child must have at least attained stage 4 to evidence gestural communication and stages 5 or 6 for expressive single-word and early multiword constructions. Table 4.2 depicts Piaget's sensorimotor substages. Again, children exhibit individual variability in this cognitive-linguistic correspondence, and this correspondence attests to a more general relationship between representational development and language acquisition. It is clear, though, that language development is related in very potent and complex ways to cognitive capacities.

There appears to be some agreement that most children prior to Piaget's sensorimotor substage 5 are not typically using verbal language in a productive way. The present authors can find no report of a child in stage 3 or 4 who uses language normally. Thus, it appears that the diagnostician would find it useful to obtain at least a "ballpark" estimate of a child's level of development in the sensorimotor period. A primary reason to do an assessment of cognitive level is to prove or disprove a child's ability to represent reality and deal with symbols.

An important notion to keep in mind is that when assessing cognitive attainments, we watch a child's behavior and *infer* his/her conceptual holdings. As Lund and Duchan (1988) point out, it is often difficult to categorize a behavior as indicating knowledge of a concept since we have no history of how a child behaves. Lund and Duchan say, for example, that a child who tries to drink from an empty cup may not be exhibiting symbolic play by pretending to drink. Rather, the child may be *trying* to drink, which is a functional use of an object and not symbolic play. Thus, in cognitive assessment we can only make inferences about what

TABLE 4.2   Piaget's Sensorimotor Stages

Stage and Age (Months)	General	Imitation	Object Concept	Causality	Means-End
Stage 1 Birth–1	Reflexive Adaptive intelligence	Notion not present	No differentiation of self from objects	Egocentric	Notion not present
Stage 2 1–4	Primary circular reactions (self-repetitions) Coordination of sensory schemata	Self-imitation of actions with unexpected results "Preimitation"	Object followed with eyes until out of view Change in perspective interpreted as change in object	No differentiation of self and moving objects	Notion not present Intentionality lacking
Stage 3 4–8	Secondary circular reactions Repetition of actions of others	Imitation of others' actions already in repertoire	Anticipation of position of moving objects; no manual search	Self as cause of all events	Repetition of events with unexpected outcomes; heightened interest in event outcome Intentionality follows initiation of behavior
Stage 4 8–12	Coordination of secondary schemata Known means applied to new problems	Imitation of behaviors different from those in repertoire Facial imitation	Manual search for object where last seen Object constancy	Some externalization of causality Realization that objects can cause action	Coordination and integration of schemata Establishment of goal prior to initiation of activity Anticipation of outcomes
Stage 5 12–18	Tertiary secondary schemata Experimentation	Imitation of behaviors markedly different from repertoire	Sequential displacements considered Awareness of object spatial relations	Realization that he/she is one of many objects in environment	New means through experimentation Tools used
Stage 6 18–24	New means through mental combination Representational thought	Deferred imitation	Representation of displacements Awareness of unseen movements	Representation of causality Able to predict cause-effect relationship	Language used to influence others Representation of outcome or end

a child knows, and we must bear this fact in mind as the assessment is completed. We should obtain as much information as possible about the child's typical play routines and object use. The parent interview is invaluable here. The failure of a child to perform a task that we set up to evaluate a particular cognitive attainment is not necessarily evidence of a lack of the concept. A child can "fail" a cognitive task because of inattention, disinterest, or some other reason that has nothing to do with his/her cognitive status.

With the above admonitions in mind, how does one perform a cognitive assessment? And what type of child undergoes the evaluation? We have found it productive to take note of cognitive development especially in children who are nonverbal and with those who are at the single-word level. Children who are currently using *productive* early multiword utterances are evidencing some representational ability and symbolic ability just by using language normally. It is not useful to routinely administer a lengthy and complex cognitive test battery initially. We recommend that the diagnostician move from general analyses to more specific ones. Table 4.3 contains references for use in cognitive assessment.

The first level of analysis can be a lengthy behavioral observation of the child while he/she is engaged in play. In our experience, children whose cognitive levels are lower will exhibit primitive play routines and perseverative use of objects. Westby (1980) outlines some useful stages to use in assessing the developmental relationship between cognitive development, language, and play. The clinician can set up a play situation and watch the child interact with objects and people. The examiner should be looking for behavior that suggests the specific cognitive prerequisites indicated above. It is optimal to videotape the play interaction for later specific analysis (Lund and Duchan 1988). The clinician must always view the specific behaviors in reference to the context in which they occurred. For instance, pretending that a block is a car can qualify as symbolic play only if the clinician did not demonstrate this activity earlier in the session. At any rate, it is important to view children's nonverbal play behaviors contextually and, if possible, obtain some historical data on their play routines. Sometimes, there is a clear cognitive deficit.

TABLE 4.3   Measures of Cognitive Development

- The Ordinal Scales of Psychological Development (Uzgiris & Hunt, 1975)
- Albert Einstein Scales of Sensorimotor Development (Corman & Escalona, 1969)
- Infant Cognitive Development Scale (Merhabian & Williams, 1971)
- A Clinical and Educational Manual for Use with the Uzgiris and Hunt Scales of Psychological Development (Dunst, 1980)
- Beyond Sensorimotor Intelligence: Assessment of Symbolic Maturity Through Analysis of Pretend Play (Nicolich, 1977)
- The Symbolic Play Test (Lowe & Costello, 1976)
- Evaluation of Cognitive Behavior in Young Nonverbal Children (Chappel & Johnson, 1976)
- Assessment of Cognitive and Language Abilities Through Play (Westby, 1980)

Case Example. Ralph was enrolled in a preschool handicapped classroom. He was two-years-old and nonverbal. He seemed to enjoy imitating the clinician when she put blocks into a coffee can. When presented with other toys, however, Ralph just persisted in putting the blocks in the can and dumping them out again. The cycle continued, putting the blocks in and dumping them out. The other toys were immediately mouthed and banged on the floor. No matter what other toys Ralph had access to, he would put them in his mouth and/or bang them on the floor. When the clinician attempted to provide a model of functional use of objects or more-productive play routines, Ralph would persist with his limited repertoire.

Subsequent to observation of play routines, the clinician should note whether a cognitive delay is suspected based on the quality of play exhibited. Sometimes, there will clearly be no representational problem owing to the sophistication of the play routines observed. At other times, as depicted above, behavior will occur that strongly suggests a rather primitive representational ability. Many cases fall between these two ends of the cognitive continuum, and these children may require further testing to determine which level of cognitive development they have attained. We recommend Westby (1980) for an account of "normal" play behavior. Sometimes, in dealing with so many disordered clients, it is easy to forget that we must also be familiar with normal behavior. Students should actively observe and play with normal children to learn what kinds of things they typically do at various ages.

The second level of analysis can involve the administration of cognitive "screening scales" and specific tasks that more closely evaluate certain conceptual prerequisites. Chappell and Johnson (1976) and Merhabian and Williams (1971) have devised rather simple scales that help the clinician to arrive at a general level of cognitive development. These scales can be administered in a short time period and involve the clinician's setting up task situations for the child to respond to. Again, we recommend proceeding to this second level of analysis primarily with children who are clearly not playing normally or whose behaviors are "suspicious" to the clinician. If the child performs at a delayed level of cognitive development on the screening scale, then further testing might be undertaken.

A final level of analysis is to administer a more detailed scale such as that developed by Uzigiris and Hunt (1975). Dunst (1980) has developed some helpful procedures for use with the Uzigiris and Hunt scales, which make the clinical administration of the tasks more streamlined. Such lengthy measures should be administered in cases where cognitive deficits are strongly suspected.

When assessing cognitive attainments associated with language, the SLP should be careful not to allow other professionals or parents to perceive this evaluation procedure as the testing of a child's intelligence. We should make no judgments about how "smart" a child is or about the child's potential for cognitive growth. Children whose play behavior and performance on cognitive scales indicate they are lacking a cognitive basis for language should be referred to other professionals (e.g., psychologist, special educator) for diagnosis of their mental ability and potential for learning. It should be emphasized that we examine cognitive attainments only because they appear to be related to the acquisition and use of abstract language systems. If we determine that a child does not possess the cognitive holdings for acquiring our normally abstract and arbitrary symbol system, we then can consider attempting to train cognitive abilities (Kahn 1984) or train a communication system that is less abstract, such as simple signs that code concrete and frequently occurring activities.

Some significant alterations to the procedures mentioned above are necessary if the clinician is evaluating an older, severely handicapped client. Most measures of sensorimotor intelligence were pioneered on normally developing children, and there are some difficulties in applying these directly to older children or adults. Snyder-Mclean, Mclean, and Etter (1988) provide many useful suggestions in evaluating the cognitive status of older, severely involved clients.

Assessment of Communicative Intent and Function

Some authorities have indicated that a frequent manifestation of early language disorder in children is their different use of language (Fey 1986; Lucas 1980; Wetherby and Prutting 1984). As mentioned previously, a prelinguistic or nonverbal child has no expressive language. This does not imply, however, that the child is not communicating. Any mother of a prelinguistic child will attest that her child communicates profusely about his/her desires, moods, and a variety of pleasing and noxious biological states. Bates (1976) studied the sensorimotor performatives of young children and determined that those children have primitive forms of imperatives or commands by which they use adults to obtain access to objects in their environment. The goal is to gain access to the object. One can initially see the child physically manipulating the adult, as in putting the adult's hand on a jar to open it. Later, the child may use pointing coupled with vocalizations to indicate to the adult what he/she wants done. Bates also noted primitive forms of the declarative in which the child uses an object to gain adult attention as the goal. There appears to be a progression that begins with the child's showing and giving objects to adults. Ultimately, the child exhibits the declarative by pointing toward objects with an alternating gaze between the adult and object. Bates (1979) reported a "gestural complex" that, in part, may be related to language development. Thus, communication is taking place quite vividly in the preverbal child.

There are also preverbal evidences of the "functions" of language alluded to by Halliday (1975) and Dore (1975). That is, children use the greeting function nonverbally by waving, they question by exhibiting a quizzical look, and they regulate adults physically before they use language for these purposes. In preverbal children, the primary evidence for their communication ability is found in gestures, facial expressions, and/or vocalizations. These phenomena can be observed by a clinician in a diagnostic session, or caretakers can be asked in an assessment interview about how the child makes his/her needs known at home and at school. A nonverbal child is also beginning to expand the phonetic inventory, and the clinician can transcribe phonetic elements present in the child's system.

Communicative intents can be realized on a gestural, vocal, or verbal level. Dore et al. (1976) noted that a prelinguistic child is not simply uttering "jargon" vocalizations. At a certain point in development, Dore et al. noted the presence of Phonetically Consistent Forms (PCF) that he termed "transitional phenomena." Phonetically consistent forms are vocalizations that are stabilized around certain situations. They are not word approximations but are fairly stable phonetic productions typically consisting of vowel or consonant-vowel combinations. They are repeatedly associated with specific situations such as showing affect (emotion), indicating or pointing to aspects of the environment, or expressing a desire to obtain an object or event. Dore et al. observed that these PCFs seem to act as a transition to words wherein certain phonetic elements must be stabilized around a specific referent. Thus, it would be important in an evaluation of communicative function not only to determine which basic functions are present, but also to determine whether those functions manifest themselves on a gestural, vocal, or verbal level. Stark, Bernstein, and Demorest (1993) report useful data on vocalizations produced for a variety of communicative functions and outline an orderly developmental sequence of vocal communication in the first eighteen months of life.

According to Chapman (1981), the clinician may adopt an existing classification scheme or change these available systems so that functions that are of interest can be coded. The two most famous systems referring to children's uses of language are the schemes developed by Halliday (1975) and Dore (1975). However, other systems might also be useful clinically (Coggins and Carpenter 1978; Folger and Chapman 1978; Lucas 1980; Tough 1977). From examining the categories in these systems, it is clear that many of the terms overlap with respect to the functions they describe. Mclean and Snyder-Mclean (1978) have suggested that functions of language may be distilled into two basic uses. One use is to influence joint attention, and the other is to influence joint activity. These functions basically correspond to the imperative and the declarative in English. Thus, as Chapman (1981) suggests, it makes little difference exactly which system is used to assess the function of language. The clinician should select a system, however, that at least contains some basic declarative and imperative operations so that the child's initiation of a response to communications can be coded.

Some additional general guidelines should be discussed. The assessment of communicative function should be carried out in a naturalistic situation. It is sometimes difficult to contrive situations in which a child will express a genuine communicative intent. The clinician should have present in the room a wide variety of toys and stimuli that would elicit a number of different conversational possibilities and expressions of need or declarations. If there are other children or adults in the situation, the clinician must remember that the functions expressed by the child are inextricably related to the behavior and utterances of other conversational participants. In addition, functions are only interpretable in light of the nonverbal context of communication. Another variable to bear in mind is the notion of sampling functions of communication in multiple settings. Our earlier example of how a child's use of language was dramatically different in the preschool setting as opposed to the clinic should illustrate the importance of multiple sampling. It would be a shame to target the regulatory function for training in the clinic when the child frequently regulates the behavior of people in other situations. It is not necessarily a communication disorder when a child does not regulate in the clinic.

Some authors have suggested using standard elicitation tasks for basic communicative functions. This has been done for imperatives and declaratives (Dale 1980; Snyder 1978, 1981; Staab 1983; Wetherby and Prizant 1993; Wetherby and Rodriguez 1992) but not as widely for more-specific functions of communication. Generally, declaratives seem to be elicited most effectively by presenting novel or discrepant events and objects in the sampling situation. The child may then comment on the novel stimulus. Imperatives are more reliably obtained than declaratives since the clinician can maintain control over the stimuli and activities in the sampling situation. The child will ask for access to toys or will ask the clinician to assist in certain operations (winding of toys, etc.).

Wetherby et al. (1988) have contributed research that practicing clinicians will find most helpful. These researchers studied normally developing children at the preverbal, single-word, and early multiword stages of development to describe their intentional communication. Rate of communicative acts increased predictably as the children increased in mean length of utterance. The communication acts were analyzed in categories of regulating behavior, social interaction, and referencing joint attention. The subjects exhibited acts in all categories and tended to initiate more than respond to communication. They tended to move from gestural modes in the prelinguistic stage to verbal modes in the early multiword stage. This report outlines specific procedures for structured and nonstructured sampling of communication acts and provides guidelines for use in discriminating potentially language-delayed clients from normally developing children. We only have preliminary normative data on the typical use of communicative functions in normally developing children, but we suspect that there is considerable variability in these functions as a product of children's individuality, differing contexts, and types of interactants. Wetherby, Yonclas, and Bryan (1989) used similar procedures on children with language impairment, Down syndrome, and autism and indicate that some of these measures (e.g., rate of intentional communication) may have potentially useful clinical value in describing these populations.

More-extensive normative data are available in the *Communication and Symbolic Behavior Scales* (Wetherby and Prizant 1993). These scales examine the areas of communicative functions, gestural communicative means, vocal communicative means, verbal communicative means, reciprocity, social-affective signaling, and symbolic behavior. The data on this measure come from caregiver questionnaires, direct sampling, and some structured elicitation tasks. Standardization data on almost 300 children are available for use by the examiner. This test is a good example of how ecologically valid behaviors can be evaluated and put into a normative developmental framework. Standardized testing does not always have to be artificial. The "communicative temptations" used in the Communication and Symbolic Behavior Scales were piloted in the earlier work of Wetherby mentioned above and are excellent examples of how clinicians can elicit imperatives and declaratives from children in clinical settings. Videotapes are also available to demonstrate administration and scoring of the Communication and Symbolic Behavior Scales.

In cases where the child is nonverbal or at the single-word level, it is feasible to analyze functions and target communicative functions in treatment (Wilcox

1984). For example, the clinician may want to increase the number of regulatory attempts in a particular child or increase the verbal realizations of regulation in a client. Brunson and Haynes (1991) provide an example of an alternating-time sampling procedure that can be used in classroom contexts to monitor the use of communicative functions in naturalistic activities. This system can also track intentional communication of teachers for possible inclusion in the treatment program.

Use of Tests and Formal Procedures with Limited-Language Children

Only two decades ago there were few assessment instruments available to the SLP for use on children with limited language. This is not necessarily because SLPs were uninterested in preschool-age children, because we have always dealt with youngsters of this age. There have been several influences on test development that have increased the construction of instruments appropriate for the preschool, or limited-language, population. First of all, passage of PL 99-457 mandates that preschool children between the ages of three and five years will be dealt with by clinicians working in the public school setting. Many school systems are currently responsible for children between birth and three. With the enactment of federal legislation, test developers have increased their efforts in devising test instruments for preschoolers. The second influence on test development has been the significant strides that we have made in communication development research in the past twenty years.

We can divide the preschool tests that deal with communication into several categories. First, there are large test batteries that include language or communication as one aspect of assessment. For example, a general test instrument often referred to is the Battelle Developmental Inventory (BDI) (see Table 4.4). This instrument is a standardized battery that includes sections on motor skill, cognition, personal-social behavior, adaptive behavior, and communication. The portion dealing with communication is necessarily incomplete and superficial since the entire battery must examine so many different domains. This general battery, however, could suggest that a child's communication development may be delayed in comparison to the norming sample, and herein lies one value of the test ("problem–no problem" issue). Certainly, the test could never tell a clinician specific aspects of communication that are delayed or that suggest treatment objectives. There are many larger batteries that include language as a subpart, and Table 4.4 provides a selected list.

On a more specific level, there are tests that focus completely on language and communication. These instruments may be helpful to the SLP in providing direction toward areas in need of probing through nonstandardized methods. Table 4.5 includes a selected list of instruments that could be applied to limited-language cases. Some of these instruments are standardized, norm-referenced tests, and others may be criterion referenced. The inclusion on this list does not suggest that the measures meet rigid psychometric standards. These measures should satisfy any administrative requirements imposed by work settings on obtaining scores in

TABLE 4.4   General Developmental Measures

Battelle Developmental Inventory
Publisher: DLM Teaching Resources

Brigance Diagnostic Inventory of Early Development
Publisher: Curriculum Associates, Inc.

Carolina Curriculum for Handicapped Infants at Risk
Publisher: Riverside

Denver Developmental Screening Test
Publisher: University of Colorado Medical Center

Developmental Programming for Infants and Young Children
Publisher: University of Michigan Press

Developmental Indicators for the Assessment of Learning (DIAL-R)
Publisher: Childcraft Education Corporation

Hawaii Early Learning Profile
Publisher: VORT Corporation

McCarthy Scales of Children's Abilities
Publisher: The Psychological Corporation

Minnesota Child Development Inventory
Publisher: Behavior Science Systems, Inc.

Vineland Adaptive Behavior Scales
Publisher: American Guidance Service

assessment. The measures also could prove useful as a beginning point for naturalistic evaluation tasks. Crais (1995) reviews many of these instruments and discusses issues related to early assessment.

Assessment of Structure and Function in Early Utterances

So far, we have briefly sketched the development of cognitive and social prerequisites to language. The present section deals with formation of the linguistic code in communicative development. Our discussion will consider two general phases: single word and early multiword. These stages are based on length of utterance, which up to about age four generally correlates with chronological age (Miller and Chapman 1981) and linguistic attainment (Brown 1973; Carrow-Woolfolk and Lynch 1982; Lund and Duchan 1988). Each stage has certain acquisitions associated with it that may indicate that the child is ready for transition to the next stage.

Single-Word Utterances
After a period of using no real words and becoming more consistent with the use of vocalizations accompanied by gestures, the child begins to use single words to code

TABLE 4.5 Communication/Language Measures

Ages and Stages Questionnaire: A Parent Completed Clinical Monitoring System
Publisher: Brookes

Assessing Prelinguistic and Early Linguistic Behaviors In Developmentally Young Children
Publisher: University of Washington Press

Assessment, Evaluation and Programming System, Measurement for Birth to Three Years
Publisher: Paul Brookes

Birth to Three Assessment and Intervention System
Publisher: DLM Teaching Resources

Bracken Basic Concept Scale
Publisher: The Psychological Corporation

Carolina Curriculum for Infants and Toddlers with Special Needs
Publisher: Paul Brookes

Cognitive, Linguistic and Social Communicative Scales
Publisher: Modern Education Corporation

Cognitive Abilities Scale
Publisher: Pro-Ed

Communication and Symbolic Behavior Scales (CSBS)
Publisher: Riverside

Early Language Milestone Scale
Publisher: Modern Education Corporation

Evaluating Acquired Skills in Communication (EASIC)
Publisher: Communication Skill Builders

Individualized Assessment and Treatment For Autistic and Developmentally Disabled Children
Publisher: Pro-Ed

Language Development Survey (Rescorla 1989)
MacArthur Communicative Development Inventories

Preschool Language Scale
Publisher: The Psychological Corporation

Preverbal Assessment-Intervention Profile (PAIP)
Publisher: ASIEP Education Co.

Program for the Acquisition of Language With the Severely Impaired (PALS)
Publisher: Charles E. Merrill

Receptive-Expressive Emergent Language Scale 2 (REEL)
Publisher: Riverside

Sequenced Inventory of Communicative Development-R
Publisher: PRO-ED

objects and events. The words are not adult productions, but typically CV or CVCV approximations of the correct production (Nelson 1973). Nelson has found that children's early lexicons represent specific categories. These one-word utterances were formerly called "holophrases," which meant a single word referring to an entire thought (e.g., "cookie" may really mean "I want a cookie") (McNeil 1970). Research has reported that subgroups of language-developing and language-disordered children are "referential" (word and object oriented) or "expressive" (social and conversation oriented). That is, the referential children use mostly nouns and refer to objects and events. They also like to play with objects and spend more time playing alone. The expressive children, on the other hand, enjoy talking to and being with people and use more personal-social words (Weiss et al. 1983). There are perhaps other ways to characterize early single-word productions, but the point is that children go through a period of talking, as Lois Bloom (1973) says, using "one word at a time." Toward the end of the single-word period, Nelson (1973) indicates that the child accrues an expressive lexicon of about fifty words and then begins to attempt word combinations.

Children in the single-word period can be examined for both the types of words they use and the apparent reasons they use them. The form of single-word utterances has been viewed in different ways by various authorities. Nelson (1973), for instance, categorized single words as members of the classes in Table 4.6. Other researchers have found similar results (Benedict, 1975). Lahey (1988) provides a lengthy discussion and examples of a system for early-utterance analysis. Ideally, single words should be paired with functions such as those discussed earlier.

Parent checklists are especially useful in obtaining data on lexicon size and content. Fenson et al. (1993) developed the MacArthur Communicative Development Inventories that provide normative data on children from eight months to thirty months of age in terms of gestures, words, and multiword utterances. Rice, Sell, and Hadley (1990) provide a system for on-line coding of children's verbal initiations and responses in natural classroom settings as a function of environmental and play variables. While the system does not examine types of single words used, it documents whether the child is using single-word, multiword, or gestural communications.

Prior to the first word combinations, Dore et al. (1976) noted another transitional phenomenon known as the Presyntactic Device (PSD). Dore stated that a syntactic utterance is one in which two words that have a meaning relationship are combined under the same intonational pattern (e.g., "Mommy go"). A presyntactic device is the combination of two elements under an intonation contour that do not have a meaning relation because one element is not a real word, or because the word combination is reduplicated or a highly learned "rote production." Thus,

TABLE 4.6   Percentage of First 50 Word Lexicon Accounted for by Grammatical Categories in Two Major Studies

Category	Nelson (1973)	Benedict (1975)	Example
General Nominal	50	51	chair, kitty
Specific Nominal	11	14	person's name
Action Word	19	14	go, eat
Modifier	10	9	dirty, big
Personal-Social	10	9	hi, no, please
Function	0	4	that, for

a child who says /WI KITI/ is combining a real word (KITI) with a nonword (WI) under an intonation contour. Other presyntactic transitional elements that have been reported are empty forms, which are consistently used productions that appear to be nonsense words (e.g., "wida," "gocking") (Bloom 1973; Leonard 1975). Bloom (1970) reports the use of two single words that have a meaning relationship, with a pause inserted between the two elements (e.g., "car . . . go"). All of the above presyntactic devices prepare a child to combine two meaningful language elements under an intonation pattern that is the essence of early multiword combinations. Bain and Olswang (1995) point out the utility of using a dynamic assessment approach to examine readiness for learning early multiword utterances. This information would add a significant dimension to the assessment of a single-word communicator.

The Case of "Late Bloomers"

Children who reach the age of two years with significant delays in expressive language despite normal cognitive, auditory, structural, and language comprehension abilities, have been the subject of much research. These children usually have less than a fifty-word lexicon and no evidence of multiword combinations at age two. Some authorities suggest that as many as 50% of these children will be at risk for the language delay's persisting beyond their third birthday, while the other 50% may "catch up" and exhibit near normal communication at age three. The latter group have been called "late bloomers" or "late talkers." One challenge of the diagnostician is to be able to distinguish children who will persist in their language impairment from those who are simply late talkers. A series of studies suggests that there are some potent variables to use in making this distinction (Paul and Jennings 1992; Rescoria and Goossens 1992; Thal and Tobias 1992; Weismer, Branch, and Miller 1994). The following are signs that research has suggested that may aid in discriminating late bloomers from those children whose language impairment will persist beyond age three:

- Children whose disorders persist may have a family history of speech and language problems.
- Late bloomers tend to have a higher frequency of communication acts.
- Children whose disorders persist tend to have less-mature syllable structure, for example, less consonants in their phonetic inventories.
- Late bloomers tend to have higher scores in language comprehension on measures such as the MacArthur Communicative Development Inventories.
- Late bloomers have higher levels of symbolic play and more evidence of combinatorial play as compared to children whose disorders persist.

The clinician should look for *patterns* of such signs and should not base a decision on one indication alone. It is notable that the majority of these symptoms are not typically addressed in most of our standardized tests for early language, and thus nonstandardized tasks can provide critical information to the well-informed clinician.

Early Multiword Utterances

Perhaps the most-researched and -reported period of language acquisition is the time when children begin to combine lexical items to form meaning relationships (semantic relations). There has been a long history of interpreting these early utterances as traditional parts of speech (e.g., noun, verb), telegraphic speech (Brown and Fraser 1963), pivot/open classes (Braine 1963), and underlying structures of transformational grammar (McNeil 1970). Currently, many authorities support a semantic view of early multiword utterances using a case grammar (Fillmore 1968) and have rendered interpretations of early utterances using semantic relations (Bowerman 1974; Bloom 1970; Bloom and Lahey 1978; Brown 1973; Leonard 1976; Schlessinger 1974). Some of the basic early multiword constructions are composed of the semantic cases (Brown 1973) in Table 4.7. Note that these basic semantic relations code aspects of the world that the child has learned about during the sensorimotor period of cognitive development, which is one reason that some authorities have indicated the strong cross-cultural similarities in early utterances (Brown 1973). There are many more "fine-grained" analyses of children's early multiword utterances (Bloom, Lightbrown, and Hood 1975; Braine 1976; Leonard 1976), and the basic relation types in Table 4.7 are included in these analyses along with some other more subtle distinctions.

Semantic relations must always be interpreted in light of the nonverbal context surrounding the utterance. The main point here is that children begin to use word combinations that code various common relationships in their environments; and if we merely assign adult, syntactic categories (e.g., noun, verb) to the utterances, we miss some of the skill that children have in coding rather subtle relations that are cognitively understood in the sensorimotor period. This skill has been termed a "rich interpretation" by Brown (1973) and gives the child credit for being able to talk about various relationships that syntactic metrics do not. As in

TABLE 4.7   Semantic Relations Reported by Brown (1973)

Nomination + X	"This ball"
Recurrence + X	"More milk"
Nonexistence + X	"Allgone egg"
Agent + action	"Mommy run"
Action + object	"Hit ball"
Agent + object	"Mommy shoe"
Action + locative	"Go outside"
Entity + locative	"Ball kitchen"
Possessor + Possession	"Mommy skirt"
Entity + attribute	"Ball red"
Agent + action + object	"Mommy hit ball"
Agent + action + locative	"Mommy run outside"

the single-word period, these semantic relations are used for various functions; that is, agent + action can be used as a comment/label (e.g., "Mommy run"—when a child points to mother jogging) or as a regulatory statement (e.g., "Mommy push"—when the child is trying to get mother to push the wagon). According to authorities, it is wise to always consider both the structure (form) and use (function) of early multiword utterances (Bloom and Lahey 1978; Mclean and Snyder-Mclean 1978). There is a more recent move toward not using a priori semantic relation categories and giving a child credit for a multiword relation only after he/she has demonstrated "productivity" of use (Howe 1976; Leonard, Steckol, and Panther 1983; Lund and Duchan 1988).

As mentioned previously, there are existing methods of viewing and analyzing early semantic relations in children's utterances (Bloom 1973; Braine 1976; Brown 1973; Leonard 1976). There are also, as discussed above, a number of systems for examining communicative functions in children (Halliday 1975; Dore 1975). Few systems, however, exist that interactively analyze structure and function in early utterances. Lahey (1988) described an analysis system that takes into account structure and function. The system suggests that the clinician transcribe the child's utterances, the adult's utterances, and the nonverbal communicative contextual events that are relevant to the communication. Lahey (1988) prefers the use of videotape in recording a sample for use in the analysis since all linguistic and contextual information can be preserved and reviewed. Lahey recommends that the beginning clinician start by gaining practice with a particular coding taxonomy through carefully scoring videotaped sessions. When speed and reliability are increased, then hand transcriptions may be easier and more accurate.

At the very least, we recommend that the clinician videotape the child in an interaction with caretakers, teachers, or children so that the former can transcribe the child's utterances and note the context of communication. We feel that the following assumptions are important in a basic early multiword assessment:

1. It is important to determine if there is a "basic" set of semantic relations or if there is a limited usage of just a few relations used by a child (Lahey 1988; Mclean and Snyder-Mclean 1978).
2. A child should be able to verbally code many relationships and aspects of the environment.
3. The clinician should obtain an inventory of communicative functions used by a child to determine if there is a "basic set" of uses of language (Wetherby et al. 1988).
4. Structure and function should be viewed interactively (Bloom and Lahey 1978; Lahey 1988; Muma 1978).
5. The clinician may find it valuable to get a feeling for the percentage of time that a child initiates language versus the percentage of adult-initiated utterances (Bloom and Lahey 1978; Wetherby et al. 1988).
6. The clinician must be able to analyze utterances from one to four words in length.

7. Early multiwords are analyzed in a way that is different from the analysis of later syntax (Bloom and Lahey 1978; Bowerman 1973; Brown 1973; Leonard et al. 1983), typically using semantic grammars.
8. The clinician should be sensitive to later developing forms present with the early multiwords (e.g., word endings, function words) to project development into later stages (Lahey 1988; Miller 1981).

Appendix B contains a suggested transcription sheet for use with the analysis. The clinician should first write down the child's utterance either phonetically or orthographically, then follow this transcription with the immediate interpretation of a semantic relation and function. Thus, the first three columns can be filled out at the time of each utterance. The videotape can be rewound to replay problematic utterances. This procedure could be used as a preliminary part of an assessment to find out basic semantic relations and functions in a child's communication (Taenzer, Harris, and Bass 1975). It also can be carried forward as a means of monitoring treatment progress. From the data, later analysis can determine the percentage of child-initiated versus adult-initiated utterances as well as the percentage of the use of each function and semantic relation in the sample. A summary sheet is presented in Appendix C. The remaining columns (4–6) of the transcription sheet can be filled out by the clinician subsequent to the evaluation session and can be used to complete the summary sheet. When a child is leaving the early multiword period, he/she has reached a mean length of utterance of over 2.25. At this point, the acquisition of a variety of syntactic conventions begins to emerge.

Assessment of Children's Early Language Comprehension

Confounding Factors: Nonlinguistic Context

Children's responses to language are multidetermined. That is, a child's correct response could be primarily in reaction to nonverbal contextual aspects of the situation. The following is a typical scenario:

> The mother says, "He can understand everything that we tell him. He just doesn't talk." The clinician leans forward and says, "Can you show me how you know he understands what you tell him?" The mother shifts uncomfortably in her chair and tells the child to "go turn off the light," as she points alternately between the light switch and the ceiling fixture. The child turns the light off and on several times. Later when the mother was told to provide only verbal stimuli, the child was not able to perform many one- and two-level commands if they were unaccompanied by gestures.

Thus, children and adults rely on the context in which language is used to aid in interpretation of what was said.

Confounding Factors: Comprehension Strategies

In 1978, Chapman discussed the notion of "comprehension strategies" exhibited by children. According to Chapman, a comprehension strategy is "a short cut, heuristic or algorithm for arriving at sentence meaning without full marshaling of the information in the sentence and one's linguistic knowledge. Thus, it sometimes yields the correct answer, although it may more usually give the appearance of understanding" (310). Clinicians who attempt to assess early language comprehension should be wary of correct responses by children that could have been generated by attention to contextual stimuli or comprehension strategies. An example would be that many children process the name of an object and then act on the object in a habitual manner. This behavior gives the appearance of knowing an entire sentence (e.g., "Throw the ball") when in actuality the child may understand only the word "ball" and simply throws it as he usually would. Chapman gives many other comprehension strategies, and we encourage clinicians to become familiar with these patterns.

We have suggested that comprehension is difficult to test without contaminating influences from the context and comprehension strategies. Understanding of single words in young children appears to us to be the easiest to test. The clinician should make sure that objects are maximally separated in the evaluation room so that it will be clear which item the child turns toward when the examiner names it. If the child directs his/her attention to or retrieves the appropriate object when its name is uttered by an examiner (with appropriate controls for contextual cues), the child probably recognizes the lexical item. We begin to run into trouble when we try to test two word utterances and larger sentences. Edmonston and Thane (1992) point out the difficulty in assessing relational words because of comprehension strategies. Some attempts have been made to remove the effects of context and comprehension strategies by using anomalous commands in the testing of children (Duchan and Siegel 1979; Kramer 1977). This technique involves giving to children commands that they are not likely to expect from their past experience. A child may be told to "Sit on the ball" or "Kiss the phone." If the child performs, he/she is said to have comprehended both elements in the command. If the child does not perform (and this is where we run into the problem again), is it that he/she has not understood? Perhaps anomalous commands are "silly" to children and are disregarded. There may be a cognitive mismatch between the command and the child's knowledge of the object's typical use. At any rate, failure to perform an anomalous command may not really mean lack of comprehension. The clinician should also not avoid more naturalistic assessment methods such as engaging the child in play or conversation and evaluating the appropriateness of verbal and nonverbal responses. Several popular instruments rely on parental reports to gauge receptive lexicon size. For example, in *MacArthur Communicative Development Inventories* (Fenson et al. 1993) normative data is provided on lexical comprehension based on parental reports.

Chapter 5 outlines some additional considerations in assessing language comprehension in older children.

Assessment of Utterances Using Length Measures

One of the most common measures recommended for use in a basic language evaluation is the mean length of utterance (MLU) (Miller 1981). Length measures are not new in speech pathology and were used historically as a mainstay of our clinical armamentarium (Johnson, Darley, and Spriestersbach 1963). There are several reasons that authorities have continued to recommend computing a length measure on utterances obtained in a language sample. First, there is a general correlation between the MLU and chronological age in many groups of children up to age four (Miller 1981). Thus, the MLU may be used as a very gross indicator of language development in children up to age four, but the clinician cannot simply rely on length measures alone in an analysis. A second important reason for computing MLU on a child is that Brown (1973) has used this length measure to demarcate his five stages of language development. Allegedly, MLU is a much better predictor of language development than chronological age is. Brown (1973) has postulated that if two children are matched on MLU a clinician may predict that the constructional complexity of their language will be similar. Brown (1973) and Miller (1981) provide suggestions for the computation of MLU (Table 4.8 is from

TABLE 4.8   Rules for Calculating Mean Length of Utterance and Upper Bound

1. Start with the second page of the transcription unless that page involves a recitation of some kind. In this latter case start with the first recitation-free stretch. Count the first 100 utterances satisfying the following rules.
2. Only fully transcribed utterances are used; none with blanks. Portions of utterances, entered in parentheses to indicate doubtful transcription, are used.
3. Include all exact utterance repetitions (marked with a plus sign in records). Stuttering is marked as repeated efforts at a single word; count the word once in the most complete form produced. In the few cases where a word is produced for emphasis or the like (*no, no, no*) count each occurrence.
4. Do not count such fillers as *mm* or *oh*, but do count *no, yeah*, and *hi*.
5. All compound words (two or more free morphemes), proper names, and ritualized reduplications count as single words. Examples: *birthday, rackety-boom, choo-choo, quack-quack, night-night, pocketbook, see saw*. Justification is that no evidence that the constituent morphemes function as such for these children.
6. Count as one morpheme all irregular pasts of the verb (*got, did, went, saw*). Justification is that there is no evidence that the child relates these to present forms.
7. Count as one morpheme all diminutives (*doggie, mommie*) because these children at least do not seem to use the suffix productively. Diminutives are the standard forms used by the child.
8. Count as separate morphemes all auxiliaries (*is, have, will, can, must, would*). Also all catenatives: *gonna, wanna, hafta*. These latter counted as single morphemes rather than as *going to* or *want to* because evidence is that they function so for the children. Count as separate morphemes all inflections, for example, possessive {s}, plural {s}, third person singular {s}, regular past {d}, progressive {in}.
9. The range count follows the above rules but is always calculated for the total transcription rather than for 100 utterances.

From: Brown, R. (1973). *A First Language: The Early Stages*, Cambridge: Harvard University Press, Used with permission. © 1973 by the President and Fellows of Harvard College.

Brown). Miller (1981) recommends a distributional analysis to insure that the MLU has a relatively normal distribution around an average length. The analysis is simply a listing of the number of utterances at each morpheme level (e.g., 1, 2, 3, 4). If the distributional analysis reveals an MLU with a small variation, perhaps an organic condition or sampling error has played a role in the length of utterance. Compared to normal-language children, Johnston et al. (1993) found that children with language impairments tended to respond to questions with higher proportions of elliptical utterances. This finding certainly could affect MLU measures by increasing sampling error. Chapman and Miller (1981) report normative data for MLU (see Table 4.9), and research on temporal reliability on older children has also been published (Chabon, Udolf, and Egolf 1982). The latter investigators report that MLU has weak temporal reliability in older children, and its use for prediction of language level may be less sensitive than previously thought.

The norms for MLU are presently reported on a rather narrow population, and further data gathering is necessary for different socioeconomic and cultural groups. The use of MLU may presently be in a state of transition; but until more conclusive data and viable alternatives are provided, we feel that MLU should be routinely calculated in a language evaluation of limited language children.

TABLE 4.9 Predicted MLU Ranges and Linguistic Stages of Children Within One Predicted Standard Deviation of Predicted Mean Length of Utterance

Age ± 1 Month	Predicted MLU[a]	Predicted SD[b]	Predicted MLU ± 1 SD (middle 68%)
18	1.31	0.325	0.99–1.64
21	1.62	0.386	1.23–2.01
24	1.92	0.448	1.47–2.37
27	2.23	0.510	1.72–2.74
30	2.54	0.571	1.97–3.11
33	2.85	0.633	2.22–3.48
36	3.16	0.694	2.47–3.85
39	3.47	0.756	2.71–4.23
42	3.78	0.817	2.96–4.60
45	4.09	0.879	3.21–4.97
48	4.40	0.940	3.46–5.34
51	4.71	1.002	3.71–5.71
54	5.02	1.064	3.96–6.08
57	5.32	1.125	4.20–6.45
60	5.63	1.187	4.44–6.82

[a]MLU is predicted from the equation MLU = -0.548 + 0.103 (AGE).
[b]SD is predicted from the equation SD MLU = -0.446 + 0.0205 (AGE).
From: Miller, J. and Chapman, R. (1981). Research note: The relation between age and mean length of utterance in morphemes. *Journal of Speech and Hearing Research*, 24, 154–161. Used with permission.

Infant, Toddler and Family Assessment

Public Law 99-457 mandates that the SLP assess and treat children between the ages of three and five. Speech-language pathologists in many states are currently serving the birth-to-five population, and this practice will no doubt become the norm before the current decade is over. The present section provides some references for SLPs who are faced with the assessment of infants and toddlers in hospital and clinical settings.

Many categories of infants and children are at risk for communication disorders. There is a host of syndromes (e.g., Turner's, 18Q, Down, Hurlers, Morquio, Goldenhar, Mohr, Treacher-Collins) with associated speech, language, and hearing problems (Clark 1989). In addition, communication disorders can result from a variety of other sources, such as environmental toxins (e.g., mercury, lead, cadmium, cocaine, fetal alcohol exposure), infections prior to birth (e.g., syphilis, rubella, congenital cytomegaloviris, toxoplasmosis), or postnatally acquired infections (e.g., herpes, otitis, streptococcus infections). Other groups such as premature infants and those suffering early respiratory distress or intracranial hemmorhages are also at high risk for communication disorders. The SLP is more frequently involved than ever before on evaluation and intervention teams working with these high-risk infants and their families. Often, this population is intimidating to those without experience in serving infants and toddlers.

Assessment of infants and toddlers must involve several components: (1) assessment of the infant, (2) assessment of the family situation, (3) assessment of the primary caregiver, and (4) assessment of caregiver-child interaction patterns.

Sparks (1989) provides some general guidelines for assessment of the infant. First, the SLP should become intimately familiar with the child's prenatal and perinatal history. We must know the medical status of the child so that we can try to predict which types of communication disorders are likely to be associated with a particular syndrome or condition. This predictive capacity allows the SLP to take preventive measures against a variety of secondary impairments. Second, we should gain a general appreciation of the infant's ability to maintain homeostasis. This means learning how individual infants cope with handling, when they lose control, and how we need to help them to maintain respiration, thermal control, and proper nutrition (Sparks 1989). Frequently used measures for this are in *Neonatal Behavioral Assessment* (Brazelton 1984) or *Assessment of Preterm Infant Behavior* (Als et al. 1982). Third, the child's oral-motor behavior is an important skill to evaluate. Proctor (1989) provides an excellent description of vocal development and a detailed assessment protocol for use in evaluation of infant oral/vocal skills. Finally, the infant's hospital environment should be examined for available stimulation and opportunities for communication. Often, these children are in neonatal intensive care units (NICU) or in other hospital units, and these environments provide the only exposure to communication to which the child has access.

Regarding the evaluation of caregiver-infant interactions, a number of potential schemes are available (Cole and St. Clair-Stokes 1984; Duchan and Weitzner-Lin 1987; Klien and Briggs 1987; Lifter et al. 1988; Wetherby et al. 1988). We are also interested in more-basic issues such as availability of the caregiver and caregiver expectations about communication. The actual analyses of caregiver-child interactions embody many behaviors discussed earlier in the present chapter. The reader should examine some of the references listed above for specific procedures.

Some team member, perhaps the SLP if he/she is the case manager, will participate in a family strength and needs assessment. Bailey and Simeonsson (1988) provide procedures and suggestions for family assessment. With infants and toddlers, the assessments of family status and interaction patterns are as important or even more significant than evaluation of the child. Without an intact family that functions adequately as a system, the planning and implementation of intervention cannot take place. In addition, PL 99-457 requires an Individualized Family Service Plan (IFSP), which specifies not only goals for the child but objectives for the family as a unit. Thus, assessment of infants and toddlers typically involves a team approach, with the SLP working closely with social workers, psychologists, medical professionals, early childhood special educators, and others.

Assessment of Special Populations

Communication is the Major Focus

Since the nature of communication/language and the model that we subscribe to does not change with the client, assessing special populations should not be dramatically different from examining children with developmental language disorders. That is, our business is still to assess the integrity of the communication system (biological, cognitive, linguistic, social, pragmatic), and this process should be in operation regardless of etiology. We feel, as Bloom and Lahey (1978) and Lahey (1988) have indicated, that the diagnostic group of which a child is a member contributes little insight into his/her language impairment. Certainly, however, there are some characteristics that are important to consider in evaluating specific populations. Lahey (1988) provides an excellent summary of the research on communication skills associated with specifically language-impaired, hearing-impaired, autistic, mentally retarded, acquired aphasia, learning-disabled, and blind populations. The clinician should be familiar with this research because it helps in parent counseling as well as in knowing what to expect in an evaluation session. It is our view that the basic assessment of the communication of any client should focus on the communicative process from an integrative vantage point.

Increased Probability of Focusing Assessment on Precommunicative Areas

Dealing with special populations increases the probability of having to focus the assessment on biological, social, and cognitive areas. Children with mental retardation and those with autism are common examples. Clearly, a child with mental retardation is, by definition, cognitively impaired (Cosby and Ruder 1983; Kamhi and Johnston 1982; Rogers 1977; Weisz and Zigler 1979). The clinician must be certain that the child possesses the cognitive ability necessary for learning a particular symbol system (objects, pictures, words, gestures, etc.). Similarly, many children diagnosed with autism also have cognitive difficulties (Curcio 1978; Rutter 1978; Clune, Paolella, and Foley 1979). Children with autism and/or mental retardation are frequently reported to be socially withdrawn, and their general nonverbal social interaction may have to be modified in treatment before they can be expected to use functional communication (Opitz 1982; Baltaxe and Simmons 1975). For children with autism, Prizant and Wetherby (1988) recommend assessment areas that are highly similar to those previously advocated for any child with a language impairment. Thus, assessment of cognitive, social, and biological areas is critical.

Increased Possibility of Recommending Augmentative Communication Modes
Another aspect involved in dealing with a special population is that the clinician has an increased probability of prescribing a nonverbal/nonvocal response mode or augmentative communication device. Children with more-severe involvement may benefit from training in gestural communication modes in addition to or as an alternative to using speech as the output modality (Silverman 1995). Thus, it may be incumbent on the diagnostician to determine the potential that a given client may have for learning a nonvocal system. Some general guidelines are available in the literature (Beukelman and Mirenda 1992; Coleman, Cook, and Meyers 1980; Owens and House 1984; Shane and Bashir 1980; Silverman 1995). Clinicians who do formal evaluations in the area of augmentative communication should have specialized training and experience in this arena prior to prescribing and introducing a nonvocal mode to a client. Unfortunately, it is beyond the scope of the present chapter to elaborate on these issues.

Prognostic Implications
Special populations, as a whole, generally have a poorer prognosis than language-impaired children without complicating difficulties. The prognosis decreases in proportion to the number of ancillary problems that the child exhibits (hearing impairment, neuromotor involvement, mental retardation, absent caretakers, etc.). In addition, the existence of ancillary problems increases the likelihood that a larger multidisciplinary team will be involved in the evaluation. The assistance of special educators, audiologists, psychologists, and medical personnel is necessary and invaluable to the clinician in making treatment recommendations for children from special populations. As dictated by federal legislation (PL 94-142; PL 99-457), the speech pathologist has the opportunity to collaborate in staffings with other professionals to discuss assessment and treatment of language-disordered children. In most cases, we have found this involvement to be stimulating and in the best interest of all concerned, especially in early language cases.

Noting Specific Characteristics
With certain types of children, the diagnostician should make an inventory of characteristic behaviors that may need to be modified in the treatment program. For instance, it has been reported that children with autism and mental retardation engage in self-stimulatory behaviors (arm flapping, rocking, etc.). Some authorities believe that new learning cannot effectively take place while the child is in a self-

stimulatory state. Thus, one goal of treatment might be to reduce the occurrence of self-stimulation, and these behaviors should be cataloged by the diagnostician. Alternatively, some self-stimulatory acts can even be used as reinforcers in more-structured types of treatment. In these populations there have also been many reports of self-abusive behaviors. These should also be noted by the clinician as potential considerations in planning treatment.

Consolidating Data and Arriving at Treatment Recommendations

To a certain degree, even if the diagnostician adheres to an integrative model of language, the assessment process tends to fragment the child and the information obtained in the evaluation. Before arriving at treatment recommendations, suggestions for further testing, and/or referral decisions, the clinician should pause and take stock of what has been done in the assessment process. We have found it useful and insightful to summarize the following areas (see Appendix D):

Data Obtained in the Evaluation
This section refers to the actual behaviors observed and procedures administered to a child in the evaluation. It does not include the different analyses of the data. For instance, a spontaneous language sample can be subjected to a variety of analyses (MLU, form-function analysis, phonological analysis, etc.). Often, at the end of an evaluation, a clinician will be struck by the need for additional data that may be obtained in the initial phase of treatment. We sometimes wonder why we cannot make clinical judgments about certain aspects of a child's language, and then we find that we did not gather all of the data necessary to make these decisions. Appendix D provides a checklist for clinicians to use in summarizing the data collected.

Analyses Performed on the Data
This section allows the clinician to summarize the analysis procedures performed on the data collected. On the surface this procedure may appear to be rather simplistic, however, since language has so many aspects that may be important to assess, it is easy to forget to gather certain data or perform certain analyses.

Areas of Concern and Strength
By examining the data and analyses of the communicative process and language development stages, the clinician will be impressed with areas of normality, strength, and concern. The clinician should look for patterns in the data that are revealed when a judgment must be made about the overall effectiveness of each area in the language model. For instance, a clinician may have concerns in the biological prerequisite area over poor motor coordination and remarkable birth and developmental histories. The same child may have performed poorly on cognitive tasks, and the clinician questions the child's conceptual bases for language development. Similarly, on social areas of the model, the child is not operating according to age

level and is not exhibiting optimal social prerequisites for communication. Adaptive behavior scales show a delay in all areas of development. In the language development area, the child turns out to be nonverbal. When the clinician checks the areas of concern and strength, the child will get a minus (–) under biological prerequisites for neurological areas and minuses for social areas of play partner and reciprocity. The child would also earn minuses on the cognitive prerequisites of play level, sensorimotor substage, and symbolic play as well. Finally, the child would receive minuses for most categories in single-word, phonology, and early multiword combination areas. By examining the summary statements, the clinician can develop a profile of areas of strength and concern for each case. If no clear-cut statement for concern or strength can be made, then the clinician should examine the data gathered and the analyses performed to determine if enough information has been accumulated. In most cases, an inability to make a general statement about areas of the model is due to insufficient information, poor-quality information, or insufficient analysis.

Recommendations

The areas that are covered in the recommendation section revolve around four topics. First, the child may require referral to other professionals to obtain further information. For instance, referral to a psychologist or special educator may be warranted to determine the child's mental ability and potential for learning. Audiometric referral may be another common need. Second, the clinician may have been unable to perform certain tests or analyses because of time constraints or lack of cooperation by the child. Before specific treatment recommendations can be made, it may be that more data are required. By examining the sections on data obtained and analyses performed, the clinician can determine this need.

Third, if enough data were obtained and analyses performed, the clinician is in a position to make treatment recommendations. By examining the child's areas of strength and weakness, the clinician can consider intervention avenues that are the most appropriate. For instance, if a child is biologically, cognitively, and socially ready for communicative development and the clinician has located the child in the language development process, an appropriate goal might be to begin concentrating on the language forms that develop next according to the acquisition literature and the child's need to communicate. If the child is normal in most respects and the major concern is intelligibility, then this carries with it a phonological treatment priority. If the child has cognitive and social problems in addition to language delay, then some of the treatment goals might revolve around these prerequisite areas (facilitating cognitive development; improving social nonverbal skills, etc.). The areas of concern and strength also carry with them prognostic implications. To date, we really have no certain method of computing a given child's prognosis for success in language treatment. There are so many variables that relate to the child's capacities, skills, motivation, environment, caretaker participation, time in treatment, and so forth. One approach to prognosis that will probably reflect reality is to regard the child who elicits fewer concerns in the major areas of the model as having a more favorable prognosis than one who has many deficiencies.

Concluding Remarks

We have attempted to show that assessment of limited-language children is no simple matter. It requires that the clinician learn a multitude of skills and read a disparate literature in order to perform it competently. The diagnosis of language disorder requires more than just a single test or procedure. It demands that the clinician examine the communicative process differently for children of varying communicative levels and cultures.

Bibliography

Als, H., Lester, B., Tronick, E., and Brazelton, T. (1982). "Toward a Research Instrument for the Assessment of Preterm Infants' Behavior (APIB)." In *Theory and Research in Behavioral Pediatrics*, Vol. 1, ed. H. Fitzgerald, B. Lester and M. Yogman (New York: Plenum Press).

Allen, D., Bliss, L., and Timmons, J. (1981). "Language Evaluation: Science or Art?" *Journal of Speech and Hearing Disorders* 46:66–68.

Anderson-Yockel, J., and Haynes, W. (1994). "Joint Book Reading Strategies in Working Class African American and White Mother-Toddler Dyads." *Journal of Speech and Hearing Research* 37:583–593.

Aram, D., and Nation, J. (1975). "Patterns of Language Behavior in Children with Developmental Language Disorders." *Journal of Speech and Hearing Research* 18:229–241.

Aram, D., and Nation, J. (1982). *Child Language Disorders*. St. Louis, MO: Mosby.

Bailey, D., and Simeonsson, R. (1988). *Family Assessment in Early Intervention*, Columbus, OH: Merrill.

Bain, B., and Olswang, L. (1995). Examining Readiness for Learning Two Word Utterances by Children with Specific Expressive Language Impairment: Dynamic Assessment Validation. *American Journal of Speech-Language Pathology* 4:81–91.

Baltaxe, C., and Simmons, J. (1975). "Language in Childhood Psychosis: A Review." *Journal of Speech and Hearing Disorders* 40:439–458.

Balthazar, E. (1973). *Balthazar Scales of Adaptive Behavior II. Scales of Social Adaptation*. Palo Alto, CA: Consulting Psychologists Press.

Bates, E. (1976). *Language in Context*, New York: Academic Press.

Bates, E. (1979). *The Emergence of Symbols: Cognition and Communication in Infancy*. New York: Academic Press.

Bates et al. (1986). *Language and Gesture Inventory*, Unpublished Vocabulary Checklist.

Beard, R. (1969). *An Outline of Piaget's Developmental Psychology for Students and Teachers*. New York: Basic Books.

Belkin, A. (1975). "Investigation of the Functions and Forms of Children's Negative Utterances." Unpublished doctoral dissertation, Columbia University.

Benedict, H. (1975). "Early Lexical Development: Comprehension and Production." *Journal of Child Language* 6:183–200.

Beukelman, D., and Mirenda, P. (1992). *Augmentative and Alternative Communication*. Baltimore, MD: Brookes.

Bloom, L. (1970). *Language Development: Form and Function in Emerging Grammars*. Cambridge, MA: MIT Press.

Bloom, L. (1973). *One Word at a Time: The Use of Single Word Utterances Before Syntax*. The Hague, Neth.: Mouton.

Bloom, L. (1974). "Talking, Understanding and Thinking." In *Language Perspectives-Acquisition, Retardation and Intervention*, ed. L. Lloyd and R. Schiefelbusch (Baltimore: University Park Press).

Bloom, L., and Lahey, M. (1978). *Language Development and Language Disorders*. New York: Wiley.

Bloom, L., Lightbrown, P., and Hood, L. (1975). "Structure and Variation in Child Language." *Monographs of the Society for Research in Child Development* 40:1–41.

Bornstein, M., Tal, J., and Tamis-Lemonda, C. (1991a). "Parenting in Cross-Cultural Perspective: The United States, France and Japan. In

Cultural Approaches to Parenting, ed. M. H. Bornstein (Hillsdale, NJ: Lawrence Erlbaum Associates).

Bornstein, M., Tamis-Lemonda, C., Pecheux, M. and Rahn, C. (1991b). "Mother and Infant Activity and Interaction in France and the United States: A comparative study. *International Journal of Behavioral Development* 14:21–43.

Bowerman, M. (1973). "Structural Relationships in Children's Utterances: Syntactic or Semantic?" In *Cognitive Development and the Acquisition of Language,* ed. T. Moore (New York: Academic Press).

Bowerman, M. (1974). "Development of Concepts Underlying Language." In *Language Perspectives: Acquisition, Retardation, and Intervention,* ed. R. Schiefelbusch and L. Lloyd (Baltimore, MD: University Park Press).

Braine, M. (1963). "The Ontogeny of English Phrase Structure: The First Phrase." *Language* 39:1–14.

Braine, M. (1976). "Childrens' First Word Combinations." *Monographs of the Society for Research in Child Development* 41:1–104.

Brazelton, T. (1984). *Neonatal Behavior Assessment Scale,* Philadelphia: Lippincott.

Brown, R. (1973). *A First Language: The Early Stages,* Cambridge: Harvard University Press.

Brown, R., and Fraser, C. (1963). "The Acquisition of Syntax." In *Verbal Behavior and Learning: Problems and Processes,* ed. C. Cofer and B. Musgrave (New York: McGraw-Hill).

Brunson, K., and Haynes, W. (1991). "Profiling Teacher/Child Classroom Communication: Reliability of an Alternating Time Sampling Procedure." *Child Language Teaching and Therapy* 7, no. 2:192–212.

Carrow-Woolfolk, E., and Lynch, J. (1982). *An Integrative Approach to Language Disorders in Children.* New York: Grune and Stratton.

Chabon, S., Udolf, L., and Egolf, D. (1982). "The Temporal Reliability of Brown's Mean Length of Utterance Measure with Post Stage V Children." *Journal of Speech and Hearing Research* 25:124–128.

Chapman, R. (1978). "Comprehension Strategies in Children." In *Speech and Language in the Laboratory, School and Clinic,* ed. J. Kavanagh and W. Strange (Cambridge, MA: MIT Press).

Chapman, R. (1981). "Exploring Children's Communicative Intents." In *Assessing Language Production in Children: Experimental Procedures,* ed. J. Miller (Baltimore: University Park Press).

Chappel, G., and Johnson, G. (1976). "Evaluation of Cognitive Behavior in Young Nonverbal Children." *Language, Speech and Hearing Services in Schools* 7:17–27.

Chomsky, N. (1957). *Syntactic Structures.* The Hague, Neth.: Mouton.

Clark, D. (1989). "Neonates and infants at risk for hearing and speech-language disorders." *Topics in Language Disorders* 10, no. 1:1–12.

Clune, C., Paolella, J., and Foley, J. (1979). "Free Play Behavior of Atypical Children: An Approach to Assessment." *Journal of Autism and Developmental Disorders* 61–72.

Coggins, T., and Carpenter, R. (1978). "Categories for Coding Prespeech Intentional Communication." Unpublished Manuscript, University of Washington, Seattle.

Cole, E., and St. Clair-Stokes, J. (1984). "Caregiver-Child Interactive Behavior: A Videotape Analysis Procedure" *Volta Review* 86:200–217.

Coleman, D., Cook, A., and Meyers, L. (1980). "Assessing Non-Oral Clients for Assistive Communication Devices", *Journal of Speech and Hearing Disorders* 45:515–527.

Corman, H., and Escalona, S. (1969). "Stages of Sensorimotor Development: A Replication Study." *Merrill Palmer Quarterly* 15:351–361.

Cosby, M., and Ruder, K. (1983). "Symbolic Play and Early Language Development in Normal and Mentally Retarded Children." *Journal of Speech and Hearing Research* 25:404–411.

Crais, E. (1995). "Expanding the Repertoire of Tools and Techniques for Assessing the Communication Skills of Infants and Toddlers." *American Journal of Speech-Language Pathology* 4:47–59.

Crais, E., and Roberts, J. (1991). "Decision Making in Assessment and Early Intervention Planning. *Language, Speech and Hearing Services in Schools* 22:19–30.

Curcio, F. (1978). "Sensorimotor Functioning and Communication in Mute Autistic Children." *Journal of Autism and Childhood Schizophrenia* 8:281–292.

Dale, P. (1976). *Language Development: Structure and Function.* New York: Holt, Rinehart, and Winston.

Dale, P. (1980). "Is Early Pragmatic Development Measureable?" *Journal of Child Language* 7:1–12.

Devilliers, J., and Devilliers, P. (1978). *Language Acquisition*. Cambridge: Harvard University Press.

Dore, J. (1975). "Holophrases, Speech Acts and Language Universals." *Journal of Child Language* 2:21–40.

Dore, J., et al. (1976). "Transitional Phenomena in Early Language Acquisition." *Journal of Child Language* 3:13–28.

Duchan, J., and Siegel, L. (1979). "Incorrect Responses to Locative Commands: A Case Study." *Language, Speech and Hearing Services in Schools* 10:99–103.

Duchan, J., and Weitzner-Lin, B. (1987). "Nurturant-Naturalistic Intervention for Language Impaired Children: Implications for Planning Lessons and Tracking Progress." *Journal of the American Speech and Hearing Association* 29, no. 7:45–49.

Dunst, C. (1980). *A Clinical and Educational Manual for Use with the Uzigiris and Hunt Scales of Infant Psychological Development*. Baltimore: University Park Press.

Edmonston, N., and Thane, N. (1992). "Children's Use of Comprehension Strategies in Response to Relational Words: Implications for Assessment." *American Journal of Speech-Language Pathology* 1:30–35.

Elder, J., and Pederson, D. (1973). "Preschool Children's Use of Objects in Symbolic Play." *Child Development* 49:500–504.

Fenson, L., et al. (1993). *MacArthur Communicative Development Inventories*. San Diego, CA: Singular Publishing.

Fey, M. (1986). *Language Intervention with Young Children*, San Diego, CA: College-Hill.

Fillmore, C. (1968). "The Case for Case." In *Universals in Linguistic Theory*, ed. E. Bach and R. Harms (New York: Holt, Rinehart, and Winston).

Flavell, J. (1977). *Cognitive Development*. Englewood Cliffs, NJ: Prentice-Hall.

Fogel, A., Toda, S., and Kawai, M. (1988). "Mother-Infant Face-to-Face Interaction in Japan and the United States: A Laboratory Comparison Using 3-Month-Old Infants." *Developmental Psychology* 24:398–406.

Folger, J., and Chapman, R. (1978). "A Pragmatic Analysis of Spontaneous Imitations." *Journal of Child Language* 5:25–38.

Gallagher, T. (1983). "Preassessment: A Procedure for Accomodating Language Use Variability." In *Pragmatic Assessment and Intervention Issues in Language*, ed. T. Gallagher and C. Prutting (San Diego, CA: College-Hill).

Garnica, O. (1974). "Some Characteristics of Prosodic Input to Young Children." Paper Presented at the SSRC Conference on Language Input and Acquisition, Boston, MA.

Ginsburg, H., and Opper, S. (1969). *Piaget's Theory of Intellectual Development: An Introduction*. Englewood Cliffs, NJ. Prentice-Hall.

Gopnik, A., and Meltzoff, A. (1987). "The Development of Categorization in the Second Year and Its Relation to Other Cognitive and Linguistic Developments." *Child Development* 58:1523–1531.

Halliday, M. (1975). *Learning How to Mean: Explorations in the Development of Language*. New York: Elsevier.

Haynes, W., and Shulman, B. (in press). *Communication Development: Foundations and Clinical Applications*, Englewood Cliffs, NJ: Prentice-Hall.

Heath, S. (1983). *Ways with words*. Cambridge, Eng.: Cambridge University Press.

Heath, S. (1989). "The Learner as a Cultural Member." In *The Teachability of Language*, ed. M. Rice and R. Scheifelbusch (Baltimore, MD: Brookes).

Hedrick, D., Prather, E., and Tobin, A. (1975). *Sequenced Inventory of Communication Development*. Seattle: University of Washington Press.

Holland, A. (1975). "Language Therapy for Children: Some Thoughts on Context and Content." *Journal of Speech and Hearing Disorders* 40:514–523.

Howe, C. (1976). "The Meanings of Two-Word Utterances in the Speech of Young Children." *Journal of Child Language* 3:29–47.

Hubbell, R. (1981). *Children's Language Disorders: An Integrated Approach*. Englewood Cliffs, NJ: Prentice-Hall.

Ingram, D. (1989). *First Language Acquisition: Method, Description and Explanation*. New York: Cambridge University Press.

Johnson, W., Darley, F. and Spriestersbach, D. (1963). *Diagnostic Methods in Speech Pathology*. New York: Harper and Row.

Johnston, J., Miller, J., Curtiss, S., and Tallal, P. (1993). "Conversations with Children Who

Are Language Impaired: Asking Questions." *Journal of Speech and Hearing Research* 36: 973–978.

Kahn, J. (1984). "Cognitive Training and Initial Use of Referential Speech." *Topics in Language Disorders* 5:14–18.

Kamhi, A., and Johnston, J. (1982). "Towards an Understanding of Retarded Children's Linguistic Deficiencies." *Journal of Speech and Hearing Research* 25:435–445.

Kirk, S. and Kirk, W. (1971). *Psycholinguisic Learning Disabilities.* Urbana: University of Illinois Press.

Klee, T., and Fitzgerald, M. (1983). "The Relation Between Grammatical Development and Mean Length of Utterance in Morphemes." Paper Presented at the Convention of the American Speech and Hearing Association, Cincinnati, OH.

Klein, M., and Briggs, M. (1987). "Facilitating Mother-Infant Communicative Interactions in Mothers of High-Risk Infants." *Journal of Childhood Communication Disorders* 10, no. 2:95–106.

Kramer, P. (1977). "Young Children's Free Responses to Anomalous Commands." *Journal of Experimental Child Psychology* 24:219–234.

Lahey, M. (1988). *Language Disorders and Language Development,* New York: MacMillan.

Lahey, M., and Edwards, J. (1995). "Specific Language Impairment: Preliminary Investigation of Factors Associated with Family History and with Patterns of Language Performance." *Journal of Speech and Hearing Research* 38: 643–657.

Lambert, N., Windmiller, M., Tharinger, D., and Cole, L. (1981). *AAMD Adaptive Behavior Scale.* Monterey, CA: Publishers Test Service.

Leonard, L. (1975). "On Differentiating Syntactic and Semantic Features in Emerging Grammars: Evidence from Empty Form Usage." *Journal of Psycholinguistic Research* 4:357–364.

Leonard, L. (1976). *Meaning in Child Language: Issues in the Study of Early Semantic Development.* New York: Grune and Stratton.

Leonard, L. (1978). "Cognitive Factors in Early Linguistic Development." In *Bases of Language Intervention,* ed. R. Schiefelbusch (Baltimore: University Park Press).

Leonard, L., Steckol, K., and Panther, K. (1983). "Returning Meaning to Semantic Relations: Some Clinical Applications." *Journal of Speech and Hearing Disorders* 48:25–35.

Lifter, K., and Bloom, L. (1989) Object Knowledge and the Emergence of Language. *Infant Behavior and Development* 12:395–423.

Lifter, K., Edwards, G., Avery, D., Anderson, S. and Sulzer-Azaroff, B. (1988). "Developmental Assessment of Children's Play: Implications for Intervention." Paper presented at the convention of the American Speech-Language-Hearing Association, Boston, MA.

Lowe, M., and Costello, A. (1976). *The Symbolic Play Test.* London: National Foundation for Educational Research Publishing.

Lucas, E. (1980). *Semantic and Pragmatic Language Disorders.* Rockville, Md.: Aspen Systems Corporation.

Lund, N., and Duchan, J. (1988). *Assessing Children's Language in Naturalistic Contexts.* Englewood Cliffs, NJ: Prentice-Hall.

MacDonald, J., and Carroll, J. (1992). "A Social Partnership Model for Assessing Early Communication Development: An Intervention Model for Preconversational Children." *Language, Speech and Hearing Services in Schools* 23: 113–124.

MCarthy, D. (1935). "The Language Development of the Preschool Child." University of Minnesota Institute of Child Welfare Monograph Series IV. Minneapolis: University of Minnesota Press.

McCathren, R., Warren, S., and Yoder, P. (1996). "Prelinguistic Predictors of Later Language Development." In *Assessment of Communication and Language,* ed. K. Cole, P. Dale, and D. Thal (Baltimore, MD: Brookes).

McCollum, J., and Stayton, V. (1985). "Social Interaction Assessment/Intervention." *Journal of the Division for Early Childhood* 9:125–135.

Mclean, J., and Snyder-Mclean, L. (1978). *A Transactional Approach to Early Language Training.* Columbus, OH: Merrill.

McNeil, D. (1970). *The Acquisition of Language: The Study of Developmental Psycholinguistics.* New York: Harper and Row.

Merhabian, A., and Williams, M. (1971). "Piagetian Measures of Cognitive Development for

Children up to Age Two." *Journal of Psycholinguistic Research* 1:113–125.

Millen, K., and Prutting, C. (1979). "Consistencies across Three Language Comprehension Tests for Specific Grammatical Features." *Language, Speech and Hearing Services in Schools* 10: 162–170.

Miller, J., and Chapman, R. (1981). "The Relation between Age and Mean Length of Utterance in Morphemes." *Journal of Speech and Hearing Research* 24:154–161.

Morehead, D., and Morehead, A. (1974). "From Signal to Sign." In *Language Perspectives-Acquisition, Retardation and Intervention,* (Baltimore: University Park Press).

Muma, J. (1973). "Language Assessment: Some Underlying Assumptions." *Journal of the American Speech and Hearing Association* 15:331–338.

Muma, J. (1978). *Language Handbook: Concepts, Assessment, Intervention.* Englewood Cliffs, NJ: Prentice-Hall.

Muma, J. (1983). "Speech Language Pathology: Emerging Clinical Expertise in Language." In *Pragmatic Assessment and Intervention Issues in Language,* T. Gallagher and C. Prutting (San Diego, CA: College-Hill Press).

Nation, J., and Aram, D. (1982). *Diagnosis of Speech and Language Disorders.* St. Louis: Mosby.

Nelson, K. (1973). "Structure and Strategy in Learning to Talk." *Monographs of the Society for Research in Child Development* 38:11–56.

Nelson, K. (1974). "Concept, Word and Sentence: Interrelations in Acquisition and Development." *Psychological Review* 81:267–285.

Newhoff, M., and Leonard, L. (1983). "Diagnosis of Developmental Language Disorders." In *Diagnosis in Speech-Language Pathology,* ed. I. Meitus and B. Weinberg (Baltimore, MD: University Park Press).

Nicolich, L. (1977). "Beyond Sensorimotor Intelligence: Assessment of Symbolic Maturity through Analysis of Pretend Play." *Merrill Palmer Quarterly* 23:89–101.

Olswang, L., Stoel-Gammon, C., Coggins, T., and Carpenter, R. (1987). *Assessing Prelinguistic and Early Linguistic Behaviors in Developmentally Young Children.* Seattle: University of Washington Press.

Opitz, V. (1982). "Pragmatic Analysis of the Communicative Behavior of an Autistic Child." *Journal of Speech and Hearing Disorders* 47: 99–108.

Owens, R. (1995). *Language Development: An Introduction.* Needham Heights, MA: Allyn and Bacon.

Owens, R., and House, L. (1984). "Decision-Making Processes in Augmentative Communication." *Journal of Speech and Hearing Disorders* 49:18–25.

Paul, R. (1995). *Language Disorders from Infancy through Adolescence: Assessment and Intervention.* St. Louis, MO: Mosby.

Paul, R., and Jennings, P. (1992). "Phonological Behavior in Toddlers with Slow Expressive Language Development." *Journal of Speech and Hearing Research* 35:99–107.

Proctor, A. (1989). "Stages of Normal Noncry Vocal Development in Infancy: A Protocol for Assessment." *Topics in Language Disorders,* 10, no. 1:26–42.

Project RHISE (1979). *Manual for Administration of the Rockford Infant Developmental Evaluation Scales,* Bensenville, IL: Scholastic Testing Service.

Prizant, B., and Wetherby, A. (1988). "Providing Services to Children with Autism (ages 0 to 2 years) and Their Families." *Topics in Language Disorders* 9, no. 1:1–23.

Rescorla, L., and Goossens, M. (1992). Symbolic Play Development in Toddlers with Expressive Specific Language Impairment (SLI-E)." *Journal of Speech and Hearing Research* 35:1290–1302.

Reynell, J. (1969). *Reynell Developmental Language Scales.* Buckinghamshire, Eng.: National Foundation for Educational Research in England and Wales.

Rice, M., Sell, M., and Hadley, P. (1990). "The Social Interactive Coding System (SICS): An On-Line, Clinically Relevant Descriptive Tool", *Language, Speech and Hearing Services in Schools* 21:2–14.

Rogers, S. (1977). "Characteristics of the Cognitive Development of Profoundly Retarded Children." *Child Development* 48:837–843.

Ruder, K., and M. Smith (1974). "Issues in Language Training." In *Language Perspectives-Acquisition, Retardation and Intervention,* ed.

R. Schiefelbusch and L. Lloyd (Baltimore: University Park Press).

Rutter, M. (1978). "Diagnosis and Definition of Childhood Autism." *Journal of Autism and Childhood Schizophrenia* 8:139–169.

Saville-Troike, M. (1986). "Anthropological Considerations in the Study of Communication. In *Communication Disorders in Culturally Diverse Populations,* ed. O. Taylor (San Diego, CA: College Hill Press).

Schieffelin, B. (1985). "The Acquisition of Kaluli." In *The Cross-linguistic Study of Linguistic Acquisition,* Vol. 1, ed. D. Slobin (Hillsdale, NJ: Lawrence Erlbaum Associates).

Schlesinger, I. (1974). "Relational Concepts Underlying Language." In *Language Perspectives-Acquisition, Retardation and Intervention,* ed. R. Schiefelbusch and L. Lloyd (Baltimore: University Park Press).

Shane, H., and Bashir, A. (1980). "Election Criteria for the Adoption of an Augmentative Communication System: Preliminary Considerations." *Journal of Speech and Hearing Disorders* 45:408–444.

Siegel, G. (1975). "The Use of Language Tests." *Language, Speech and Hearing Services in Schools* 6:211–217.

Silverman, F. (1995). *Communication for the Speechless.* Neeham Heights, MA: Allyn and Bacon.

Snow, C. (1972). "Mother's Speech to Children Learning Language." *Child Development* 43: 549–565.

Snow, C. (1977). "The Development of Conversation between Mothers and Babies." *Journal of Child Language* 4:1–22.

Snyder, L. (1978). "Communicative and Cognitive Disabilities in the Sensorimotor Period." *Merrill Palmer Quarterly* 24:161–180.

Snyder, L. (1981). "Assessing Communicative Abilities in the Sensorimotor Period: Content and Context." *Topics in Language Disorders* 1:31–46.

Snyder-McLean, L., McLean, J., and R. Etter (1988). "Clinical Assessment of Sensorimotor Knowledge in Nonverbal, Severely Retarded Clients." *Topics in Language Disorders* 8:1–22.

Sparks, S. (1989). "Assessment and Intervention with At-Risk Infants and Toddlers: Guidelines for the Speech-Language Pathologist." *Topics in Language Disorders* 10, no. 1: 43–56.

Sparrow, S., Balla, D., and Cicchetti, D. (1984). *Vineland Adaptive Behavior Scales.* Circle Pines, MN: American Guidance Service.

Staab, C. (1983). "Language Functions Elicited by Meaningful Activities: A New Dimension in Language Programs." *Language, Speech and Hearing Services in Schools* 14:164–170.

Stark, R., Bernstein, L., and Demorest, M. (1993). "Vocal Communication in the First 18 Months of Life." *Journal of Speech and Hearing Research* 36:548–558.

Steckol, K., and Leonard, L. (1981). "Sensorimotor Development and the Use of Prelinguistic Performatives." *Journal of Speech and Hearing Research* 24:262–268.

Taenzer, S., Harris, L., and Bass, M. (1975). *Assessment in a Natural Context.* Paper presented at the American Speech and Hearing Association National Convention, Washington, DC.

Thal, D., and Tobias, S. (1992). Communicative gestures in children with delayed onset of oral expressive vocabulary. *Journal of Speech and Hearing Research* 35:1281–1289.

Toffler, A. (1981). *The Third Wave.* New York: Bantam Books.

Tough, J. (1977). *The Development of Meaning.* New York: Halsted Press.

Trantham, C., and Pedersen, J. (1976). *Normal Language Development.* Baltimore, MD: Williams and Wilkins.

Uzigiris, I., and Hunt, J. (1975). *Assessment in Infancy.* Urbana: University of Illinois Press.

Watson-Gegeo, K., and Gegeo, D. (1986). "Calling Out and Repeating Routines in Kwara'ae Children's Language Socialization." In *Language and Socialization across Cultures,* ed. B. Schieffelin and E. Ochs Cambridge, Eng: Cambridge University Press.

Weismer, S., Branch, J., and Miller, J. (1994). "A Prospective Longitudinal Study of Language Development in Late Talkers." *Journal of Speech and Hearing Research* 37:852–867.

Weiss, A., Leonard, L., Rowan, L., and Chapman, K. (1983). "Linguistic and Nonlinguistic Features of Style in Normal and Language-Impaired Children." *Journal of Speech and Hearing Disorders* 48:154–163.

Weisz, J., and Zigler, E. (1979). "Cognitive Development in Retarded and Nonretarded Persons: Piagetian Tests of the Similar Sequence Hypothesis." *Psychological Bulletin* 86:831–851.

Westby, C. (1980). "Assessment of Cognitive and Language Abilities through Play." *Language, Speech and Hearing Services in Schools* 11:154–168.

Wetherby, A., Cain, D., Yonclas, D., and Walker, V. (1988). "Analysis of Intentional Communication of Normal Children from the Prelinguistic to the Multiword Stage." *Journal of Speech and Hearing Research* 31:240–252.

Wetherby, A., and Prizant, B. (1992). "Profiling Young Children's Communicative Competence. In *Causes and Effects in Communication and Language Intervention*, ed. S. Warren and J. Reichle (Baltimore, MD: Brookes).

Wetherby, A., and Prizant, B. (1993). *Communication and Symbolic Behavior Scales*. Chicago, IL: Riverside.

Wetherby, A., and Prutting, C. (1984). "Profiles of Communicative and Cognitive-Social Abilities in Autistic Children." *Journal of Speech and Hearing Research* 27:364–377.

Wetherby, A., and Rodriguez, G. (1992). "Measurement of Communicative Intentions in Normally Developing Children During Structured and Unstructured Contexts." *Journal of Speech and Hearing Research* 35:130–138.

Wetherby, A., Yonclas, D., and Bryan, A. (1989). Communicative Profiles of Preschool Children with Handicaps: Implications for Early Intervention. *Journal of Speech and Hearing Disorders* 54:148–158.

Wilcox, M. (1984). "Developmental Language Disorders: Preschoolers." In *Language Disorders in Children: Recent Advances*, ed. A. Holland (San Diego, CA: College-Hill).

Wolfus, B., Moscovitch, M., and Kinsbourne, M. (1980). "Subgroups of Developmental Language Impairment." *Brain and Language* 10: 152–171.

Wood, B. (1981). *Children and Communication: Verbal and Nonverbal Language Development*. Englewood Cliffs, NJ: Prentice-Hall.

Zimmerman, I., Steiner, V., and Evatt, R. (1969). *Preschool Language Scale*. Columbus, OH: Merrill.

Chapter 5

Assessment of School-Age and Adolescent Language Disorders

The model by MacDonald and Carroll (1992) that was presented in Chapter 4 dealt with specific competencies required for communication development. Specifically, we talked about becoming *play partners*, *turn-taking partners*, and the beginning of developing a role as a *communicative partner* through the use of early multiword utterances. The present chapter rounds out the last two components in the model by discussing the period when the child becomes a *language partner* through the use of semantic and grammatical rules. Finally, we will consider the child's becoming a *conversational partner* as pragmatic rules are developed to regulate the social use of language in a conversational context.

The present chapter focuses on school-age and adolescent students who are speaking at the sentence level and who may well have difficulty with syntactic rules and who may also have deficiencies in semantics, pragmatics, metalinguistics, morphology, reading, writing, cognitive abilities, and general language processing. Thus, the reader will find that the assessment targets, tasks, and measurements we discuss in the present chapter differ dramatically from those mentioned in Chapter 4.

Table 5.1 lists some common symptoms of language disorder in school-age and adolescent students. One can see that these symptoms span all areas of language and include comprehension as well as production impairments. There are also phonological disorders in this population that are addressed more fully in Chapter 6. It should be noted that some of the symptoms in Table 5.1 are rather gross linguistic errors that would be easily detected in conversation (e.g., syntac-

TABLE 5.1   Common Symptoms of Language Disorders in Older Students

Semantics

- Word finding/retrieval deficits
- Use of a large number of words in an attempt to explain a concept because the name escapes them (circumlocutions)
- Overuse of limited vocabulary
- Difficulty recalling names of items in categories (e.g., animals, foods)
- Difficulty retrieving verbal opposites
- Small vocabulary
- Use of words lacking specificity (thing, junk, stuff, etc.)
- Inappropriate use of words (selection of wrong word)
- Difficulty defining words
- Less comprehension of complex words
- Failure to grasp double word meanings (e.g., can, file)

Syntax/Morphology

- Use of grammatically incorrect sentence structures
- Simple, as opposed to complex, sentences
- Less comprehension of complex grammatical structures
- Prolonged pauses while constructing sentences
- Semantically empty placeholders (e.g., filled pauses, "uh," "er," "um")
- Use of many stereotyped phrases that do not require much language skill
- Use of "starters" (e.g., "You know . . . ")

Pragmatics

- Use of redundant expressions and information the listener has already heard
- Use of nonspecific vocabulary (e.g., thing, stuff) and the listener cannot tell from prior conversation or physical context what is referred to
- Less skill in giving explanations clearly to a listener (lack of detail)
- Less skill in explaining something in a proper sequence
- Less conversational control in terms of introducing, maintaining, and changing topics (may get off the track in conversation and introduce new topics awkwardly)
- Rare use of clarification questions (e.g., "I don't understand," "You did what?")
- Difficulty shifting conversational style in different social situations (e.g., peer vs. teacher; child vs. adult)
- Difficulty grasping the "main idea" of a story or lecture (preoccupation with irrelevant details)
- Trouble making inferences from material not explicitly stated (e.g., "Sally went outside. She had to put up her umbrella." Inference: It was raining.)

From: Haynes, W., Moran, M. and Pindzola, R. (1990), *Communication Disorders in the Classroom* (Dubuque, IA: Kendall-Hunt).

tic rule violations), while some errors are rather subtle and discernible only with specialized communication sampling. We should reinforce the point here that standardized tests may not reveal a subtle linguistic impairment in a school age child (Plante and Vance 1995). It is not unusual for an elementary-level student to pass many of our formal language tests and yet exhibit a significant linguistically based communication disorder. Many of these errors would only be seen in non-standardized probing and conversational sampling. Similar difficulties have been found with some standardized language-screening instruments (Sturner et al. 1993). Interestingly, some surveys have indicated that the majority of public school SLPs routinely use a combination of formal (standardized) and informal (non-standardized) methods of assessment (Hux, Morris-Friehe, and Sanger, 1993; Wilson et al. 1991).

Students with Language Problems: The "High-Risk" Groups

There are several specific groups of school-age students that have an increased likelihood of being diagnosed with a language disorder:

1. *History of language impairment as a preschooler.* Longitudinal studies of children who had language delays as preschoolers have shown a strong tendency for the emergence of academic and language problems as these youngsters get older (Aram and Nation, 1980; Bashir et al. 1983; Hall and Tomblin, 1978; King, Jones, and Lasky 1982; Strominger and Bashir, 1977). Many of these studies suggest that over 50% of preschoolers with a history of language difficulties are at risk for academic and language problems. This is not just because of their "weakness" in the area of language but also because of increased academic difficulty and teacher language complexity as the child moves up the grade levels. In the opinion of the present authors, the evidence suggests strongly that parents of preschoolers enrolled in language treatment, when they are dismissed from therapy, should be counseled about the possible reemergence of language-based problems as the child is faced with increasing academic and linguistic complexity after entering school.

2. *Students with Learning and/or Reading disabilities.* The literature on learning disabilities has consistently supported the notion that the largest percentage of children diagnosed with reading and learning problems have either a history of language impairment or current linguistic difficulties (Maxwell and Wallach 1984; Wiig and Semel 1976). Most recent publications have referred to this population as "language-learning disabled," emphasizing the pivotal role of language in their impairment. If a student is receiving services for reading problems or a learning disability, there is an increased risk that some form of language disorder may be present as well.

3. *Students who are "Academically at-risk".* Simon (1989) refers to a group of children who have "fallen between the cracks" of the educational system. These are students who have not been diagnosed as having a language problem but who are floundering academically on a consistent basis. Simon suggests that a significant percentage, maybe as many as 50%, of these students exhibit linguistic problems in addition to their academic difficulties. Simms-Hill and Haynes (1992) studied fourth-grade students who were rated "academically at risk" by their teachers.

These children consistently earned grades lower than "C." These students were not receiving any remedial services in speech/language or in any other area and had no history of language delay. Simms-Hill and Haynes (1992) found that over 50% of these students scored low enough on three different language tests to warrant clinical concern.

Thus, one mechanism of detecting school-age children with language disorders is to carefully examine students from the three high-risk groups mentioned above. This survey could be done through teacher referral, screening, or formal testing as part of a team evaluation of problematic children.

Use of Standardized Tests with Syntax-Level Children

As we indicated in Chapter 3, formal tests are best suited to comparing performance on some measure to that of same age peers who took the test under similar conditions. Formal tests, as Muma (1973a) stated, address the issue of whether or not a problem exists. These measures are not particularly good at defining the nature of the problem or helping in the selection of treatment targets. We recommend that clinicians always use a standardized test to document the existence of a language disorder, and most work settings require the use of such instruments as part of determining eligibility for services. It is important to note, however, that just because a child "passes" a standardized test, it does not mean that a language-based communication disorder does not exist. Many children's language disorders are not exposed until an actual conversational sample is elicited by the clinician or until the children's language abilities are challenged by increased difficulty on academic tasks. Appendix E lists some instruments that are commonly available. The fact that we have compiled this list does not suggest that we are recommending these tests or even the notion of formal testing in general. We provide the list simply as an informational tool to demonstrate that there are many formal tests in the area of language disorders. Each year a plethora of new tests become available to the SLP. No doubt, by the time you are reading this chapter, there will be many new tests, and some of the ones on our list will be out of print. Especially in the area of language, it is almost impossible to remain abreast of all recent test developments. Another problem, of course, is that no single individual, clinical setting, or training program can afford to purchase every test instrument that is published. Some of our information in Appendix 5.A comes from examining the actual test instruments themselves; however, in other cases we had to rely on reviews, catalogs, or flyers that advertise the tests. Thus, we make no attempt to critically analyze or detail these tests. Other sources provide substantial reviews and descriptions of many of these instruments (Aram and Nation 1982; Conoley and Impara 1995; Darley 1979; Peterson and Marquardt 1990).

The reader will note that the tests are calculated to tap a variety of language skills (expression, vocabulary, comprehension, imitation, cognition, pragmatics, syntax, etc.), are targeted for use with a wide spectrum of age ranges, and represent a number of different theoretical points of view. The older tests obviously do not take into account current advances in thinking about language acquisition or assessment. Chapter 3 of the present textbook outlines major considerations that the clinician should take into account relative to the psychometric properties of assessment instruments. Owens et al. (1983) provide a summary of specific grammatical forms examined by a wide variety of tests. This information might be helpful to a clinician who wishes to probe only selected grammatical forms. Rarely, however, will formal tests include enough items to thoroughly evaluate a particular linguistic structure, and some forms (e.g., derivational morphology) are not adequately dealt with on standardized tests (Moats and Smith 1992).

Wilson et al. (1991) surveyed clinicians in the state of California to determine which modes of assessment were used most in the public school systems. They also obtained data on specific standardized tests used by SLPs. Table 5.2 shows that most clinicians use a combination of standardized and nonstandardized methods to test both comprehension and production in the public school population. As we stated in Chapter 1, assessment embodies both elements of art and science. It makes sense that working clinicians find that they must go beyond formal standardized testing and probe behaviors in more informal ways to gain adequate insight into a child's language system. Table 5.3 lists some specific instruments that were reported by the clinicians, and most readers will recognize these familiar tests from the shelves of their own clinical facilities. It is somewhat comforting to realize that there is a small core of highly used instruments that clinicians tend to rely on at any one point in time. Some of these instruments have a long history of use, and others are newer. As you read this, there are no doubt more recent instruments that have either replaced some of those in Table 5.3 or that are used in addition to the tests listed.

The bulk of the instruments in Appendix 5.A focus on structural aspects of language (syntax, semantics, literal meaning of sentences), although there are several that deal with other areas as well (e.g., pragmatics, metalinguistics, concepts).

TABLE 5.2   Reported Methods of Assessing Child Language

Expressive Language

Published formal instruments/informal methods	53%
Published clinician-devised methods	22%
Published formal instruments	16%
Clinician-devised informal methods	9%

Receptive Language

Published formal instruments/informal methods	47%
Published formal instruments	41%
Published clinician-devised methods	12%

Adapted from Wilson et al. (1991).

TABLE 5.3 Most Frequently Used Formal Tests

Expressive	Receptive
Expressive One-Word Picture Vocabulary Test	PPVT-R
	CELF
Test of Language Development	Test of Language Development
Clinical Evaluation of Language Functions	TACL-R
	Boehm Test of Basic Concepts
ITPA	ITPA
PLS	Receptive One-Word Picture Vocabulary Test
The Word Test	
Structured Photographic Expressive Language Test	PLS
	Token Test for Children
Test of Problem Solving	Detroit Test of Learning Aptitude
Detroit Test of Learning Aptitude	ACLC
TEEM	Bracken Basic Concepts Scale
Language-Processing Test	

Adapted from Wilson et al. (1991).

Some of these tests may well be used by the SLP to gain *preliminary* insights into selected aspects of language performance, and the tests certainly can fulfill institutional expectations for obtaining scores on formal instruments.

Nonstandardized Testing

Sometimes clinicians are interested in eliciting particular syntactic structures from a child as opposed to administering an entire standardized test. This occasion would arise if the clinician wanted to probe the child's use of certain constructions, such as question forms in spontaneous speech. Mulac, Prutting, and Tomlinson (1978) suggest that a variety of tasks could be used to elicit a particular construction. They found that the most-effective tasks for eliciting the "is interrogative" were those tasks that required intent, had contextual referents, and some inherent structure to the activity. One example was a guessing game in which children had to guess what was in a bag (e.g., "Is it a—?"). The notion of using several different informal elicitation tasks to evaluate certain syntactic structures has been supported by others as well (Leonard et al. 1978; Lund and Duchan 1993; Musselwhite and Barrie-Blackley 1980).

If one were to examine the host of standardized tests that are available to examine the comprehension and production of language, a striking observation would be that many of these instruments have more similarities than differences because there are only a certain number of ways that expressive and receptive

TABLE 5.4   Elicitation Procedures Used in Nonstandardized Assessment

Comprehension	Production
Identification (pointing to, touching)	Elicited immediate imitation
Acting out (following directions)	Elicited delayed imitation
Judgment task (right, wrong, silly, polite)	Nonimitative modeling
Conversation (requests for repair)	Cloze task (carrier phrase)
	Spontaneous evoked (naming, picture description, barrier)
	Story retelling (paraphrase)
	Narratives
	Conversation (legitimate)
	Free play

language can be sampled. It is instructive to move from thinking about "tests" toward thinking about "tasks" that are used to sample language by means of these instruments. For example, many tests involve asking a child to point at pictures when the clinician gives a verbal stimulus (e.g., "Show me airplane flying"). When all tests are examined from the perspective of the types of tasks they use in assessing comprehension and production of language, the tests appear highly similar. Even research projects that examine language use specific tasks to elicit responses to study comprehension and production of language. Decades ago, Leonard et al. (1978) studied formal tests and research protocols to determine which types of tasks were used to gain insight into child language. Table 5.4 illustrates some of the common threads they saw running through tests and research projects. There are no doubt other assessment methods not included in Table 5.4, but most are probably there. Clinicians who want to informally probe language comprehension and production in children have a relatively finite number of ways to do it. This is both comforting and disturbing at the same time. When clinicians use nonstandardized methods to assess language, they must design stimuli and tasks that will give them information beyond that provided by standardized instruments. As stated in Chapter 3, just because nonstandardized methods are used, the clinician is not absolved from having to be systematic in the way data are gathered.

Language Sampling: A General Look at the Process

A common thread that has woven its way through the text thus far has been the notion of ecological validity. When done appropriately, language sampling of a spontaneous conversation is perhaps the closest we come to evaluating real communication. As Miller (1981) says, we must broaden our definition of what we mean by sampling. Perhaps a better name for this process would be "communication sampling" rather than "language sampling" because a child can use flawless syntax and yet not communicate effectively if a pragmatic disorder is present.

Spontaneous sampling is the only way to hold content, form, and use intact; thus, it is one of our most-powerful tools.

Most SLPs have had the opportunity to sit in a small room with a child and attempt to fill a cassette with a representative sample of language. Most of us also have experienced the despair and humiliation (if observed) of harvesting a string of one-word utterances and elliptical responses. Faced with this, we begin to put the pressure on the child for longer utterances and ask questions about the obvious. "What is in this picture?" we ask, when both the child and the clinician know the answer. "Tell me about what you did at school today," we cajole, and the child shrugs his/her shoulders, saying, "Nuthin'." A very wise observation was made by Hubbell (1981) after he studied spontaneous talking in young children. When children feel they are being interrogated and there is a great deal of pressure for them to talk, they tend to clam up. One of the worst liabilities the clinician can have is a mother who says to her child in the waiting room, "Now we're here to get your speech evaluated. So be sure to talk." This is, in many cases, the "kiss of death" for a decent language sample. Children need to feel at ease and not pressured to talk. Clinicians also should try to resist the very strong urge to "interrogate" school-age children and, worst of all, to question them about the obvious. As we mentioned earlier, all communication is affected by the context in which it occurs, and language sampling is no different. Since each sampling session is a product of an individual student, clinician, and communicative environment, it is impossible to provide guidelines that will work with all cases. All we can do is play the probabilities and provide some suggestions that may facilitate spontaneous talking in most cases.

For detailed treatments of language-sampling procedures the reader is referred to the ample sources dealing with the topic (Barrie-Blackley, Musselwhite, and Rogister 1978; Miller 1981). Some general watchwords are as follows:

1. Always tape-record the sample. We tend to subjectively fill in utterances that are incomplete if we transcribe during the sample. Additionally, it is distracting if you are attempting to carry on a legitimate conversation while scribbling on a tablet. Either we are engaging in a real conversation or we are not. We typically transcribe the communication sample so that a permanent record is available for comparison at a later date. Paul (1995) has suggested that some analyses can be done with less time commitment if the clinician simply listens to the taped sample while taking specific data on errors. This allows the clinician an opportunity to replay the tape in cases where the client's productions are less intelligible.

2. Use a good-quality tape recorder and position it in such a way as to promote optimal recording. This is one of the most-often-overlooked aspects of sampling language. It is a real disappointment when a clinician has done a masterful job of eliciting natural conversation from a child only to have the speech rendered unintelligible by a poor recording.

3. Minimize the use of yes/no questions. Remember, as soon as you ask these questions, you know the answer will be "Yes," "No," or "I don't know." Beginning clinicians typically bombard the child with yes/no questions, and the sample may be so loaded with single-word utterances that the child's MLU is severely under-estimated because of sampling error (see Miller 1981).

4. An attempt should be made to minimize questions that can be answered with one word (e.g., "What color is your dog?"). Although you have to ask some of these questions in the normal course of conversation, they do elicit single word responses.

5. Try to ask broad-based questions such as, "What happened?" "What happened next?" "Can you tell me about . . . ?" "Why?" "How?" and so forth.

6. Do not be afraid to make contributions to the conversation. One of the most common errors in beginning clinicians is that they want the child to do all the talk-ing. This is not a natural conversational situation. Furthermore, the child's utter-ances are typically in the role of responder. Think back to the last language sample you took and ask yourself if the child had opportunities to initiate conversation instead of merely respond to your interrogations. In addition, ask yourself if you were a legitimate conversational participant. Did you tell the child some of your feelings and experiences? Did you talk mostly about things that were obvious or trivial? As Hubbell (1981) states, a facilitator of conversation is a good conversa-tional model. It has been our experience, that as soon as we stop the barrage of questions and begin to make some observations about what is going on in the ses-sion and what we think about things, the child begins to make some contributions to the conversation.

7. As Miller (1981) says, try not to "play the fool" during a language sample, with an older child especially. We have heard clinicians say, "I don't know what's in this picture, can you tell me?" Another example is a clinician who says, "Tell me how to make a sandwich. I don't know how." Give the child credit for the intelligence to know that you could easily describe pictures or that you know how to do sim-ple, everyday tasks.

8. Learn to tolerate periods of silence or pauses. Beginning clinicians seem to feel that they have to fill up all the communicative space with verbalizations. Give the child an opportunity to initiate conversation.

9. Stay on a topic long enough to converse about it. Do not change topics after the child says one utterance on the issue. This approach encourages a series of "one-liners" from children, and the clinician is again placed in the position of having to interrogate. It also interferes with the clinician's ability to gather a sample that is appropriate for analyzing conversational mechanisms, such as topic maintenance.

10. Finally, be aware of children's cognitive levels when you ask questions. The clinician should be aware that children have differing conceptual frameworks from those of adults, as well as altered perspectives of time and space. We have heard clinicians ask three-year-olds questions such as, "Why do you think the truck goes so fast?" Conversely, we do not want to ask questions that are cogni-tively too simple for older students.

There are variables that appear to affect the length and complexity of language samples obtained by researchers and examiners. First, the racial/cultural backgrounds of the participants could have a potential influence on a child's conversation. Several studies have suggested that young Black children may engage in style shifting or code switching when confronted with a White, adult examiner (Cazden, 1970; Labov 1970). Cazden (1970) has stated that Black children speak in a school register (for teachers and administrators) and a street register (for peers and family). Interestingly, the school register is different in content, has a shorter MLU, is less complex, and is more disfluent than the street register. Similarly, Harris (1985) reviewed the literature on assessing language in Native American children and reports that "Indian children tend to be nonverbal in totally teacher-directed activities, especially activities in which verbal responses are demanded of the participants" (48). Of course, everyone style shifts to some degree when conversing with another person from different social, cultural, educational, and economic backgrounds. This certainly has implications for language sampling. Clinicians should realize that the samples they obtain from young children from a cultural group different from their own may underestimate linguistic abilities.

Verbalizations of the examiner also may affect language sampling. Lee (1974) suggests that the clinician attempt to speak with a variety of syntactic structures when sampling a child's language. The modeling literature has shown that children, in as little as a single session, can use language that is roughly similar in complexity to an adult model, whether the model uses extremely simple sentences or complex sentences involving embedding and conjoining (Haynes and Hood 1978). Children are also sensitive to pragmatic aspects of a communicative situation. If they are placed in a play situation with younger children, their language will be simpler than it would be if they were talking to adults (Sachs and Devin 1976).

Presupposition also may play a role in the length and complexity of samples obtained from children. Like adults, children will elaborate linguistically about objects and events that are not present in the current communicative context (Strandberg and Griffith 1969). If a child does not share visual access to the stimuli with the clinician, he/she will tend to elaborate linguistically to a greater degree (Haynes, Purcell, and Haynes 1979).

Several studies have shown that children provide longer and more-complex language samples if they are engaging in conversation as opposed to performing picture description tasks (Haynes, Purcell, and Haynes 1979; Longhurst and File 1977; Longhurst and Grubb 1974). Picture description tends to lend itself to the naming of elements in a picture rather than elaborating linguistically about a topic unknown to the clinician. These are typically single-word responses or elliptical answers. Most important, if the clinician views the picture with the child, the task becomes not one of conversing but of naming aspects of pictures. In the studies mentioned above, the children evidenced longer and more-complex language samples when they were engaging in conversation than when they were describing pictures or objects. Conversation, of course, carries with it an element of presupposition because the clinician does not know what the child will talk about and there is no contextual support for things removed in time and space. Thus, the child is forced to linguistically elaborate since the clinician is not aware of the conversational aspects that the child is attempting to convey. Picture description, however, is a viable method of sampling language for some children. Certainly, some children will not readily engage in conversation, and picture description is needed to elicit some language for analysis (Atkins and Cartwright 1982). Evans and Craig (1992) have found an interview approach that elicits more language than a free-play scenario does.

We have seen that obtaining a language sample is a critical part of doing a language evaluation. There are a host of variables that can affect the size and quality of the sample obtained by the examiner. These variables, and their effect on sample size, may play a major role in the clinician's interpretation of the student's language sample and must be considered when analyzing the client's communicative ability.

Later Language Development: Emerging Data

Structural analysis of a language sample can compare the child's production to the growing stockpile of normative data on youngsters between the ages of nine and eighteen years of age (Nippold 1988, 1993). During the period from late elementary through high school there are slow but systematic changes in measurements, such as sentence length (Klecan-Aker and Hedrick 1985; Loban 1976; Morris and Crump 1982), use of subordinate clauses (Scott 1988), understanding of cohesive devices (Nippold, Schwarz, and Undlin 1992), and use of the literate lexicon and figurative language (Nippold 1993). These measurements may be sensitive to discourse genre (conversation, narrative, formal speech) and modality (speaking vs. writing) and the clinician must be mindful of such influences. However, some of the studies mentioned above provide concrete measurements that a clinician could use in documenting the existence of language impairment or clinical changes as the result of treatment.

Testing Language Comprehension

Bransford and Nitsch (1978) point out that comprehension involves a situation plus an input. A human organism is not a static system but has a current state of excitation, a history, and background knowledge. A given input of language is placed in this situation along with the nonverbal context of communication. Many variables come to bear on the understanding of an input, not the least of which are the person's background, as well as the linguistic and nonlinguistic contexts. Rees and Shulman (1978) have written an article in which they indicate that most tests of language comprehension measure only the literal meanings of utterances. For example, if asked to point to a picture of a boy who is running, the child can choose the correct picture and not point to one of a boy who is standing. Thus, the child understands the notions of "boy" and "run" and can discriminate them from other literal meanings, such as "standing." But comprehension involves so much more than the literal meaning of utterances. Miller and Paul (1995) provide several examples of other types of comprehension knowledge, as illustrated in Table 5.5. As another example, the skill of inferencing is used in almost every interaction and certainly many times during a school day. To fully comprehend an utterance such as "It's supposed to rain today, but I forgot my umbrella," one must infer that the person may get wet, although this is never specifically stated. Another broader notion of comprehension has to do with understanding the main point in a narrative, lecture, or conversation. If a child cannot comprehend the main point in a lecture, this is certainly as much of a comprehension problem as not understanding literal meanings. Comprehension of figurative language such as idioms and metaphors involves more than just literal meaning. If a teacher says, "This science project should really shine," the child should know that the teacher does not mean that the project requires lights (Simon, 1987).

We must go past the idea of assessing literal meanings when dealing with comprehension assessment. Most comprehension tests are quite artificial when compared

TABLE 5.5 Selected Types of Comprehension Knowledge (adapted from Miller and Paul 1995)

- **Knowledge of literal meaning:** "Show me the picture of the monkey."

  A correct response would be to point to the monkey to show literal knowledge of the requested item.

- **Social knowledge:** "Do you want to be sent to your room without supper?"

  This is not a question from a mother to a child. It is actually a threat and requires knowledge of the situation to interpret appropriately.

- **Knowledge of sincerity conditions:** "Is the Pope Catholic?"

  When someone produces this question, we know that this is just another way of saying "Yes" in a conversation and is not a query about the religious affiliation of the Pontiff.

- **Knowledge of cohesive devices:** "He fixed the car."

  One cannot comprehend this sentence correctly unless information from outside the utterance is considered. The listener must be able to figure out who "he" is and whose vehicle was repaired.

- **Knowledge of presupposition:** "They managed to sell their house."

  A listener must know not only that the people sold their home, but that it was done with some difficulty because of the word "managed."

- **General world knowledge:** "It's raining."

  Miller and Paul (1995) give an example of poll workers who know that rainy weather often results in low voter turnout, and thus the above utterance takes on special meaning beyond simply talking about the weather.

- **Specific background knowledge:** "I'm the Michael Jordan of soccer."

  Unless the listener knew about the prowess of this famous basketball player, it would be difficult to know that the utterance refers to playing soccer exceptionally well.

to the richness of language comprehension in a natural situation. The typical comprehension assessment situation involves presenting a child with test plates containing pictures. The child is asked to point to the picture that best represents some verbal stimulus uttered by the examiner. The pictures are often line drawings, and the verbal stimuli are not discursively related to one another (in one case the child is asked to point to a "monkey," and in the next plate the topic is "shopping"). In these tests there is no temporal sequence of events that would allow a child to be able to predict what will be said, as in real language comprehension. Naturalistic situations also give the child the opportunity to ask for clarification or repetition in the face of information loss. The notion of comprehension monitoring implies that we are always scanning to determine if we are understanding someone's utterances; and if we do not understand, we initiate repair sequences that can clarify information that we do not comprehend. We do not afford children this chance in comprehension testing. In fact, we are often forbidden by the examiner's manual from presenting a stimulus a second time, even if the child asks for a repetition! The above statements are meant only to reinforce the notion that real language comprehension is a highly complex phenomenon and cannot be assessed easily.

Millen and Prutting (1979) studied three language comprehension tests for consistency of response on specific grammatical features. They found that on the Northwestern Syntax Screening Test (NSST), Assessment of Children's Language Comprehension (ACLC), and Bellugi Comprehension Test there was general agreement in the overall scores generated by the measures. There were, however, significant differences among the tests for more than half of the specific grammatical features evaluated. The investigators logically suggest that the tests are not equivalent and not clinically sound for generating specific remediation targets. Other stimulus, task, and subject variables have been studied in comprehension tests. Haynes and McCallion (1981) found that on the Test of Auditory Comprehension of Language (TACL) children with a reflective cognitive tempo, or long decision time, performed significantly better than impulsive children with a short decision time. Further, these researchers reported that scores on the TACL improved significantly over standard administration when the subjects were given two stimulus presentations or if the test was administered imitatively.

Thus, it appears that variables other than language comprehension enter into test performance, and failure to do well on a comprehension test could be explained by other factors. Attentional set, hearing impairment, ambiguous pictures, test administration procedures (Shorr 1983), cognitive style, and unrelated stimuli—all could account for poor performance on a standardized test of language comprehension. Additionally, Gowie and Powers (1979) showed that a child's expectations about what a sentence was going to say significantly influenced their performance on a comprehension task. Gowie and Powers observed that "knowing a word involves a set of expectations about the referents and about the types of messages in which the word is likely to occur" (40).

We have suggested that comprehension is difficult to test in limited-language cases without contaminating influences from the context and the child's use of comprehension strategies. Further, we have said that failure to perform well on a test of comprehension does not necessarily indicate the presence of a comprehension disorder. Based on the current literature, about all we can say with some conviction is that adequate performance on a standardized test of language comprehension probably means that the child is capable of comprehending some language in a highly artificial situation. This does not necessarily represent comprehension ability in natural situations. Failure of a comprehension test, on the other hand, does not necessarily mean that the child is incapable of comprehending language either in the contrived testing situation or the natural environment.

Currently, language comprehension is tested in four ways by SLPs. First, there are a number of standardized tests of comprehension (See Appendix 5.A). Second, some researchers have tested comprehension by having children act out certain commands (Leonard et al. 1978). Third, several investigators have used a decision task in which the child makes judgments such as "good or bad" or engages in a preference task to say which of two sentences was the best. Finally, similar to the standardized tests, clinicians have used pictures and/or objects and have engaged children in an informal pointing task. Miller and Paul (1995) have developed an impressive series of nonstandardized comprehension assessment tasks for use with clients from under twelve months of age to those over ten years old. Each task is directly related to a developmental level, and detailed instructions are provided for administration, scoring, and interpretation. Perhaps the "best" method of comprehension testing would be to examine it via several methods, both formal and informal. The clinician should utilize more naturalistic assessment methods such as engaging the child in play or conversation and evaluating the appropriateness of verbal and nonverbal responses. Observation in the classroom combined with teacher and parent interviews can provide valuable insight into comprehension in everyday situations. It also should be noted if the child uses requests for clarification or repetition in conversation. Research has shown that these clarification/repetition requests can be successfully elicited by the clinician by using informal probes (Brinton and Fujiki 1989).

When a child does not comprehend an utterance, the clinician should systematically determine where the process of understanding begins to break down. Unfortunately, no single test is presently available to solve this dilemma; however, several researchers have made progress in this area (Miller and Paul 1995). For older children, clinicians can systematically experiment with the variables listed in Table 5.6 to determine where the breakdown occurs.

Assessment of Syntax by Using Elicited Imitation

Elicited imitation has been used in psycholinguistic research on language development for decades (Slobin and Welsh 1971). There is a correlation between age, on the one hand, and the ability to imitate sentences of increasing length and complexity, on the other (Brown 1973). Elicited imitation, as an assessment procedure, carries with it certain assumptions that the SLP user must believe to be true about language and linguistic processing. A basic assumption of imitative techniques is

TABLE 5.6   Selected Evaluation Areas to Determine Source of Comprehension Breakdown

Input Variables

- *Complexity of vocabulary (semantics).* Does comprehension break down when the vocabulary increases in complexity? Does the child lack knowledge of the literal meanings of words?
- *Syntactic complexity.* Does comprehension break down as sentences become more complex?
- *Sentence length.* Does comprehension break down as sentences become longer?
- *Context.* Does comprehension improve when there is a clear physical context to support the utterance? Does comprehension break down in decontextualized utterances?

Internal Variables

- *Auditory acuity.* Does comprehension break down because of hearing impairment?
- *Attentional abilities.* Does comprehension improve when a child is given a "set" to attend or when there is less distractions in the context?
- *Comprehension monitoring.* Does comprehension improve when a child is asked to continuously judge whether he/she understands utterances and to ask for repairs?

Specific Problems

- *Intersentence relations.* Does comprehension break down when meaning must be derived from analysis of multiple sentences?
- *Cohesion.* Does comprehension break down when the listener must derive the meaning of cohesive devices (e.g., pronouns) from prior discourse?
- *World or specific knowledge.* Does comprehension break down when the topic requires general or when it requires specific types of world knowledge?

---

that children will repeat only those structures for which they have linguistic competence. If a child omits or misuses a syntactic element in a sentence imitation task, the examiner must suspect that the child does not have that element in his/her repertoire. Conversely, if the child does imitate an item, it is assumed that the youngster has that structure. This basic assumption of elicited imitation has been challenged during the last decade, and investigators have explored variables that affect the elicited imitation response other than linguistic competence.

Some studies have shown that nonlinguistic context (e.g., use of pictures or objects) in conjunction with elicited imitation may increase correct performance (Haniff and Siegel 1981; Nelson and Weber-Olsen 1980). A context may assist children in remembering elements presented in a model sentence or may allow them to focus on more-obscure aspects of a sentence since the major subject-verb-object elements are depicted for them. One study, however, does not support the finding that context improves imitative performance (Connell and Myles-Zitzer 1982).

Elicited imitation also is affected by stress patterns present in the model sentence (Blasdell and Jensen 1970; Slobin and Welsh 1971). Two studies have suggested a trial or practice effect in elicited imitation (Haynes and Haynes 1979; Lang and Moore 1977). Haynes and Haynes (1979) gave children a sentence imitation task two times separated by two days. They found that over 52% of the children's errors on the first trial had been corrected on the second trial even though only two days separated the performances. Interestingly, 22% of the children's errors remained the same, and 25% of the errors on the second day were new ones that had not occurred at all on the first trial. Fujiki and Brinton (1983) reported that sampling reliability for elicited imitation may not stabilize until a syntactic structure is repeated over three trials. This certainly gives one pause when contemplating the administration of an elicited imitation test in a single trial.

Bonvillian, Raeburn, and Horan (1979) found that there were significantly more errors on longer sentences, those sentences presented at faster speech rates, and less errors on the longer sentences when normal intonation patterns were used as compared to a monotone presentation.

Several investigators have expressed concern about the validity of elicited imitation as being representative of spontaneous grammatical performance (Connell and Myles-Zitzer 1982; Daily and Boxx 1979; McDade, Simpson, and Larnt 1982; Prutting, Gallagher, and Mulac 1975; Werner and Kreseck 1981). Bloom (1974) has reported a case of a child who was incapable of effectively imitating his own spontaneous utterances that were recorded and transcribed from a prior session. Bloom attributed this performance decrement to a lack of context during the imitative task.

From the above general review, it can be seen that performance on an elicited imitation task is affected by many variables. If this is true, then we cannot be certain what elicited imitation is measuring. Further, many studies have shown that elicited imitation performance can agree with or differ from spontaneous speech performance. As Prutting and Connolly (1976) so aptly state: "Elicited imitations alone may underestimate, overestimate or accurately describe the child's language performance" (420). On a theoretical plane, elicited imitation violates the integrative model of language because it separates structure from function and uses unrelated utterances with no communicative intent. There are several advantages to the use of elicited imitation, however. First, an imitative task can be administered in a short time, usually under fifteen minutes. Second, with imitation, the clinician can assess specific structures instead of waiting for them to appear spontaneously in a language sample. Third, some tests (Carrow 1974) include normative data for comparing children's performance in order to solve the problem/no problem issue. There are several tests that have been constructed in an elicited imitation format (Carrow 1974; Zachman et al. 1978). The present authors feel that elicited imitation is a useful procedure, but clinicians should never rely solely on an imitative assessment. Treatment targets should only be selected from spontaneous language samples; and if imitative techniques are used, they should always be supplemented by spontaneous performance.

Assessment of Syntax by Using Analysis Packages

After the SLP has obtained a language sample, judgments must be made regarding the syntactic development of the child. Analysis of syntax can be conceptualized on a continuum. On the left end of the continuum is the administration of formal tests. These measures can give the clinician some insight into general syntactic development. In the middle of the continuum, the clinician can analyze a language sample in accordance with specific packaged assessment procedures (Lee 1974) and obtain more precise information than is available from standardized tests. Finally, on the right end, the clinician can analyze the sample by using knowledge of linguistics and language development and does not have to rely on a step-by-step package analysis procedure (Hubbell 1988; Kahn and James 1980; Lund and Duchan 1993; Muma 1973b; Retherford 1993). The left end of the continuum requires less expertise than does the right end in terms of clinician experience and training. The left end of the continuum takes less time for the analysis than does the right, but also provides less clinically relevant information. Thus, the clinician must make a decision as to the time available for the analysis, training and expertise in linguistics, and the depth of information desired.

It is beyond the scope of the present chapter to instruct clinicians in performing an analysis of a child's syntax. The best way to learn an analysis system is to obtain a sample and follow the guidelines provided by authors of complexity analysis packages. Typically, the authors provide explicit instructions for obtaining a sample, segmentation, and analysis. Beginning clinicians should realize that any syntactic analysis method requires practice in order to be used effectively. The most widely known analysis procedures are listed in Table 5.7.

Muma (1978) points out that descriptive procedures have greater power than normative ones do because they help the clinician to describe individual differences. Descriptive procedures, because they are based on spontaneous language samples, also provide the clinician with more-relevant intervention targets since these procedures do not fracture the integrity of the content-form-use model as imitative and standardized tests do. Thus, there are advantages to performing a descriptive analysis, and package systems provide the clinician with guidelines for

TABLE 5.7   Selected Language Sample Analysis Procedures

- Assessing Children's Language in Naturalistic Contexts (Lund and Duchan 1993)
- Assigning Structural Stage (Miller 1981)
- Co-Occurring and Restricted Structures Analysis (Muma 1973b)
- Developmental Sentences Analysis (Lee 1974)
- Indiana Scale of Clausal Development (Dever and Bauman 1974)
- Language Assessment, Remediation and Screening Procedure (Crystal, Fletcher, and Garman 1976)
- Language Sampling, Analysis and Training (Tyack and Gottsleben 1974)
- Length Complexity Index (Miner 1969)
- Length of T-Unit or Communication Unit (Loban 1976)
- Linguistic Analysis of Speech Samples (Engler, Hannah, and Longhurst 1973)
- Mean Length of Utterance and Distributional Analysis (Miller 1981)
- Method for Assessing Use of Grammatical Structures (Kahn and James 1980)
- Structural Complexity Score (McCarthy 1930)

From: Owens, (1996) *Language Development: An Introduction* (Needham Heights, MA).

completing such an analysis. We should, however, remember that each analysis procedure reflects the author's bias regarding language, and that most systems look at a language sample in only limited ways.

Consumers who intend to use an analysis package should be aware that the procedures differ importantly. These differences may determine whether or not a clinician finds it appropriate to use a particular package. We will use the Developmental Sentence Scoring (DSS) procedure in our examples since this methodology is widely known and is still regarded as a viable assessment procedure some twenty years after its development (Hughes, Fey, and Long, 1992). Using this procedure in our discussion is not meant to be a criticism or an endorsement of this particular approach.

1. Some package systems recommend obtaining a specific sample size before subjecting the language to analysis. For instance, Lee (1974) recommends using 50 subject-verb utterances for computation of the DSS. A later study, however, stated that a sample of 150 utterances may be more appropriate for reliable scoring. If the clinician does not have a large enough sample, perhaps a different procedure would be more appropriate.

2. The analysis packages vary considerably in the time required for completion. This may be due to several influences. First, some procedures are quite detailed and lengthy (Bloom and Lahey 1978; Crystal, Fletcher, and Garman 1976). Other procedures use very specific terminologies and vocabulary or have complicated scoring systems that require much time and practice in order for the clinician to use the procedure economically.

3. The procedures differ in terms of how they segment or separate utterances obtained in the sample. The DSS, for instance, analyzes subject-verb utterances and does not score sentence fragments. Some clinicians, however, feel that there is much useful information in sentence fragments (e.g., elliptical responses) that may be important to analyze.

4. Some systems are recommended by their authors as ideal for use with particular treatment approaches. Lee, Koenigsknecht, and Mulhern (1975) use the DSS as an input to their interactive language teaching strategy and continue to monitor progress by using the system.

5. Another way that evaluation systems differ is in terms of the structures they do or do not analyze. For example, the DSS does not specifically analyze certain forms (e.g., prepositions and articles) and accounts for their presence or absence by assigning a "sentence point" to an utterance if it is grammatical. Other systems specifically analyze most structural elements of English, even structures that may not be of interest to the clinician.

6. Analysis packages differ in their provision of normative data. The DSS has normative data, while some other packages are purely descriptive and make no attempt to gather numerical scores on normal and disordered children.

7. Finally, the analysis procedures are not uniform in applying the results to a normal-language-development progression. That is, some procedures are designed to examine linguistic elements without locating the child on a language development continuum. Others apply their results to the normal developmental progression

(Crystal, Fletcher, and Garman 1976; Lahey 1988; Lee 1974; Miller 1981). Research has shown that many aspects of syntactic and morphological acquisition in children with language impairments develop in an order similar to that found in normally developing children (Paul and Alforde 1993).

Several investigations have shown that some of the package analysis procedures appear to be capable of documenting language changes in children, at least in a general way (Hughes, Fey, and Long 1992; Longhurst and Schrandt 1973; Sharf 1972). Furthermore, any method that a clinician selects will require specific training and practice in order to use it effectively. It should be remembered that any method used depends to a significant degree on the quality of the sample obtained and typically analyzes only the structural elements of language independent of pragmatics. Thus, any analysis package procedure will take the clinician time and practice to learn, and in the end will look at language only from a specific point of view (Miller 1981). It is the preference of the present authors that if clinicians are going to spend time learning about analysis of the structural aspects of language, their time would be better spent learning linguistics and language acquisition instead of one specific analysis package that probably would not be appropriate for all clients. An analysis package could always be learned later to supplement the clinician's linguistic knowledge and would probably be learned more easily owing to the experience with linguistics. A knowledge of linguistics would allow the clinician to generally analyze samples for structures that are present, absent, and inconsistent and to still choose treatment targets that are relevant, instead of trying to find a package analysis procedure that is of "best fit" for the child. There are a number of fine textbooks that provide information on sentence structure and one of them should be a reference in the professional library of every SLP (Hubbell 1988; Quirk and Greenbaum 1975). We feel that, ultimately, the clinician must determine (1) which structures the child appears to have acquired, (2) which structures are absent in obligatory contexts, (3) which structures are inconsistently used, and (4) which contexts seem to be associated with use and nonuse of the inconsistent structures. Muma (1973b) and Kahn and James (1980) have advocated such descriptive procedures that focus on determining present, absent, and inconsistent syntactic elements, and we view this as a commonsense approach to analysis that has direct clinical application. It also does not involve the clinician's commitment of time to learning one or two package procedures and their unique scoring systems. Tables 5.8 and 5.9 provide a hypothetical sample and analysis.

Recently, computer analyses of language samples have come to the fore. Software programs are available that provide detailed information about a language sample; however, the clinician must remember that some time is typically invested in coding the transcript into the computer. In some cases, this may take more time than a paper-and-pencil analysis, if the clinician merely wants to define treatment targets. In addition, the computer analyses may provide the clinician with more information than is really needed. The output from these programs is truly phenomenal. For example, Lingquest 1 (Mordecai, Palin, and Palmer 1982) performs a lexical analysis that includes specific assessment of nouns, verbs, modifiers, con-

TABLE 5.8   General Guidelines for Syntactic Analysis of Language Sample

- Obtain a converstional sample.
- Transcribe the sample orthographically (or in phonetics if the client has misarticulations).
- Locate errors in sample:
  Find sentences containing errors and highlight them.
  Mark specific errors within the highlighted sentences (circle them).
- Make a list of forms/structures the child uses correctly.
- Make a list of forms/structures the child consistently misuses (never correct).
- Make a list of forms/structures the child inconsistently misuses.
- For inconsistently misused forms/structure make a list of contexts:
  List contexts where form/structure is correct.
  List contexts where form/structure is incorrect.
- Common variables to consider regarding contextual influence:
  Syntactic complexity of sentence
  Semantic complexity of lexical items used in sentence
  Type of sentence (e.g., question, declarative)
  Phonological complexity of sentence
  Pragmatic variables (e.g., listener uncertainty; narrative)
- Look for possible patterns using above variables that account for when error occurs and does not occur.

junctions, prepositions, negation, interjections, and WH words, as well as over eighty subcategories of parts of speech. A type-token ratio also is computed. In analyzing grammatical structure, a variety of phrase and sentence types are identified as well as an analysis of verb tense. Mean length of utterance in words and morphemes is also computed. Computerized Profiling (Long and Fey 1993) is a most useful program that does detailed phonological analysis, semantic analysis, LARSP (Crystal, Fletcher, and Garman 1976), DSS (Lee 1974), conversational acts profile, prosodic analysis, single-word analysis, and early multiword analysis. The outputs from this program are quite complex and it is reasonably priced and user friendly. The Systematic Analysis of Language Transcripts (SALT) program (Miller and Chapman 1995) also provides analyses of specific grammatical classes and computes numerical indices similar to the other programs mentioned above. Additionally, SALT contains a very flexible search program that allows the user to address specific questions regarding specific words or constructions. The above programs probably represent the most comprehensive and detailed applications to date; and by the time the present text is published, there will no doubt be others.

The advantage of the computer would appear to lie in the multiple analyses that could be performed once the sample is inputted. That is, a clinician can take the same transcript and analyze it for insight into the child's semantic system, phonological system, syntactic system, and occurrence of speech acts (if appropriately coded). An important point to emphasize is that these programs are only as good as the coding of the language sample that they analyze. Some of the programs mentioned above

TABLE 5.9   Transcript Analysis Example

1. Grant got one of them.	17. Him go to the hospital.
2. Him go flop flop.	18. Thats a hospital.
3. It go like that.	19. They are too big.
4. They have a wagon.	20. I running fast.
5. Jay is my brother.	21. They boys are driving a car.
6. Somebody drop a glass on the floor.	22. The cat is sleeping.
7. Him live at that house.	23. Her feed the baby.
8. Him the boy that live next door.	24. Her have a cold.
9. They are going to town.	25. We have to let him in car.
10. Him riding a bike.	26. We ride in car and go fast.
11. It is at home	27. A boy on the rocker and one in house.
12. Her going fast.	28. They in parking lot while the boy sleep.
13. I don't know	29. The cat is running up the drapes.
14. Smudge is a boy cat.	30. The girl is holding her ears.
15. I four years old and I live in Eufaula.	31. Him carrying a box of apples.
16. It brown and brick.	

Selected Forms Used

Proper noun	Uncontractible copula
Irregular verb	Personal pronoun ("my," "I")
Cardinal number	Prepositions
Plural pronoun	Definite article
Verbs	Auxillary ("are")
Demonstrative ("that")	Present progressive
Adverbial of manner	Auxillary ("do")
Indefinite pronoun ("somebody")	Adjective
Verb "have"	Conjunctions ("and," "while")
Nondefinite article	Plural ("boys")
Nouns	

Errors	*Errors Consistently Misused*
"him"/"he" (objective for subjective pronominal case)	"him"/"he"
	3rd person "-s"
"go"/"goes"; "live"/"lives"; "feed"/"feeds"; "sleep"/"sleeps" (3rd person sing.)	Regular past "-ed" (1 instance)
	Omitted copula "am"
"drop"/"dropped" (regular past "-ed")	"have"/"has"
Omitted copula "is"	
Omitted auxillary "is"	
Omitted copula "am"	
"have"/"has"	
Omitted definite article	
Omitted copula "are"	

automatically classify lexical items or grammatical forms based on internal algorithms. Most programs allow the clinician to change these a priori classifications of transcript items if they are incorrect. That is, sometimes a program will not identify a word or grammatical construction correctly, and the clinician needs to check how the computer has classified transcript items. There is no substitute for close

TABLE 5.9 *Continued*

Errors Inconsistently Misused	*Context When Inconsistent Error Was Absent*
Omitted copula "is"	Copula "is":
Omitted auxillary "is"	#8 high complexity, embedding,
Omitted definite article	"him"/"he" substitution
Omitted copula "are"	#16 complex, conjoining and deleting
	#27 complex, conjoining
	Auxillary "is":
	#10 "him"/"he" substitution
	#12 "her"/"she" substitution
	#31 "him"/"he" substitution
	Copula "are":
	#28 complex, conjoining
	Definite article:
	#25 complex, embedding
	#26 complex, embedding
	#27 complex, embedding
	#28 complex, embedding

Context of Inconsistent Errors When Present

Copula "is":	Definite article:
#5 simple, "Jay is . . ."	#6 simple
#11 simple, "It is . . . "	#17 simple
#14 simple, "Smudge is . . . "	#21 simple
#18 "That is . . . "	#22 simple
Auxillary *is*:	#23 simple
#22 simple, "The cat is . . . "	#27 complex, conjoining
#29 simple, "The cat is . . . "	#28 complex, conjoining
#30 simple, "The girl is . . . "	#29 simple
Copula *are*:	#30 simple
#9 simple, *They are* . . .	
#19 simple, *They are* . . .	
#21 simple, *The boys are* . . .	

clinician monitoring when using these programs. Just because the computer pumps out a profile or summary of a child's performance, does not mean that the clinician should not at least spot-check the analysis for correctness. It is easy to be seduced into relying on complex summaries without checking on validity.

No doubt we will learn much in the next decade from these procedures about patterns of error and subtypes of language disorder. No single procedure can tell a clinician all he/she needs to know about a child's language. Again, ultimately it is the clinician's judgment that must be applied to a particular case, whether it is a decision to choose among several package analysis systems, computer-assisted analysis, or to simply focus on a more specific descriptive linguistic analysis.

Assessment of Conversational Pragmatics

Many reports exist in the literature that attest to pragmatic differences in children with language impairments. Some investigations report that these children have difficulty organizing narratives and staying on a topic (Johnston 1982; Lucas 1980). Fey and Leonard (1983) have hypothesized that there may be subgroups of language-impaired children who exhibit a variety of pragmatic problems. There have been reports of children with language disorders who have difficulty taking listener perspective into account (Muma 1975). Unfortunately, there are no tests that tap all relevant aspects of conversational pragmatics. While there are some formal measures that focus on limited facets of pragmatic ability (Blagden and McConnell 1983; Shulman 1986), it would be difficult to develop a broader assessment device because of the many aspects included under the rubric of pragmatics. Conversational abilities are also difficult to tap by using artificial tasks, limited samples, or contrived topics of discourse. If the clinician is interested in conversational abilities, there is no substitute for legitimate conversation. When the clinician focuses on conversation and discourse, it is necessary to obtain a sample of the child's conversational performance and to transcribe both the utterances of the child and of the interlocuter. This transcription is a time-consuming task; however, if the clinician is to obtain data on the child's conversational performance, the contributions of both participants cannot be ignored. There are several measures that the clinician might elect to use to analyze conversation, depending on which aspects of the discourse are of interest. Some of these measures may overlap to a certain degree. The present authors recommend beginning at a general level and then progressing to more-specific analyses.

Evaluation of General Parameters: Identification of a Potential Problem

Prutting and Kirchner (1987) developed a pragmatic protocol that gives an overall communicative index for children, adolescents, and adults. It includes thirty pragmatic aspects of language in the broad groupings of verbal, paralinguistic, and nonverbal skills. There are specific definitions for each parameter used in the system, and they provide preliminary data on both adults and children with normal and disordered language. This approach to evaluating a child's pragmatic abilities begins with a molar view of conversational performance to determine if certain types of errors are especially obvious to the clinician. Prutting and Kirchner (1987) rated children's conversation on the thirty parameters. The most-inappropriate pragmatic parameters found in forty-two children with language impairments involved turn taking, specificity/accuracy, cohesion, repair/revision, topic maintenance, and intelligibility. Use of the protocol described above at the very least forces the clinician to consider the relevant parameters of pragmatics and to make a judgment regarding each. Then more-concentrated evaluation tasks can be applied to the case that might define the nature of the conversational errors more specifically. Similarly, Damico (1985) has developed a screening tool that has been used successfully by teachers in identifying children with pragmatic disorders. This instrument includes a rating scale, to be completed by teachers, that focuses on common symptoms of pragmatic disorders as well as academic skills. Another more detailed system is recommended by Bedrosian (1985). Again, this type of approach moves from general to more specific in terms of evaluating language in older students. More molecular analyses can be initiated after a student is identified by a general procedure.

Narrowing the Focus: Assessment of Narrative Production

Narratives give an "account of happenings," as in telling a story, and adhere to some definable conventions or rules in the children's generation (Liles 1993). Educational research has suggested that narratives are a bridge between oral language and literacy since their structure resembles written text. Narrative skills have been shown to reliably predict academic success in children who are normally developing as well as those with learning disabilities and a specific language disorder (Owens 1995; Paul 1995). Narratives are seen repeatedly in our daily discourse as we talk to others about weekend experiences, tell jokes, explain a process to a teacher, relate anecdotes, gossip, and describe our activities and possessions to impress our listeners. Thus, narratives are important academically as well as socially and communicatively. The narrative has been a topic of research interest over the past decade because it synthesizes a variety of abilities in order to be effective. For example, the ability to tell a story involves skill in sequencing events, creative cohesive text, use of precise vocabulary, nonreliance on contextual support, and understanding of universal story grammar to structure the narrative production. According to Liles (1993):

> There is a consistency across investigators regarding the structural limitations of young children's narratives and the apparent acceleration in development around age 5. Researchers analyzing the structure of narratives in older children have generally agreed that by age 6 children can produce an ideal (e.g., adult) structure, but development continues in 9- and 10-year old children. The development of narrative structure in older children is evidenced by both an increased number of episodes and the children's growing ability to link them together in complex ways (e.g., embedding one episode within another). More recent studies investigating narrative structure in older children (Purcell & Liles, 1992; Roth & Speckman, 1986) found that the number of complete episodes continued to increase in the narratives of children aged 8 to 16 years. (875)

As narrative productions develop in children and become more complex, increasingly more elements of story grammar are incorporated into the narrative (Applebee 1978; Johnston 1982; Paul 1995). For example, story grammar typically includes a description of the *setting*, which includes the environmental context as well as the main characters. Another component is the *initiating event*, which is some action, event, or change in the environment that affects the characters. This is often a "problem" of some sort (e.g., eruption of a volcano). Characters generally have an *internal response* to the initiating event, which may include emotions, goals, thoughts, and intentions leading to a plan of action. This plan of action leads to *attempts* or actions directed toward resolving the situation/problem or attaining a goal. Next, the attempts will result in *consequences,* which will either result in the resolution of the problem or the attainment of the goal or in the failure to deal adequately with the situation. Finally, the character will have a *reaction* to the consequence mentioned above, which includes internal states (e.g., feelings, thoughts). As narratives become more complex, the child will include more of the above elements in the production.

Studies of children with a specific language disorder have revealed narratives with some of the following characteristics (Merritt and Liles 1989; Owens 1995):

- Fewer total words
- Fewer different words
- Fewer story grammar components
- Fewer complete episodes
- Fewer protagonist plans and internal responses
- Fewer conventional story openings/closings
- Improper amounts of information (too much/little)
- Fewer successful repairs
- Fewer accommodations to listeners
- Fewer complete cohesive ties and more incomplete/erroneous ties

Clinicians who wish to analyze narratives in children with language impairments might look for some of the differences mentioned above. As children become older, their language disorders often take on more-subtle characteristics. The impairment may not be revealed in structural errors, but may become obvious on a pragmatic-conversational level. Narrative analysis is a valuable adjunct to our assessment repertoire and is regarded as an important diagnostic consideration by most current authorities (Paul 1995; Owens 1995). We must also remember that narrative production may vary according to a person's culture. Gutierrez-Clellen and Quinn (1993) indicate that narratives are influenced by a child's information and organization abilities, world knowledge/experience, the type of elicitation task, interactional style, and use of paralinguistic conventions.

Looking for Specific Errors: Clinical Discourse Analysis

Damico (1980, 1985) has taken a different approach and has advocated the analysis of specific discourse errors in children's language. He provides a listing of nine discourse errors that can be detected in conversation and computed into a percentage of utterances containing pragmatic difficulties. He recommends obtaining 180 utterances over two sessions in conversational interaction about home and school activities. The goal of the analysis is to describe specific discourse errors that exist in the interaction. Damico has gathered data on many normal and language-disordered children and proposes some error percentage ranges for determining very generally the existence and severity of a discourse problem and its severity.

Assessment of Contingency

Bloom, Rocissano, and Hood (1976) provide us with guidelines regarding the assessment of contingency, the evaluation of which is also recommended by Gallagher (1982). Contingency is the extent to which a speaker's contribution to a conversation reflects the effect of a previous utterance. Bloom, Rocissano, and Hood (1976) define three types of adjacent utterances: (1) contingent speech, which shares the same topic with the preceding statement and adds new information; (2) imitative speech, which shares the same topic but does not add new information; and (3) noncontingent utterances, which do not share the same topic as prior utterances. Bloom et al. have shown that contingent speech increases between Brown's (1973) language development Stages I and V, while imitative and noncontingent speech decreases. Early in Stage I, children are not particularly contingent and they become progressively more able to stay on a topic and make additional contributions. Obviously, a person cannot be contingent all of the time owing to topic shifts. Children in Stage V were about 50% contingent in their utterances. Thus, one method of analyzing a child's conversational participation is to obtain a molar view of the contingency of the utterances. A child who is not capable of a reasonable degree of contingency will have trouble maintaining topics and perpetuating interactions with others.

Assessment of Topic Manipulation

Topic manipulation is another area that overlaps with contingency, but an analysis of topic may give the clinician slightly different information (Keenan and Schiefflin 1976). Topics may use general knowledge shared by interactants, information physically present in the context or previous discourse. According to Keenan and Schiefflin (1976) much conversational space is taken up by communicators to establish a topic. Once the topic is established, an interactant can use a turn to either maintain the topic (continuous discourse) or change the topic (discontinuous discourse). When speakers continue a discourse topic by corroborating a previous utterance with a related statement, or incorporating information in a prior utterance into their statement, the topic is maintained. When a speaker discontinues a discourse topic, it is either by introducing a topic that is unrelated to previous utterances or by reintroducing a prior topic ("Getting back to what we said about . . ."). Thus, topic-maintaining utterances corroborate a prior statement or incorporate it into a new statement that is still on the topic. Developmentally, the length of continuous discourse increases with age. In assessment, we need to determine how a child is able to secure the attention of a listener in order to initiate a topic (by crying, yelling, gesturing, and tugging, or with loudness, prosody, or an introduction such as "Know what?"). We can measure the length of the topic unit in terms of number of turns taken per topic. We also can measure the topic-maintaining and -shifting utterances used by a child. It is important in assessment to examine a child's ability not only to continue topics but also to initiate them. In sampling, as mentioned previously, we may not often provide for this. Some of the most productive work on in-depth analysis of topic manipulation has been done by Brinton and Fujiki (1984). Brinton and Fujiki (1989) provide detailed procedures for evaluation of all relevant aspects of topic manipulation in clinical work. We need further research to more specifically define the normal development of topic manipulation in both normal and language-impaired children. Some language-impaired children clearly have difficulty with these skills (Prutting and Kirchner 1987), while other subgroups of children with linguistic impairment appear to manipulate topics normally (Edmonds and Haynes 1988; Ehlers and Cirrin 1983). We also need to know more about topic manipulation throughout the lifespan to determine changes in these skills in aging normal subjects since there is some evidence that differences exist among age groups (Stover and Haynes 1989).

Assessment of Repairs: The Contingent Query

Another major category of measurement of conversational competence is the contingent query. A number of studies (Garvey 1977a, 1977b) show that contingent queries are used by adults and children to achieve cohesion in conversation. Children as young as three years use contingent queries. Basically, the queries serve multiple functions in conversation, many of which have to do with repair procedures that allow the conversation to continue. For instance, a contingent query can be used to request a general repetition ("Huh?"), a specific repetition ("A what?"), a request for confirmation ("A tape recorder?"), and elaboration ("We have to go where?"). There are more-complex aspects of contingent queries that are explained in the above references. One can see, however, that these queries are important mechanisms of conversational competence and that a child who does not know how to ask for clarification, for instance, will have difficulty continuing a particular topic with an interactant. The term *conversational repair* has been used most often in association with contingent queries. Clinically, it would be important to determine if a child can both respond to and produce requests for conversational repair (Brinton and Fujiki 1989). For example, we would like to see if a child can adjust an utterance to a listener's request for repetition, clarification or elaboration. On the other hand, we would like to determine if a child would ask for clarification if a clinician asks for a "ferbis" or makes a statement violating truth constraints in a particular context. Brinton and Fujiki (1989) provide many helpful suggestions for both assessment and intervention with conversational repair mechanisms.

Assessment of Cohesive Adequacy

Some children produce narratives or conversational turns that lack adequate cohesion. Cohesion refers to the relationships or ties between elements in discourse that are dependent upon one another (Halliday and Hasan 1976). Stover and Haynes (1989) provide an example:

> *Wash the* dirty dishes *that are in the sink. Dry* them *and then put* them *in the cabinet. In the second sentence* them *refers directly back to the* dirty dishes *thus forming a cohesive tie. Of course, the cohesive marker may extend far beyond the immediately preceding sentence to an utterance produced earlier in the conversation. . . . In a complete tie, the referent to which a cohesive marker refers is easily found in a prior utterance with no ambiguity as in the above example. In an incomplete tie, a cohesive marker refers to something not mentioned in prior utterances (e.g., I like ice cream. He* does too). *In this example* he *cannot be associated with a particular person mentioned previously in the sentence. In an erroneous tie, there is ambiguity or error in interpreting who a referent is (e.g., Tom and Jerry live in the city. He* likes it). *In this example, we do not know if* he *refers to Tom or Jerry.* (140)

Liles (1985) provides specific procedures for cohesion analysis. One can readily see that this type of analysis would be useful in cases that do not take into account the listener's perspective in discourse and that are not aware of the requirements of conversational rules (Grice 1975). Some recent studies suggest that there may be subgroups of children with cohesion difficulties. For example, Craig and Evans (1993) found that children with both receptive and expressive language impairments produced significantly more incomplete, erroneous, and ambiguous cohesive ties compared to children with disorders exclusively in expressive language. Further research is needed on this issue.

Evaluation of Metalinguistic Ability and School Curriculum

As we mentioned at the beginning of this chapter, there are several groups of youngsters that are at high risk to develop a language disorder during the school years. First, children with a history of preschool language delay are likely to experience subtle language disturbances throughout their school years and be at risk for academic problems (Aram and Nation 1980; Bashir et al. 1983; Hall and Tomblin 1978; King, Jones, and Lasky 1982; Strominger and Bashir 1977). These children were often dismissed from language treatment and then later rediagnosed as being reading or learning disabled. Most of these children exhibited low academic achievement throughout school because the curricular demands increase significantly in terms of language and communicative expectations while the child's linguistic abilities may not improve to meet these challenges. A second group of children that is likely to demonstrate subtle language impairments consist of those children diagnosed as being reading or learning disabled. Wiig and Semel (1976) have suggested that the majority of learning-disabled students have experienced language delays and that some of these problems continue into adulthood. Finally, children who are considered to be "academically at risk" because of poor school performance are also likely to have gaps in their ability to perform linguistic tasks (Simon 1989). It is now clear that children with speech-language impairments tend to perform poorly on reading comprehension (Catts 1993). The SLP should carefully evaluate youngsters from the groups mentioned above, especially when referred by classroom teachers. Many of the specific language symptoms likely to be seen in these groups were listed in Table 5.1. A variety of formal tests and nonstandardized assessment procedures have been discussed in the present chapter, and these should serve well in appraising the communication abilities in these children. One aspect that has not been emphasized, however, is specifically examining the types of language and communication abilities that are important for classroom success.

If a school-age child has some subtle language impairments and shows poor academic performance, part of a thorough evaluation should include (1) assessment of the child's knowledge of successful strategies to perform well in the school culture, (2) an evaluation of the teacher's communication while instructing the child, and (3) an assessment of the curriculum and materials that the child is expected to learn. You may wonder why an SLP would be interested in assessing these factors when they are peripheral to the child's abilities. A school-age child is part of a complex system that is constantly changing its expectations for academic performance. The child may have to deal with differing types of educational content and a variety of teaching styles throughout the school day. The school-age child must use language in both comprehension and production for a variety of academic tasks that often involve complex metalinguistic ability and the learning of abstract concepts presented verbally by a teacher. Teachers and SLPs should remember that metalinguistic abilities appear to be acquired in a general developmental order (Table 5.10). Additionally, the child must be aware of the expectations of the school culture and must know how to study, memorize, and effectively learn classroom material upon which he/she will be thoroughly tested. If the child has no effective study skills or strategies for remembering and understanding information, failure will occur. The child's teacher could talk at a rapid rate during instruction or use figurative language and complex sentence types. The teacher could be quite adept at using audio and visual media as aids to instruction or could exclusively rely on the lecture modality. The reading curriculum could have a heavy emphasis on phonics or other metalinguistic tasks that may make the learning of reading extremely difficult or impossible for a child with metalingistic problems. Conversely, the curriculum might emphasize a "whole language" approach with little emphasis on phonics for a child whose phonological awareness is desperately in need of remedial work. In some cases, an alternative approach could help a child learn a particular skill. What we are saying here is that the diagnostician cannot fully understand the language-impaired child unless he/she is familiar with the child's learning environment. Sometimes, the most potent treatment recommendations include curricular, instructional, and learning strategy modifications. Without examining these areas in a thorough assessment, a clinician cannot hope to make effective suggestions for remediation. Obtaining input from teachers and the older child is an important factor in evaluation. Larson and McKinley (1995) and Paul (1995) provide examples of

TABLE 5.10   Development of Metalinguistic Abilities

Stage One (ages 1½ to 2):

- Distinguishes print from nonprint
- Knows how to interact with books: right side up, page turning from left to right
- Recognizes some printed symbols, e.g., TV character's name, brand names, signs

Stage Two (ages 2 to 5½ or 6):

- Ascertains word boundaries in spoken sentences.
- Ascertains word boundaries in printed sequences.
- Engages in word substitution play.
- Plays with the sounds of language.
- Begins to talk about talking (speech acts).
- Corrects own speech/language to help the listener understand the message (spontaneously or in response to listener request).
- Self-monitors own speech and makes changes to more closely approximate the adult model: phonological first, lexical and semantic speech style last.
- Believes that a word is an integral part of the object to which it refers (word realism).
- Able to separate words into syllables.
- Inability to consider that one word could have two different meanings.

Stage Three (ages 6 to 10):

- Begins to take perspective and use language form to match.
- Understands verbal humor involving linguistic ambiguity, e.g., riddles.
- Able to resolve ambiguity; lexical first, as in homophones; deep structures next, as in ambiguous phrases ("Will you join me in a bowl of soup?"); phonological or morphemic next (Q: "What do you have if you put three ducks in a box?" A: "A box of quackers.").
- Able to understand that words can have two meanings, one literal and the other nonconventional or idiomatic, e.g., adjectives used to describe personality characteristics such as *hard, sweet, bitter*.
- Able to resequence language elements, as in pig Latin.
- Able to segment syllables into phonemes.
- Finds it difficult to appreciate figurative forms other than idioms.

Stage Four (ages 10+):

- Able to extend language meaning into hypothetical realm (e.g., to understand figurative language such as metaphors, similies, parodies, analogies).
- Able to manipulate various speech styles to fit a variety of contexts and listeners.

Wallach, G., and Miller, L. (1988), *Language Intervention and Academic Success* (Boston: Butterworth & Heineman), p. 33.

protocols to use in obtaining information from teachers and students with language impairments.

Another area of interest is to assess the child's ability to deal with the types of communication and linguistic tasks typically encountered in the classroom. Some useful measures that focus on classroom communication abilities and/or metalinguistics in older students (e.g., upper elementary through junior high) are Evaluating Communicative Competence (ECC) (Simon 1987), Classroom Communication

Screening Procedure for Early Assessment (CCSPEA) (Simon 1989), and Analysis of the Language of Learning (ALL) (Blodgett and Cooper 1987). These procedures will provide insight into a child's ability to perform classroomlike tasks and will pinpoint specific difficulties. The clinician also can experiment with any facilitating procedures that make difficult tasks more easily accomplished and can mention these in the examination report for teacher use.

A Final Note On Multicultural Variation

Brown (1973) has noted that there are striking similarities in children's language acquisition cross-culturally. That is, children from a variety of cultures tend to develop the same types of early word combinations, presumably because these semantic relations rest on concepts developed in the sensorimotor period of cognitive development. While we may not find differences in word combinations across cultures, there may certainly be variations in prelinguistic and single-word development in various groups. In older children, however, there have been significant differences reported in the development of grammatical morphemes, phonology, vocabulary, specific sentence types, and pragmatics (Dillard 1972; Gutierrez-Clellen 1996; Hester 1996; Hyter and Westby 1996; Mount-Weitz 1996; Quinn, Goldstein, and Pena 1996; Taylor 1986a, 1986b; Williams and Wolfram 1977; Wyatt 1996). We are only beginning to understand the specifics of multicultural variation in later language development, but we are certain that these differences exist. Especially when assessing school-age and adolescent students, it is of paramount importance that the SLP consider cultural differences. While we have not yet developed widely accepted specific procedures for evaluation of clients from a variety of cultures, most authorities suggest that multiple assessment measures should be used (Hamayan and Damico 1991; Stockman 1996; Vaughn-Cooke 1983; Washington 1996). The most promising avenues appear to be criterion-referenced testing, use of ethnographic techniques, and more nonstandardized as opposed to standardized procedures (Lidz and Pena 1996; Robinson-Zanartu 1996; Stockman 1996). It is beyond the scope of the present chapter to outline all the possible linguistic variations produced by the various cultural groups in the United States (e.g., African American, Native American, Hispanic, Asian). The references cited above will provide a good beginning for the clinician in learning about cultural influences on language. It is the ethical responsibility of each SLP to at least become familiar with the dialects spoken in his/her geographical area. Dialectal differences *must* be considered in making judgments about the existence of a disorder, in selecting evaluation procedures, and in recommending treatment goals.

Conclusion

One can easily see that the diagnosis and evaluation of school-age and adolescent clients is a complex activity. The SLP must work closely with teachers, parents, and other professionals in successfully dealing with these cases. The interplay between linguistic, metalinguistic, conversational, and academic areas is great, and the work of the SLP can potentially reap benefits in a child's educational performance.

Bibliography

Applebee, A. (1978). *The Child's Concept of a Story: Ages 2 to 17*. Chicago: University of Chicago Press.

Aram, D., and Nation, J. (1980). "Preschool Language Disorders and Subsequent Language and Academic Difficulties." *Journal of Communication Disorders* 13:159–170.

Aram, D., and Nation, J. (1982). *Child Language Disorders*. St. Louis, MO: Mosby.

Atkins, C., and Cartwright, L. (1982). "An Investigation of the Effectiveness of Three Language Elicitation Procedures on Headstart Children." *Language, Speech and Hearing Services in Schools* 13:33–36.

Barrie-Blackley, S., Musselwhite, C., and Rogister, S. (1978). *Clinical Oral Language Sampling*. Danville, IL: Interstate.

Bashir, A., Kuban, K., Kleinman, S., and Scavuzzo, A. (1983). "Issues in Language Disorders: Considerations of Cause, Maintenance and Change." In *ASHA Report No. 12*, ed. J. Miller, D. Yoder, and R. Shiefelbusch (Rockville, MD: American Speech, Hearing, Language Association.)

Battle, D., et al. (1983). "Position Paper on Social Dialects." *Journal of the American Speech-Language-Hearing Association* 25:23–24.

Bedrosian, J. (1985). "An Approch to Developing Conversational Competence." In *School Discourse Problems*, ed. D. Ripich and F. Spinelli (San Diego: College-Hill Press).

Blagden, C., and McConnell, N. (1983). *Interpersonal Language Skills Assessment*. Moline, IL: Linguisystems.

Blasdell, R., and Jensen, P. (1970). "Stress and Word Position Determinants of Imitation in First Language Learners." *Journal of Speech and Hearing Research* 13:193–202.

Blodgett, E., and Cooper, E. (1987). *Analysis of the Language of Learning: The Practical Test of Metalinguistics*. Moline, IL: Linguisystems.

Bloom, L. (1974). "Talking, Understanding and Thinking." In *Language Perspectives-Acquisition, Retardation and Intervention*, ed. R. Schiefelbusch and L. Lloyd (Baltimore, MD: University Park Press).

Bloom, L., and Lahey, M. (1978). *Language Development and Language Disorders*. New York: Wiley.

Bloom, L., Rocissano, L., and Hood, L. (1976). "Adult-Child Discourse: Developmental Interaction between Information Processing and Linguistic Knowledge." *Cognitive Psychology* 8:521–552.

Bonvillian, J., Raeburn, V., and Horan, E. (1979). "Talking to Children: The Effects of Rate, Intonation and Length on Children's Sentence Imitation." *Journal of Child Language* 3:459–467.

Bransford, J., and Nitsch, K. (1978). "Coming to Understand Things We Could Not Previously Understand." In *Speech and Language in the Laboratory, School and Clinic*, eds. J. Kavanagh and W. Strange (Cambridge, MA: MIT Press).

Brinton, B., and Fujiki, M. (1984). "Development of Topic Manipulation Skills in Discourse." *Journal of Speech and Hearing Research* 27:350–358.

Brinton, B., and Fujiki, M. (1989). *Conversational Management with Language-Impaired Children*. Rockville, MD: Aspen.

Brown, R. (1973). *A First Language: The Early Stages*, Cambridge: Harvard University Press.

Carrow, E. (1974). *Carrow Elicited Language Inventory*. Austin, TX: Learning Concepts.

Catts, H. (1993). "The Relationship between Speech-Language Impairments and Reading Disabilities." *Journal of Speech and Hearing Research* 36:948–958.

Cazden, C. (1970). "The Neglected Situation of Child Language Research and Education." In *Language and Poverty: Perspectives on a Theme*, ed. F. Williams (Chicago, IL: Rand-McNally).

Connell, P., and Myles-Zitzer, C. (1982). "An Analysis of Elicited Imitation as a Language Evaluation Procedure." *Journal of Speech and Hearing Disorders* 47:390–396.

Conoley, J., and Impara, J. (1995). *Twelfth Mental Measurements Yearbook.* Lincoln, Neb.: Buros Institute of Mental Measurements, University of Nebraska.

Craig, H., and Evans, J. (1993). "Pragmatics and SLI: Within-Group Variations in Discourse Behaviors." *Journal of Speech and Hearing Research* 36:777–789.

Crystal, D., Fletcher, P., and Garman, M. (1976). *The Grammatical Analysis of Language Disability: A Procedure for Assessment and Remediation.* London: Edward Arnold.

Daily, K., and Boxx, J. (1979). "A Comparison of Three Imitative Tests of Expressive Language and a Spontaneous Language Sample." *Language, Speech and Hearing Services in Schools* 10: 6–13.

Damico, J. (1980). "Clinical Discourse Analysis." Miniseminar presented at the convention of the American Speech-Language-Hearing Association, Detroit, MI.

Damico, J. (1985). "Clinical Discourse Analysis: A Functional Approach to Language Assessment." In *Communication Skills and Classroom Success: Assessment of Language-Learning Disabled Students,* ed. C. Simon (San Diego, CA: College-Hill).

Darley, F. (1979). *Evaluation of Appraisal Techniques in Speech and Language Pathology.* Reading, MA: Addison-Wesley.

Dever, R., and Bauman, P. (1974). "Scale of Children's Clausal Development." In *Linguistic Analysis of Children's Speech,* ed. T. Longhurst (New York: MSS Information Corporation).

Dillard, J. (1972). *Black English.* New York: Random House.

Edmonds, P., and Haynes, W. (1988). "Topic Manipulation and Conversational Participation as a Function of Familiarity in School-Age Language-Impaired and Normal Language Peers." *Journal of Communication Disorders* 21:209–228.

Ehlers, P., and Cirrin, F. (1983). "Topic Relevancy Abilities of Language-Impaired Children." Paper presented at the annual convention of the American Speech, Language and Hearing Association, Cincinnati, OH.

Engler, L., Hannah, E., and Longhurst, T. (1973). "Linguistic Analysis of Speech Samples: A Practical Guide for Clinicians." *Journal of Speech and Hearing Disorders* 38:192–204.

Evans, J., and Craig, H. (1992). "Language Sample Collection and Analysis: Interview Compared to Free-play Assessment Contexts." *Journal of Speech and Hearing Research* 35:343–353.

Fey, M. (1986). *Language Intervention with Young Children.* San Diego, CA: College-Hill.

Fey, M., and Leonard, L. (1983). "Pragmatic Skills of Children with Specific Language Impairment." In *Pragmatic Assessment and Intervention Issues in Language,* ed. T. Gallagher and C. Prutting (San Diego, CA: College-Hill).

Fujiki, M., and Brinton, B. (1983). "Sampling Reliability in Elicited Imitation." *Journal of Speech and Hearing Disorders* 48:85–89.

Gallagher, T. (1982). "Pragmatics." Workshop presented at Auburn University, Alabama.

Garvey, C. (1977a). "The Contingent Query: A Dependent Act in Conversation." In *Interaction, Conversation, and the Development of Language,* Vol. 5, ed. M. Lewis and L. Rosenblum (New York: Wiley).

Garvey, C. (1977b). "Play with Language and Speech." In *Child Discourse,* ed. S. Ervin-Tripp and C. Mitchell-Kernan (New York: Academic Press).

Gowie, C., and Powers, J. (1979). "Relations among Cognitive, Semantic and Syntactic Variables in Children's Comprehension of the Minimal Distance Principle: A Two-Year Developmental Study." *Journal of Psycholinguistic Research* 8:29–41.

Grice, H. (1975). "Logic and Conversation." In *Studies in Syntax, Semantics and Speech Acts,* Vol. 3, ed. P. Cole and J. Morgan (New York: Academic Press).

Gutierrez-Clellen, V. (1996). "Language Diversity: Implications for Assessment." In *Assessment of Communication and Language,* ed. K. Cole, P. Dale, and D. Thal (Baltimore, MD: Brookes).

Gutierrez-Clellen, V., and Quinn, R. (1993). "Assessing Narratives in Diverse Cultural/Linguistic Populations: Clinical Implications." *Language, Speech and Hearing Services in Schools* 24:2–9.

Hall, P., and Tomblin, J. (1978). "A Follow-Up Study of Children with Articulation and Language Disorders." *Journal of Speech and Hearing Disorders* 43:227–241.

Halliday, M., and Hasan, R. (1976). *Cohesion in English*. London: Longman.

Hamayan, E., and Damico, J. (1991). *Limiting Bias in the Assessment of Bilingual Students*. Austin, TX: Pro-Ed.

Haniff, M., and Siegel, G. (1981). "The Effect of Context on Verbal Elicited Imitation." *Journal of Speech and Hearing Disorders* 46:27–30.

Harris, G. (1985). "Considerations in Assessing English Language Performance of Native American Children." *Topics in Language Disorders* 5:42–52.

Haynes, W., and Haynes, M. (1979). "Pragmatics and Elicited Imitation: Children's Performance on Discursively Related and Discursively Unrelated Sentences." *Journal of Communication Disorders* 12:471–479.

Haynes, W., and Hood, S. (1978). "Disfluency Changes in Children as a Function of the Systematic Modification of Linguistic Complexity." *Journal of Communication Disorders* 11:79–93.

Haynes, W., and McCallion, M. (1981). "Language Comprehension Testing: The Influence of Cognitive Tempo and Three Modes of Test Administration." *Language, Speech and Hearing Services in Schools* 12:74–81.

Haynes, W., Purcell, E., and Haynes, M. (1979). "A Pragmatic Aspect of Language Sampling." *Language, Speech and Hearing Services in Schools* 10:104–110.

Hester, E. (1996). "Narratives of Young African American Children." In *Communication Development and Disorders in African American Children*, ed. A. Kamhi, K. Pollock, and J. Harris (Baltimore, MD: Brookes).

Hubbell, R. (1981). *Children's Language Disorders: An Integrated Approach*. Englewood Cliffs, NJ: Prentice-Hall.

Hubbell, R. (1988). *A Handbook of English Grammar and Language Sampling*. Englewood Cliffs, NJ: Prentice-Hall.

Hughes, D., Fey, M., and Long, S. (1992). "Developmental Sentence Scoring: Still Useful after All These Years." *Topics in Language Disorders* 12:1–12.

Hux, K., Morris-Friehe, M. and Sanger, D. (1993). "Language Sampling Practices: A Survey of Nine States." *Language, Speech and Hearing Services in Schools* 24:84–91.

Hymes, D. (1971). "Competence and Performance in Linguistic Theory." In *Language Acquisition: Models and Methods*, ed. R. Huxley and E. Ingram (New York: Academic Press).

Hyter, Y., and Westby, C. (1996). "Using Oral Narratives to Assess Communicative Competence." In *Communication Development and Disorders in African American Children*, ed. A. Kamhi, K. Pollock, and J. Harris (Baltimore, MD: Brookes).

Johnston, J. (1982). "Narrative: A New Look at Communication Problems in Older Language-Disordered Children." *Language, Speech and Hearing Services in Schools* 13:144–155.

Kahn, L., and James, S. (1980). "A Method for Assessing the Use of Grammatical Structures in Language-Disordered Children." *Language, Speech and Hearing Services in Schools*. 11: 188–197.

Keenan, E., and Schiefflen, B. (1976). "Topic as a Discourse Notion: A Study of Topic in the Conversations of Children and Adults." In *Subject and Topic*, ed. C. Li (New York: Academic Press).

King, R., Jones, C., and Lasky, E. (1982). "In Retrospect: A Fifteen-Year Follow-Up Report of Speech-Language Disorders in Children." *Language, Speech and Hearing Services in Schools* 13:24–32.

Klecan-Aker, J., and Hedrick, D. (1985). "A Study of the Syntactic Language Skills of Normal School-Age Children." *Language, Speech and Hearing Services in Schools* 16:187–198.

Kramer, C., James, S., and Saxman, J. (1979). "A Comparison of Language Samples Elicited at Home and in the Clinic." *Journal of Speech and Hearing Disorders* 44:321–330.

Labov, W. (1970). "The Logic on Nonstandard English." In *Language and Poverty: Perspectives on a Theme*, ed. F. Williams (Chicago, IL: Rand-McNally).

Lahey, M. (1988). *Language Disorders and Language Development*. New York: Macmillan.

Lang, M., and Moore, W. (1977). "Some Variables Affecting Sentence Imitation of Normal Children." Unpublished research, Auburn University, Alabama.

Larson, V., and McKinley, N. (1995). "Language Disorders in Older Students." EauClaire, WI: (1974). *Developmental Sentence Analysis*, ed. L. Thin Lee (Evanston, IL: Northwestern University Press).

Lee, L. (1974). *Developmental Sentence Analysis*. (Evanston, IL: Northwestern University Press).

Lee, L., Koenigsknecht, R., and Mulhern, S. (1975). *Interactive Language Development Teaching*. Evanston, IL: Northwestern University Press.

Leonard, L., Prutting, C., Perozzi, C., and Berkley, R. (1978). "Nonstandardized Approaches to the Assessment of Language Behaviors." *Journal of the American Speech and Hearing Association* May:371–379.

Lidz, C., and Pena, E. (1996). "Dynamic Assessment: The Model, Its Relevance as a Nonbiased Approach and Its Application to Latino American Preschool Children." *Language, Speech and Hearing Services in Schools* 27:367–372.

Liles, B. (1993). "Narrative Discourse in Children with Language Disorders and Children with Normal Language: A Critical Review of the Literature." *Journal of Speech and Hearing Research* 36:868–882.

Liles, B. (1985). "Cohesion in the Narratives of Normal and Language-Disordered Children." *Journal of Speech and Hearing Research* 28: 123–133.

Loban, W. (1976). *Language Development: Kindergarten through Grade Twelve*." Research Report No. 18. Urbana, IL: National Councils of Teachers of English.

Long, S., and Fey, M. (1993). *Computerized Profiling*. San Antonio, TX: The Psychological Corporation.

Longhurst, T., and File, J. (1977). "A Comparison of Developmental Sentence Scores for Headstart Children in Four Conditions." *Language, Speech and Hearing Services in Schools* 8:54–64.

Longhurst, T., and Grubb, S. (1974). "A Comparison of Language Samples Collected in Four Situations." *Language, Speech and Hearing Services in Schools* 5:71–78.

Longhurst, T., and Schrandt, T. (1973). "Linguistic Analysis of Children's Speech: A Comparison of Four Procedures." *Journal of Speech and Hearing Disorders* 38:240–249.

Lucas, E. (1980). *Semantic and Pragmatic Language Disorders*. Rockville, MD: Aspen.

Lund, N., and Duchan, J. (1993). *Assessing Children's Language in Naturalistic Contexts*. Englewood Cliffs, NJ: Prentice-Hall.

MacDonald, J., and Carroll, J. (1992). "A Social Partnership Model for Assessing Early Communication Development: An Intervention Model for Preconversational Children. *Language, Speech and Hearing Services in Schools* 23:113–124.

Maxwell, S., and Wallach, G. (1984). "The Language-Learning Disabilities Connection: Symptoms of Early Language Disability Change over Time." In *Language Learning Disabilities in School Age Children*, ed. G. Wallach and K. Butler (Baltimore, MD: Williams and Wilkins).

McDade, H., Simpson, M., and Larnt, D. (1982). "The Use of Elicited Imitation as a Measure of Expressive Grammar: A Question of Validity." *Journal of Speech and Hearing Disorders* 47:19–24.

Merritt, D., and Liles, B. (1989). "Narrative Analysis: Clinical Applications of Story Generation and Story Retelling." *Journal of Speech and Hearing Disorders* 54:438–447.

Millen, K., and Prutting, C. (1979). "Consistencies across Three Language Comprehension Tests for Specific Grammatical Features." *Language, Speech and Hearing Services in Schools* 10:162–170.

Miller, J. (1981). *Assessing Language Production in Children: Experimental Procedures*. Baltimore: University Park Press.

Miller, J., and Chapman, R. (1995). *SALT: Systematic Analysis of Language Transcripts*. Madison, WI: Language Analysis Laboratory, University of Wisconsin.

Miller, J., and Paul, R. (1995). *The Clinical Assessment of Language Comprehension*. Baltimore, MD: Brookes.

Miner, L. (1969). "Scoring Procedures for the Length-Complexity Index: A Preliminary Report." *Journal of Communication Disorders* 224–240.

Moats, L., and Smith, C. (1992). "Derivational Morphology: Why It Should Be Included in Language Assessment and Instruction." *Lan-*

guage, Speech and Hearing Services in Schools 23:312–319.

Mordecai, D., Palin, M., and Palmer, C. (1982). *Lingquest 1.* Napa, CA: Lingquest Software.

Morris, N., and Crump, W. (1982). "Syntactic and Vocabulary Development in the Written Language of Learning Disabled and Non-Disabled Students at Four Age Levels." *Learning Disability Quarterly* 5:163–172.

Mount-Weitz, J. (1996). "Vocabulary Development and Disorders in African American Children." In *Communication Development and Disorders in African American Children,* ed. A. Kamhi, K. Pollock, and J. Harris (Baltimore, MD: Brookes).

Mulac, A., Prutting, C., and Tomlinson, C. (1978). "Testing for a Specific Syntactic Structure." *Journal of Communication Disorders* 11:335–347.

Muma, J. (1973a). "Language Assessment: The Co-Occurring and Restricted Structure Procedure." *Acta Symbolica* 4:12–29.

Muma, J. (1973b). "Language Assessment: Some Underlying Assumptions." *Journal of the American Speech and Hearing Association* 15:331–338.

Muma, J. (1975). "The Communication Game: Dump and Play." *Journal of Speech and Hearing Disorders* 40:296–309.

Muma, J. (1978). *Language Handbook: Concepts, Assessment, Intervention.* Englewood Cliffs, NJ: Prentice-Hall.

Musselwhite, C., and Barrie-Blackley, S. (1980). "Three Variations of the Imperative Format of Language Sample Elicitation." *Language, Speech and Hearing Services in Schools* 11:56–67.

Nelson, L., and Weber-Olsen, M. (1980). "The Elicited Language Inventory and the Influence of Contextual Cues." *Journal of Speech and Hearing Disorders* 45:549–563.

Nippold, M. (1988). "Figurative Language." In *Later Language Development: Ages Nine through Nineteen,* ed. M. Nippold (Austin, TX: Pro-Ed).

Nippold, M. (1993). "Developmental Markers in Adolescent Language: Syntax, Semantics and Pragmatics." *Language, Speech and Hearing Services in Schools* 24:21–28.

Nippold, M., Schwarz, I., and Undlin, R. (1992). "Use and Understanding of Adverbial Conjuncts: A Developmental Study of Adoles-

cents and Young Adults." *Journal of Speech and Hearing Research* 35:108–118.

Olswang, L., and Carpenter, R. (1978). "Elicitor Effects on the Language Obtained from Young Language-Impaired Children." *Journal of Speech and Hearing Disorders* 43:76–86.

Owens, R. (1995). *Language Development: An Introduction.* Neeham Heights, MA: Allyn and Bacon.

Owens, R., Haney, M., Griesow, V., Dooley, L., and Kelly, R. (1983). "Language Test Content: A Comparative Study." *Language, Speech and Hearing Services in Schools* 14:7–21.

Paul, R. (1995). *Language Disorders from Infancy through Adolescence: Assessment and Intervention.* St. Louis, MO: Mosby.

Paul, R., and Alforde, S. (1993). "Grammatical Morpheme Acquisition in 4 Year Olds with Normal, Impaired and Late Developing Language. *Journal of Speech and Hearing Research* 36:1271–1275.

Peterson, H., and Marquardt, T. (1990). *Appraisal and Diagnosis of Speech and Language Disorders.* Englewood-Cliffs, NJ: Prentice-Hall.

Plante, E., and Vance, R. (1995). "Diagnostic Accuracy of Two Tests of Preschool Language." *American Journal of Speech-Language Pathology* 4:70–76.

Prutting, C., and Connolly, J. (1976). "Imitation: A Closer Look." *Journal of Speech and Hearing Disorders* 41:412–422.

Prutting, C., Gallagher, T., and Mulac, A. (1975). "The Expressive Portion of the NSST Compared to a Spontaneous Language Sample." *Journal of Speech and Hearing Disorders* 40:40–48.

Prutting, C., and Kirchner, D. (1987). "A Clinical Appraisal of the Pragmatic Aspects of Language." *Journal of Speech and Hearing Disorders* 52:105–119.

Quinn, R., Goldstein, B., and Pena, E. (1996). "Cultural/Linguistic Variation in the United States and Its Implications for Assessment and Intervention in Speech-Language Pathology: An Introduction." *Language, Speech and Hearing Services in Schools* 27:345–346.

Quirk, R., and Greenbaum, S. (1975). *A Concise Grammar of Contemporary English.* New York: Harcourt Brace Jovanovich.

Rees, N., and Shulman, M. (1978). "I Don't Understand What You Mean by Comprehension." *Journal of Speech and Hearing Disorders* 43: 208–219.

Retherford, K. (1993). *Guide to Analysis of Language Transcripts.* Eauclaire, WI: Thinking Publications.

Robinson-Zanartu, C. (1996). "Serving Native American Children and Families: Considering Cultural Variables." *Language, Speech and Hearing Services in Schools* 27:373–384.

Sachs, J., and Devin, J. (1976). "Young Children's Use of Age Appropriate Speech Styles in Social Interaction and Role Playing." *Journal of Child Language* 3:81–98.

Scott, C. (1988). "Spoken and Written Syntax." In *Later Language Development: Ages Nine through Nineteen,* ed. M. Nippold (Austin, TX: Pro-Ed).

Sharf, D. (1972). "Some Relationships between Measures of Early Language Development." *Journal of Speech and Hearing Disorders* 37:64–74.

Sheppard, A. (1980). "Monologue and Dialogue of Speech and Language-Impaired Children in Clinic and Home Settings: Semantic, Conversational and Syntactic Characteristics." Masters thesis, University of Western Ontario.

Shorr, D. (1983). "Grammatical Comprehension Assessment: The Picture Avoidance Strategy." *Journal of Speech and Hearing Disorders* 48:89–92.

Shulman, B. (1986). *Test of Pragmatic Skills, Revised.* Tucson, AZ: Communication Skill Builders.

Simms-Hill, S., and Haynes, W. (1992). "Language Performance in Low-Achieving Elementary School Students." *Language, Speech and Hearing Services in Schools* 23:169–175.

Simon, C. (1987). "Out of the Broom Closet and into the Classroom: The Emerging SLP." *Journal of Childhood Communication Disorders* 11:41–66.

Simon, C. (1989). *Classroom Communication Screening Procedure for Early Adolescents (CCSPEA).* Tempe, AZ: Communi-Cog Publications.

Slobin, D., and Welsh, C. (1971). "Elicited Imitation as a Research Tool in Developmental Psycholinguistics." In *Language Training in Early Childhood Education,* ed. C. Lavatelli (Urbana: University of Illinois Press).

Stein, A. (1976). "A Comparison of Mothers and Fathers Language to Normal and Language Deficient Children." Unpublished doctoral dissertation, Boston University, MA.

Stockman, I. (1996). "The Promises and Pitfalls of Language Sample Analysis as an Assessment Tool for Linguistic Minority Children." *Language, Speech and Hearing Services in Schools* 27: 355–366.

Stover, S., and Haynes, W. (1989). "Topic Manipulation and Cohesive Adequacy in Conversations of Normal Adults between the Ages of 30 and 90." *Clinical Linguistics and Phonetics* 3:137–149.

Strandberg, T., and Griffith, J. (1969). "A Study of the Effects of Training in Visual Literacy on Verbal Language Behavior." *Journal of Communication Disorders* 2:252–263.

Sturner, R., Heller, J., Funk, S., and Layton, T. (1993). "The Fluharty Preschool Speech and Language Screening Test: A Population-Based Validation Study Using Sample-Independent Decision Rules." *Journal of Speech and Hearing Research* 36:738–745.

Strominger, A., and Bashir, A. (1977). "A Nine-Year Follow-Up of Language-Delayed Children." Paper presented at the convention of the American Speech-Language Hearing Association, Chicago, IL.

Taylor, O. (1986a). *Nature of Communication Disorders in Culturally and Linguistically Diverse Populations.* San Diego: College-Hill.

Taylor, O. (1986b). *Treatment of Communication Disorders in Culturally and Linguistically Diverse Populations.* San Diego: College-Hill.

Tyack, D., and Gottsleben, R. (1974). *Language Sampling, Analysis and Training: A Handbook for Teachers and Clinicians.* Palo Alto, CA: Consulting Psychologists Press.

Vaughn-Cooke, F. (1983). "Improving Language Assessment in Minority Children." *Journal of the American Speech, Language, Hearing Association* 25, no. 9:29–34.

Wallach, G., and Butler, K. (1994). *Language Learning Disabilities in School-Age Children and Adolescents: Some Principles and Applications.* Needham Heights, MA: Allyn and Bacon.

Wallach, G., and Miller, L. (1988). *Language Intervention and Academic Success.* Boston: College-Hill Press.

Washington, J. (1996). "Issues in Assessing the Language Abilities of African American Children." In *Communication Development and Disorders in African American Children*, ed. A. Kamhi, K. Pollock, and J. Harris (Baltimore, MD: Brookes).

Watson, L. (1977). "Conversational Participation by Language-Deficient and Normal Children." Paper presented to the Convention of the American Speech and Hearing Association, Chicago, IL.

Werner, E., and Kreseck, J. (1981). "Variability in Scores, Structures and Errors on Three Measures of Expressive Language." *Language, Speech and Hearing Services in Schools* 12: 82–89.

Wiig, E., and Semel, E. (1976). *Language Disabilities in Children and Adolescents*, Columbus, OH: Merrill.

Williams, R., and Wolfram, W. (1977). *Social Differences vs. Disorders*. Washington, DC: American Speech and Hearing Association.

Wilson, K., Blackmon, R., Hall, R., and Elcholtz, G. (1991). "Methods of Language Assessment: A Survey of California Public School Clinicians." *Language, Speech and Hearing Services in Schools* 22:236–241.

Wyatt, T. (1996). "Acquisition of the African American English Copula." In *Communication Development and Disorders in African American Children*, ed. A. Kamhi, K. Pollock, and J. Harris (Baltimore, MD: Brookes).

Zachman, L., Hulsingh, R., Jorgensen, C., and Barrett, M. (1978). *Oral Language Sentence Imitation Test*. Moline, IL: Linguisystems.

Chapter 6

Assessment of Articulation and Phonological Disorders

In the early portion of this century, articulation was conceptualized by most clinicians as being primarily a motor act. This sensorimotor aspect of articulation was studied, and it was not uncommon for articulation treatment to emphasize almost exclusively the movements of the oral musculature through an emphasis on diagrams, models, and motoric drills (Scripture and Jackson 1927). In the mid-1970s, however, SLPs became highly interested in the work of linguists (e.g., Ingram 1976) who examined sound production differences from the perspective of phonological theory. With the advent of greater attention to linguistics (e.g., phonology) it was noted that articulation had more components than simply motoric activity. It is now well accepted that linguistic activity contributes significantly to the articulatory process (Elbert 1992; Fey 1992; Schwartz 1983; Shelton and McReynolds 1979; Shriberg and Kwiatkowski 1982a).

Multiple Components Contributing to Sound Production

Many events contribute to the final motor act of articulating. First, the biological component provides the basic structures for articulation, such as the vocal tract and the articulators, as well as the intact nervous system, which allows us to perform the sensory (auditory, tactile, kinesthetic, proprioceptive) and the motor functions necessary for controlled movement. Second, there is a cognitive-linguistic component wherein the speaker conceives of "something to say." This thought then undergoes linguistic processing whereby semantic elements are selected, words are arranged in proper syntactic order, and the utterance is appropriately tailored to the communicative situation by the speaker, taking pragmatics into consideration. The selection of phonemic elements and their order is then accomplished by applying phonological rules of our language. The details of linguistic processing of an utterance are not fully understood. It is enough to say, however, that linguistic processing involving semantic, syntactic, pragmatic, and phonological areas must occur at some point prior to expressing an utterance. Third, there is a sensorimotor-acoustic component that includes motor programming and motor learning of actual sequences of physical movement in a wide variety of phonetic contexts. Much research has been directed toward determining the basic unit of articulatory motor programming, and we do not presently know its size or identity. The motor production in the vocal tract then gives rise to acoustic vibrations that travel through a medium of air and arrive at the ears of our listeners. This brief sketch of the processes that result in articulatory production is highly simplified.

It is the view of the present authors that this gross division of the articulatory process into biological, cognitive-linguistic, and sensorimotor components carries with it several important implications. First, the diagnostician must be prepared to assess and treat any or all aspects of the process in a given client. Some authorities (Bernthal and Bankson 1993) differentiate "articulation disorders" from "phonological disorders." Bernthal and Bankson (1988) indicate, for instance, that articulation disorders can be "motorically based errors (the ability to produce a target sound is not within the person's repertoire of motor skills) . . . or cognitively or linguistically based (the client can produce a sound but does not use the sound in appropriate contexts)" (3). They further state that differentiating a motoric from a linguistically based disorder is not always an easy task. If the client exhibits primarily a linguistically based problem (e.g., a phonological simplification such as deletion of certain final consonants), we should be able to examine a sample of speech for patterns of error that represent these phonological reductions. Oral-peripheral, motoric, audiological, and ultimately medical/neurological evaluation procedures can pinpoint difficulties with the biological/sensorimotor foundations of articulation. The implication, then, is that a client can have difficulties with one or several parts of the process and the diagnostician should be equipped to assess these.

There are several ways of categorizing misarticulations. Historically, speech pathologists have used the traditional classifications of (1) substitution of one sound for another ("thoup" for "soup"), (2) omission of a sound ("kool" for "school"), (3) distortion of a sound (nonstandard production of a sound), and (4) addition of a sound ("puhlease" for "please"). These historical classifications have persisted because they do describe most articulatory deviations. If there is any fault with the categories, it is that they are not specific enough. The diagnostician must say more than "the child has substitutions and omissions in his speech." We need to know which sounds are substituted for others, how often, and in what contexts. The same could be said for distortions, omissions, and additions. Another example of the superficiality of the historical categories is that they do not imply what part of the articulatory process is affected. That is, we cannot discern from the category of "substitution" whether the error is related to deficiencies in the client's sensorimotor or linguistic/phonological systems. The traditional classifications, however, are a good place to begin the articulatory assessment. We can then assess further and attempt to determine the variability of performance in specific phonetic contexts as well as the ways in which misarticulation varies in utterances of different linguistic complexities.

Articulatory errors can also be divided into categories of *organic* (some physical cause for the misarticulation) and *functional* (no demonstrable organic cause). The latter term has come under criticism for quite some time. Powers (1971) has called the term *functional* a "diagnosis by default." This is because the diagnosis of *organic* requires some positive proof of organicity, while the diagnosis of *functional* requires no positive evidence. The classification of *functional* is made only when a lack of evidence of organicity exists. The words most frequently associated with the *functional* classification are "learned" or "habit." Thus, although the classification of *functional* has been justifiably criticized, it is still widely held that the vast majority of articulation disorders have no significant, maintaining, organic basis and that the treatment is behavioral in nature. However, future research may yet uncover subtle organic or behavioral differences in these individuals (Bernthal and Bankson 1993). Assessment of organically based articulation disorders such as dysarthria and apraxia will be dealt with in our chapter on motor speech disorders. The present chapter focuses on misarticulations that have no obvious organic component. For the remainder of the chapter we will use the term *phonological disorder* to refer to these functional cases that involve multiple phoneme errors. The term *articulation disorder* will be reserved for clients that misarticulate only one or two phonemes.

Another implication of a multicomponent conception of articulation is that no single measure is presently capable of adequately examining all parts of this complex process. It is naive to believe that administration of a traditional articulation test and an oral-peripheral examination are all that is necessary to perform a complete assessment of articulatory behavior. The articulatory process is just too complex and the disordered population too heterogeneous to rely on one or two standard tests. We support the point of view stated by Stoel-Gammon and Dunn (1985) that both independent and relational analyses should be done to provide complementary perspectives on a child's phonological system. Independent analysis simply describes a child's productions in terms of features, segments, and syllable shapes that actually occur in the speech sample. Relational analysis attempts to gloss a child's productions and compare them to adult models, resulting in an assessment of "correct and incorrect" productions. In this chapter, we are emphasizing the importance of knowing "where to go" and "what to do" to gain insight into aspects of articulation that are revealed to be problematic by the initial testing. As with any disorder area, no single chapter can possibly tell a student how to do everything well. Our goal is simply to make clinicians aware of the possibilities in articulatory assessment and refer the reader to the appropriate literature.

Seven Important Knowledge Areas for Evaluation of Articulation and Phonological Disorders

Before we discuss assessment of articulation disorders, there are several important bodies of literature that the clinician should be familiar with. In actuality, there are more areas that could be considered, but these seven seem to us to be critical pre-requisites to performing a diagnostic evaluation.

1. *Knowledge of the anatomy and physiology of the speech mechanism.* Before attempt-ing to deal with an articulatory evaluation, the clinician should be fully familiar with the normal oral mechanism. Most students obtain this knowledge in their un-dergraduate training. There are many textbooks that provide this information (Daniloff, Schuckers, and Feth 1980; Dickson and Maue-Dickson 1982; Kahane and Folkins 1984; Palmer 1984; Zemlin 1993).

2. *Knowledge of Phonetics.* It is one thing to know about the anatomy and physi-ology of the vocal mechanism, but it is quite another to be aware of how that ap-paratus actually produces the variety of consonant and vowel sounds in English. References have described sound productions and articulatory movements asso-ciated with them (Carrell and Tiffany 1960; Shriberg and Kent 1982; Van Riper and Smith 1979). Aside from knowing articulatory phonetics, the clinician must have well-developed skills in phonetic transcription. This expertise is important in order to record a client's productions accurately for later analysis. Reliable pho-netic transcription abilities are especially important in order to accomplish phono-logical analyses (Shriberg and Kwiatkowski 1980).

3. *Knowledge of phonological development.* A major goal in diagnosis is to compare a child's articulatory performance to the behavior of other children in the same age range. In this way we can tell if a child's misarticulations are developmental in na-ture or clinically significant. There are at least three interpretations of articulatory development that the clinician should be familiar with prior to doing an assessment.

The most abundant normative data available are traditionally oriented stud-ies of children's phoneme production of words with the target sound in the initial, medial, and final positions (Poole 1934; Templin 1957; Wellman et al. 1931). Al-though the procedures and criteria for acquisition in these studies differ (Smit 1986), they provide ages at which children master phonemes. More recent data (Sander 1972; Smit 1993a; Smit et al. 1990; Irwin and Wong 1983; Prather, Hedrick and Kern 1975) suggest earlier development of speech sounds and provide age ranges of development of "customary production" (two of three word positions) and mastery. The data provided by Irwin and Wong (1983) deal with sound pro-duction in connected spontaneous speech as opposed to the typical single-word responses reported in other traditional studies. Figure 6.1 is an example of nor-mative consonant development data. Most misarticulations in phonologically dis-ordered children involve consonants, so only consonant development data are presented here. Vowels are typically developed by age three (Bernthal and Bank-son 1993). This does not mean that vowels are never involved in phonological dis-order (Hodson 1980) or that vowels are easily acquired (Davis and MacNeilage 1990).

A second type of developmental data involves distinctive feature acquisition. Several sources report a developmental order in distinctive feature acquisition (Blache 1978; Singh 1976). These data could be used when analyzing a child's dis-tinctive feature system as opposed to more traditional norms.

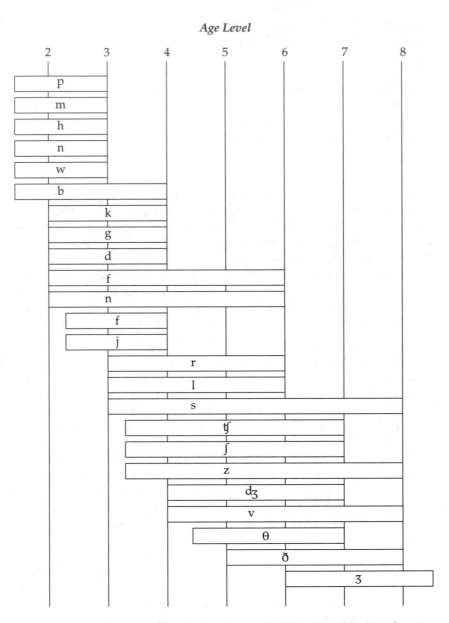

FIGURE 6.1 Average Age Estimates and Upper Age Limits of Customary Consonant Production. The solid bar corresponding to each sound starts at the median age of customary articulation; it stops at the age level at which 90 percent of all children are customarily producing the sound.

(Sander 1972, 62. © 1972, the American Speech-Language-Hearing Association, Rockville, MD.)

Finally, data are available regarding the occurrence of phonological reduction processes or patterns of error in normally developing children (Ingram 1976; Shriberg and Kwiatkowski 1980; Smit 1993b). These data provide some general age cutoffs for certain phonological processes and give the SLP a view of a child's error pattern not found in traditional norms. If a clinician sees a child who is deleting final consonants, for instance, the clinician cannot use traditional norms to determine when this tendency diminishes in normal children. Most studies have focused on children's phonological development between the ages of three and eight years. More-recent investigations have concentrated on children from one to three years in response to the emphases on early intervention and increased interest in early normal development (Dyson 1988; Grunwell 1988; Kahn and Lewis 1986; Stoel-Gammon 1987). Figure 6.2 provides an example of normative data developed within the phonological process perspective.

Bernthal and Bankson (1993) point out that there are very little longitudinal developmental data and that most of the above information was gleaned from cross-sectional investigations. No doubt, as in other aspects of development, a variety of articulatory acquisition strategies will eventually be found. A major point we wish to make here is that the clinician can look at an articulatory sample from a variety of perspectives. Traditional as well as phonological norms provide a reference point to use in assessment and treatment.

4. *Knowledge of factors related to articulation disorders.* Whenever a clinician undertakes a phonological evaluation, the clinician can expect that parents will often ask questions regarding the etiology of the problem. The clinician, then, must be familiar with the pertinent literature dealing with research on etiological factors, as well as skills and abilities of articulation-disordered children. Questions may be asked about language development, reading, spelling, educational performance, dentition, oral structures, gross and fine motor skills, intelligence, auditory abilities, and much more. Several sources summarize this research handily and should assist clinicians in answering any questions (Bernthal and Bankson 1993; Powers 1971; Winitz 1969).

5. *Knowledge of dialectal variation.* Many sources have reported articulatory differences as a product of regional dialect (Carrell and Tiffany 1960; Van Riper and Smith 1979). Other authorities report phonological differences from a multicultural perspective (Dillard 1972; Stoller 1975). According to the American Speech, Language, and Hearing Association the clinician performing an articulatory evaluation must be able to differentiate a communication disorder from a dialectical variation (Battle et al. 1983). Since there are so few tests that take dialect into account, the clinician must become familiar with this material and must routinely consider it when evaluating misarticulations.

African American English (AAE) has been sampled in isolated word contexts (Bleile and Wallach 1992; Cole and Taylor 1990; Haynes and Moran 1989; Seymour and Seymour 1981; Simmons 1988; Washington and Craig 1992) and in connected speech (Seymour, Green, and Huntley 1991; Stockman 1993; Stockman and Stephenson 1981; Vaughn-Cooke 1976; Wolfram 1989). Most research has shown more

FIGURE 6.2   **Chronology of Phonological Processes**

	2:0–2;6	2;6–3;0	3;0–3;6	3;6–4;0	4;0–4;6	4;6–5;0	5;0 →
Weak Syllable Deletion				--------			
Final Consonant Deletion		---------					
Reduplication	--------						
Consonant Harmony		--------					
Cluster Reduction (Initial) obstruent-approximant		--------	--------	---			
/s/ + consonant			--------	--			
Stopping /f/	--------	-----					
/v/							
/θ/		-----	θ → [f]			--------	
/ð/				/ð/ → [d] or [v]		--------	
/s/	-----	-----					
/z/		----	-----				
/ʃ/		Fronting '[s] type'					
/tʃ, dʒ/			Fronting [ts, dz]			--	
Fronting k, g, n/		--------	----				
Gliding r → [w]			--------	--------	--------	--------	---
Context-Sensitive Voicing		--- --------					

SOURCE: Adapted by permission from Grunwell, P. (1987), *Clinical Phonology* (Baltimore, MD: Williams and Wilkins). Used with permission. © 1987 William & Wilkins Co., Baltimore, MD.

similarities than differences between Standard English and AAE (Stockman 1996a). We know that AAE, like other dialects, changes with age and geographical region. Most differences in AAE are reported in medial and final word positions, and the initial word position shows the fewest alterations. Deletion of final consonants is one of the most frequently studied features of AAE. Moran (1993) has shown that when final consonants are deleted in AAE, the preceding vowel is systematically lengthened, which demonstrates knowledge of the deleted segment and not simply an "open syllable."

Typically, there are only a few specific classes of phonological differences between Standard English and AAE reported in the literature (Williams and Wolfram 1977; Wolfram 1991, 1994). These differences mainly center on the /TH/ and /r/ phonemes, final cluster reductions, and final consonant deletions. While there are many subtleties to be noted across word positions, canonical shapes, and word boundaries, it is clear that phonological differences are not numerous.

The difficulty of obtaining a valid communication assessment of children from different cultural groups is almost universally acknowledged. Most authorities have suggested that using a variety of assessment tasks provides the clinician with the best chance of making a valid clinical decision (Hamayan and Damico 1991; Lidz and Pena 1996; Stockman 1996a, 1996b). Criterion-referenced and ethnographic techniques may prove to be particularly helpful.

6. *Knowledge of Coarticulation.* For at least thirty years, researchers have known that speech is produced in a parallel fashion as opposed to a serial, discrete manner (Winitz 1975). This means that speech sounds are not isolated entities but that they overlap motorically and acoustically in time. Put simply, sounds are influenced by other phonemes that surround them. This influence of one sound on another is called *coarticulation* and is one of the most basic facts about the articulatory process. The phonetic environment or phonetic context in which a sound is produced influences the production of that phoneme. There are two major types of coarticulation that can be described in terms of the direction of the influence of one sound on another. Left-to-right coarticulation refers to a preceding sound's having an affect on a following sound (the "t" in "boots" is produced with some lip rounding because of the rounding /u/ vowel that precedes it). This type of coarticulation is perceived by some to be a type of "overflow" of movement from the first sound to the second. Thus, the left-to-right coarticulation is thought to be primarily the result of mechanical-inertial factors. The other type of coarticulation is right to left. This means that a sound later in the speech sequence affects a sound earlier in the stream of speech. For example, the "t" sound in the word "tea" is produced differently from the "t" in the word "too." The difference in the two situations is that in the word "tea" the sound is followed by a vowel that is not produced with rounded lips. Thus, the "t" sound in "too" might be produced with lip rounding because the following vowel is rounded. Note that in both of these cases the sound that influences the "t" occurs after the "t" has been uttered. Researchers and theorists have suggested that the right-to-left influence is probably the result of articulatory preprogramming. That is, early sounds in a sequence are produced differently in anticipation of sounds that are yet to be said. This implies some sort of motor planning.

There are many studies of coarticulation that have used cineflurorography, electromyography, and spectrographic analyses. These investigations have shown conclusively that coarticulation does, in fact, occur in speech sequences. Since it is a fact that coarticulation will be present in any utterance, it is a phenomenon that the speech pathologist can choose to use as a tool in assessment and treatment.

Whether we use coarticulatory influences in assessment and treatment to increase the efficiency of our clinical work or not, the effects will still occur. Most authorities feel that as long as coarticulation exists, we might as well use it to the best interest of the client.

The implications of the existence of coarticulation for articulatory assessment are significant. One implication is that testing sounds in isolation is an unrealistic and artificial enterprise. What a child can do with a sound in isolation may be totally different from the child's production in connected speech. Another implication has to do with testing in single words. When we speak, we typically do not put oral pauses or "spaces" between our words, as in the ones you are reading right now. The speech stream has been called an "unsegmentable whole" (Kent and Minifie 1977). Research on coarticulation has shown that the effects of one sound on another can cross both word and syllable boundaries (Amerman, Daniloff, and Moll 1970; Daniloff and Moll 1968; McClean 1973; Moll and Daniloff 1971). Thus, sounds located in two adjacent words can have an affect on one another. This means that testing sound production on the single word level may not be representative of sound production in spontaneous speech, because connected words may provide different coarticulatory effects as compared to single words alone (Faircloth and Faircloth 1970). We have known for some time that specific phonemes are misarticulated less often in consonant cluster contexts as opposed to CV environments (McCauley and Skenes 1987).

Yet another implication has to do with possible facilitating and sabotaging effects of phonemes surrounding a particular target sound. For instance, a misarticulated /r/ sound may be produced correctly by a child if it is preceded by a /k/ (e.g., /kræk/), perhaps because both sounds require grossly similar positioning of the tongue in the vocal tract (Hoffman, Schuckers, and Ratusnick 1977). Conversely, an /r/ might be misarticulated as a /w/ if words surrounding the target sound contain a lip-rounded phoneme (e.g., /row/) (Winitz 1975). Therefore, the effects of coarticulation can be either positive or negative, facilitating or sabotaging, and this finding is especially important for the clinician to consider in assessment and treatment.

Perhaps the most important implication of coarticulation is in accounting for articulatory inconsistency. Most misarticulations are notoriously inconsistent, and if the clinician analyzes these productions, he/she can find that this "inconsistency" may actually be quite consistent indeed. Phonetic context is often the common denominator among errors that appear inconsistent on the surface. We need not only think of the notion of phonetic context as a purely motoric phenomenon. In performing linguistic phonological analyses, a consideration of context is critical. In evaluating assimilation processes (e.g., nasal assimilation), the clinician may note than nonnasal sounds in the initial word position are changed to nasals only when there is a nasal phoneme in the final or medial position of the words.

7. *Knowledge of the Linguistic-Articulatory Connection.* An important postulate in discussing articulatory assessment is the intimate relationhsip between language and articulation. This connection has been shown in several ways in the literature.

a. Phonology is a component of language. Theoretically, phonology has been considered a classical component of language models. Chomsky (1957), for instance, includes phonological rules in his model of transformational grammar along with semantics and syntax.

b. Many bound morphemes are single sounds. Many bound morphemes (e.g., "-ed," plural "-s," possessive "-s") are realized through a rule-governed system in speech as single phonemes. The "-ed" in the word "walked" is really pronounced as a /t/ sound in a consonant blend at the end of the word /wkt/. Thus, a single sound makes a difference in word meaning, and that same single unit is a grammatical morpheme. A sound, therefore, is much more than merely a phonetic unit; it makes a difference in word meaning and carries linguistic value.

c. Syntactic complexity affects misarticulations. Several studies have shown that misarticulations are affected by linguistic complexity (Haynes, Haynes, and Jackson 1982; Panagos, Quine, and Klich 1979; Schmauch, Panagos, and Klich 1978). That is, more misarticulations will occur as syntactic complexity increases. Here is a clear relationship between articulation and language.

d. Semantic complexity affects misarticulations. Shriberg and Kwiatkowski (1980) have suggested that even the word's syntactic class may affect sound productions. They found, for instance, that blends may be reduced differently in verbs as compared to the same blend in nouns. In early language development there appear to be more misarticulations on action words as opposed to object words in the first lexicon. This observation has been made with normally developing as well as phonologically delayed children (Camarata and Schwartz 1985).

e. Pragmatics and communicative value affect misarticulations. Pragmatics has also been implicated as affecting sound productions in several investigations (Campbell and Shriberg 1982; Leonard 1971; Weiner and Ostrowski 1979). That is, children may produce sounds more correctly in conditions of increased information load and may misarticulate more frequently when the communicative value is lessened. This means that when there is a greater chance of being misunderstood, the child may articulate more correctly.

f. Language and phonological disorders typically co-occur. A relationship between language and articulation can be inferred from the high co-occurrence of the two disorders in children. Generally, children who have articulation problems are high risk for language disorders and vice versa. Somewhere between 50 and 80% of children with phonological problems have concomitant language disorders (Shriberg and Kwiatkowski 1988; Shriberg et al. 1986).

The implications of the above connections between articulation and language are significant for assessment. First, routine assessment of articulation with an exclusively sensorimotor orientation is not appropriate. Language and articulation are hopelessly intertwined when a person speaks spontaneously (Locke 1983). Second, when the speech pathologist is looking for sources of inconsistent phoneme production, he/she may find significant effects not only from phonetic context but also from semantic, syntactic, or pragmatic variables. The clinician can see that the most productive view would be to consider both sensorimotor and linguistic components in the assessment repertoire (Schwartz 1983).

Screening for Phonological Disorders

Speech-language pathologists in private practice may screen day-care facilities or private schools to detect children with phonological problems. While many clinicians in the public schools may rely exclusively on referrals for case detection, screening is sometimes warranted depending on school system policies or special circumstances. The purpose of screening is to select children with significant communication problems by assessing a total population with a brief but discriminating testing procedure. The objective, then, is detection, not description, of persons with disordered speech. A screening test must be swift, yet discerning. The examiner must be able to detect individuals with impaired speech while rapidly passing over all the normal speakers. Although brief, the detection process should provide a sufficient sample of each person's oral communication to permit critical judgment of articulation and also voice, fluency, and language abilities. Since screening procedures and materials differ with various age groups, we shall briefly describe methods for various target populations.

1. *Preschool and Early-Elementary Children.* There are essentially five ways to screen the speech of a young child. In cases of very young children it is quite possible that they will not talk to the clinician at all, especially if they are taken to a strange setting with an unfamiliar adult. With children who simply will not speak, it is prudent to recommend a rescreening or a diagnostic evaluation after all attempts at obtaining direct and indirect samples have failed. One way to obtain information about the communication of a reluctant child is to interview the parents or teachers, if they are available. Much important information can be provided by people who interact with the child day after day. These people can provide "ballpark" data on the child's mean length of utterance, types of word combinations, fluency, vocal quality, and intelligibility and can summarize the occasions when the child communicates most. This interview process is no substitute for observing the child's communication firsthand, but it certainly can pinpoint significant problems in any area and can be the basis for recommending a diagnostic evaluation.

A second way of obtaining information about a young child is to observe the child during free play, perhaps with other children. This procedure is very effective, but time consuming. One advantage of this process is that the child is not taken away from his/her environment and isolated with a strange adult. The clinician can also interact with the child as he/she performs schoolroom tasks and can involve other children to stimulate diverse interactions.

A third method of screening young children is to obtain a short sample of conversational speech. Research has found that screening judgments made by an experienced clinician from a two-to-three minute sample were as good or better than formal measures (Eveleigh and Warr-Leeper 1983). This finding is similar to the high correspondence between formal and informal measures in language assessment (Allen, Bliss, and Timmons 1981).

Another method of screening is to ask the child to repeat words, phrases, or sentences. The examiner's model may tend to influence the child's speech and thus may not provide a representative sample. Stimulation tends to increase correct productions (Winitz 1969). If the clinician must screen large numbers of children rapidly, however, an imitative protocol may be the most expedient method of obtaining the information in the shortest amount of time.

A fifth technique to use in screening is to ask the child to name colors, to count, and to identify pictures or objects. This is a common method used, especially with low-functioning children, since it is easy and takes little time and since children seem to respond well to the task. Many published diagnostic inventories cited later in this chapter are designed for use as screening tests for children (Bryant and Bryant 1983; Fluharty 1974; Monsees and Berman 1968; Riley 1971; Rogers 1972; Templin and Darley 1969).

2. *Later-Elementary Children.* Speech pathologists may use reading passages and conversation to screen children in grades four through eight who are typically referred by classroom teachers. The clinician may choose from among several published reading passages for later-elementary children (Avant and Hutton 1962; Eisenson and Ogilvie 1977).

To obtain a sample of spontaneous speech, questions about favorite hobbies and interests are useful. Actually, later-elementary children are often rather engaging conversationalists; they are sufficiently mature to enjoy relating to a new adult, but not old enough to resent being scrutinized. Indeed, they are often intrigued with the screening test and want to know how they have done. It is usually wise to provide a brief explanation of any noted articulation errors.

3. *Older Groups.* Reading passages, sentences loaded with consonant sounds most frequently defective, and conversations are commonly used to obtain speech samples in screening programs for older individuals. The clinician can construct a reading passage or use any of the several published versions that include "My Grandfather" (Van Riper 1963), "Arthur the Young Rat" (Johnson, Darley, and Spriestersbach 1963), "The Rainbow Passage" (Fairbanks 1960), and "Directions" (Anderson 1973). In addition to an oral reading, some questions are asked to elicit a sample of spontaneous speech. Queries such as "What are you majoring in and how did you select that field?" or "If I were to come to your home area as a tourist, what are some things I might want to see?" are good examples of starters.

Predictive Screening

A significant number of children entering kindergarten and first grade will not have acquired the normal complement of consonant sounds (Pendergast et al. 1984). This places the clinician in a dilemma. Some of the children's speech differences are merely the result of late maturation and do not require treatment. But how do you separate the normal speakers from the potentially permanent misarticulators? Operating on an ad hoc basis, some clinicians select certain children and not others. They then find it difficult to explain their selection process to teachers, parents, and administrators. The opposite extreme is to work with all first-grade children who present articulation errors.

In an effort to provide some "objective" means of determining which children should be enrolled in treatment, several test instruments have been developed that attempt to "predict" which children are "high risk" for articulation disorders (McDonald 1968; Templin and Darley 1969; Van Riper and Erickson 1969). These tests vary in terms of whether they are administered imitatively or spontaneously, and they differ in the distribution of phonemes tested. Recently, Ritterman et al. (1982) compared the McDonald Screening Deep Test, the Templin-Darley Screening Test and the Predictive Screening Test of Articulation in terms of the pass/fail judgments indicated on ninety-one first-grade children and found that there was a "poor correspondence among the tests as to the individuals failed. That is, only three subjects were failed by more than a single test" (432). The three instruments evaluate either consistency of sound production (McDonald Screening Deep Test) or the total number of correctly produced spontaneous or imitative productions (Templin-Darley Screening Test, Predictive Screening Test of Articulation).

Certainly, a child who is dramatically delayed in articulatory development would fail all three of these tests, but this type of child is not particularly problematic to the clinician. It is the child who is on the borderline that presents difficulties. Clinicians should not rely exclusively on such measures to determine if a child requires enrollment in treatment. Ultimately, it comes down to a clinical judgment that must be made for each case, based upon normative data; and although a formal screening test might be considered in concert with other variables, it cannot be the sole determiner of enrollment. Ritterman et al. (1982) state that

> research has indicated that each of the underlying variables on which the Templin Darley Screening Test of Articulation, The Predictive Screening Test of Articulation and The Screening Deep Test of Articulation are based have some degree of merit as pass/fail selection criteria. The results of the present study, however, would seem to indicate that these variables are not well correlated in that different children failed for different reasons on the three tests. (432)

A test developed more recently is the Coarticulation Assessment in Meaningful Language (CAML) (Kenney and Prather 1984). This test uses more-meaningful sentences in a delayed imitation paradigm with pictures to obtain responses (e.g., "Look, the mouse fell and the cup fell. What happened here?"). The Coarticulation Assessment in Meaningful Language and the Screening Deep Test of Articulation were compared in kindergarten subjects, and the two tests were found to be similar in general results; however, the former yielded a greater total number of errors.

Other variables that might enter into decision making for a particular case might be (1) the child's perception of himself/herself as communication disordered,

(2) the parent and teacher perceptions and desires, (3) the presence of concomitant disorders (e.g., language), and (4) the existence of characteristically resistant articulatory deviations (e.g., lateral sibilants, vocalic /r/ distortions, omissions of consonants).

Traditional Assessment Procedures

Subsequent to failure of an articulatory screening, a child may be scheduled for a complete assessment of phonological ability. There are a variety of types of articulatory assessments that differ in their theoretical assumptions, method of sample elicitation, the type of information obtained, and their therapeutic implications. Perhaps the most common type of assessment is what we will call "traditional." The theoretical orientation of traditional testing is that each English phoneme must be evaluated in the initial, medial, and final positions of words. These words are typically elicited from the client by means of pictures, word lists, sentences, or conversational sampling. Many studies examining articulation from a "traditional" perspective have shown that children tend to produce more singleton consonants correctly in single-word sampling contexts (Dubois and Bernthal 1978; Faircloth and Faircloth 1970; Healy and Madison 1987; Johnson, Whinney, and Pederson 1980; Kenney and Prather 1984; Paden and Moss 1985). On the other hand, when performance is examined from a phonological process perspective, some studies have shown no significant differences between single-word and connected-speech sampling conditions (Bowman, Parsons, and Morris 1984; Dyson and Robinson 1987; McLeod et al. 1994; Paden and Moss 1985). Even though the data for the analysis might range from words to connected speech, the orientation of the clinician is to determine omissions, substitutions, and distortions of phonemes in differing word positions. Many tests are available for use in traditional assessment (Bryant and Bryant 1983; Edmonson 1969; Fisher and Logemann 1971; Fudala 1989; Goldman and Fristoe 1986; Hejna 1963; Ingram 1971; Pendergast et al. 1984; Templin and Darley 1969). Some of these inventories include stimulus pictures for testing children, and structured sentences for older clients to read. Several tests provide norms against which a child may be compared.

Traditional diagnostic procedures have in common other basic operations. Most traditional assessments accrue a phonetic inventory from the client. This is a listing of all phonemes produced in the sample. One reason for obtaining a phonetic inventory is to compare to normative data on articulatory development the sounds produced correctly by a given client. As mentioned earlier, most normative studies are based on traditional notions and report phoneme productions of sounds in the three word positions (Poole 1934; Prather, Hedrick, and Kern 1975; Sander 1972; Templin 1957; Wellman et al. 1931).

Another traditional procedure is the testing of a client's stimulability, or response to stimulation. In other words, we evaluate the impact that the examiner's model has upon the client's production. Is there some modification in the direction of normalcy? Or is there no change in the articulatory behavior? Testing for stimulability (Milisen et al. 1954) is an extremely useful diagnostic procedure. If a client can produce the error correctly by imitating a standard model, either in isolation, in nonsense syllables, or in words, then there may be no serious organic obstacles that would prevent the eventual acquisition of the sound (Darley 1964). Stimulability is also a useful prognostic sign; clients who can modify their articulation errors by imitating the examiner's standard production have a place to start the treatment process. Stimulability has also been implicated as a potential predicter of whether children will develop normal speech through maturation (Farquhar 1961). Stimulability is frequently given "short shrift" by practicing clinicians and students in training. Sometimes it is totally omitted. Often, we see students hurry through the stimulability testing, frequently giving inadequate instructions and rather imprecise models to the client. The spirit of stimulability testing is to see how the client performs under maximal, multimodality stimulation. This is why most tests recommend that the model be presented two or three times after the client has been given a strong attentional set. Students sometimes indicate that the client was not stimulable for error phonemes after rather cursory testing. Subsequent stimulability trials, done more intensively, may reveal that the client, in fact, can produce the target sound. Prior to making negative stimulability statements in a clinical report, the clinician should be certain that the stimulation task was administered effectively.

It is our contention that traditional testing is a good starting point in an articulatory assessment. In many cases, a traditional assessment may be all that is needed, especially when the client has only a few articulatory errors and is stimulable. In cases like this, the clinician knows what the errors are and how often they occur in a test and in spontaneous speech if analyzed traditionally. Further, the clinician has a place to start production of the target sound, since the client can make it correctly with stimulation. Probe tasks that focus on particular productions can also be used as a follow-up procedure. For example, specific probing techniques have been developed for use with consonant clusters (Powell 1995). In the majority of cases, however, traditional testing does not go far enough. For instance, our discussion of coarticulation suggested that sounds will be produced differently in different phonetic environments. Most traditional tests examine only a limited number of these phonetic contexts. If a child or adult is not stimulable, the clinician may want to rely on experimentation with different coarticulatory transitions to determine if there is a facilitating context. Most traditional tests are just not equipped to do this. Another example is that traditional testing procedures are not directed toward detecting patterns of error in a client's speech. In order to define patterns of error, a phonological analysis is the most efficient method to use. Traditional analyses do not systematically examine the effects of stress, syllable complexity (Panagos, Quine, and Klich 1979) linguistic complexity, and pragmatics on misarticulation. Finally, traditional analyses do not focus on certain parameters that may be relevant to certain cases, such as distinctive feature acquisition and use. In short, no one method can do everything, and so it is with the traditional approach. The traditional test, however, is a viable instrument to use generically. If other analyses are required, they should be done when appropriate.

It is far easier to describe articulation testing than it is to administer an articulation test. A student's first attempt is generally a confusing situation that requires careful listening, attention to visual cues, recording the client's responses appropriately, and maintaining a positive client-clinician relationship. We recommend that the beginning clinician listen for only one sound at a time. When possible, have the child repeat the test words a number of times. Tape-record, or better yet, videotape the child's responses to assist in later scoring of the test. Experienced speech pathologists are able to save time by testing more than one sound simultaneously (Fristoe and Goldman 1968).

It is especially true with articulation assessment that the clinician is really the "test." Commercial articulation tests are nothing more than stacks of pictures bound together with metal or plastic. Since articulatory responses are so transient and fleeting, clinicians must listen carefully, practice frequently, and, above all, check their reliability. Studies have shown that speech pathologists are fairly reliable when the judgments they make are rather molar, such as "correct" or "incorrect" (Winitz 1969). When judgments become more "fine grained" as in determining the nature of specific substitutions in certain word positions, our reliability tends to deteriorate. One can easily see that very complex analysis procedures such as those used in distinctive features and phonology are even more susceptible to misjudgments on the part of the clinician. The clinician must always strive to improve his/her reliability through practice and by rechecking his/her results. A clinician's evaluation results are only as good as his/her ability to perceive the reality of the client's responses. No one, as an old professor said, has immaculate perception. Chapter 3 discusses interjudge reliability and provides a formula for its calculation.

Test Procedures that Evaluate Phonetic Context Effects

Subsequent to a traditional assessment, a client may be judged not stimulable. Procedures then need to be initiated to determine if a facilitating phonetic context can be found. As we mentioned in the section on coarticulation, phonemes are significantly influenced by other sounds that surround them. This phenomenon results in the existence of facilitating contexts that can encourage the correct production of a target consonant. The concept that certain phonetic environments can be facilitory of correct production was suggested in the early writings of Van Riper and Irwin (1958) where they indicated there were "key words" in which a phoneme could be produced more effectively. If certain key words were discovered for a nonstimulable client, then treatment could commence in these contexts. In 1964, Eugene McDonald devised the Deep Test of Articulation, which, among other things, is based on the idea that phonemes will be produced differently depending on the sounds that precede and follow them. By systematically permuting a variety of consonants before and after a specific phoneme, the contexts in which correct production is observed can be noted by the clinician and can serve as a starting point for treatment. In the Deep Test of Articulation, each phoneme can be observed forty or more times as the initiating or terminating sound in a syllable.

Since it is the basic unit of speech, it seems appropriate that the focus of testing should be the syllable. Here is a part of a session in which the examiner is administering the /s/ portion of the McDonald instrument to a second-grade boy with a distorted /s/:

> *Clinician: Okay, Tony, you understand now that you are to make a funny "big word" from the names of the objects on the two pictures, like we did in the example "tubvase," without stopping between the words? Here is the first one:*

1.	*housepipe*	*no change*
2.	*housebell*	*no change*
3.	*housetie*	*improvement*
4.	*housedog*	*improvement*
5.	*housecow*	*no change*
6.	*housegun*	*no change*

Note that the word "house," with a final /s/, is tested as it precedes all other phonemes. The examiner listens carefully to identify any changes in the child's misarticulations. Then, the examiner reverses the procedure so that /s/ follows all other phonemes ("cupsun," "tubsun," "kitesun," etc.). In the above example, the /s/ improved when it preceded a lingua-alveolar stop, which may represent a facilitating context for lessening the distortion of the target sound. For older clients, McDonald has prepared a series of sentences to be read aloud. The diagnostician will want to be familiar with this test.

The McDonald Deep Test has certain limitations. For instance, when we combine two lexical items into one nonsense word, we are no longer dealing with sound production in real linguistic units. In addition, as the test progresses, some children find the big words neither "funny" nor interesting. Some children also experience considerable difficulty in blending the two test items into one large word (Goda 1970). If there is a pause between the two words, the purpose of the test is defeated (McDonald 1964). Finally, depending on the child's pattern of misarticulation, many of the intended phonetic contexts are altered (e.g., "housecow" becomes "housetow"). This alteration changes the ability of the instrument to really evaluate all the contexts it is designed to elicit. We prefer to use the test during the initial stages of treatment, exploring with the client for loci of improved, or at least altered, sound production. Additionally, researchers find the McDonald Deep Test invaluable for charting improvement during the course of treatment because it deals with many contexts.

The evaluation of a variety of phonetic contexts provides an interesting contrast to the limited number of environments evaluated by traditional measures. Schissell and James (1979) compared the evaluation of articulatory abilities in children by using a more traditional test (Arizona) and the McDonald Deep Test. It was found that the traditional test missed some of the children who did not have consistent control of certain sounds, and it was also noted that the traditional test failed children on certain sounds when in actuality the children performed the sound productions well in a significant number of contexts on the McDonald Deep

Test. One interpretation of the disparity in results between these two measures is that the traditional test evaluated a limited number of phonetic contexts; for some children the environment happened to be facilitative, and for others it did not. The implication, of course, is that the more phonetic contexts examined, the more realistic the picture obtained of the clients' articulatory performance. In addition, we might find a place to begin our treatment.

Another way to examine phonetic context effects in children and adults is the use of sound-in-context sentences (Haynes, Haynes, and Jackson 1982; Mazza, Shuckers, and Daniloff 1979). These sentences can be read spontaneously by adults or imitated by children. Most work with these sentences has been done in research projects directed toward finding facilitating contexts for particular target consonants (mainly the /s/ and /r/ phonemes). The use of these sentence stimuli has shown that there are, in fact, facilitating contexts for /r/ and /s/ that occur for many clients. The essence of these sentences is that a clinician can ask the client to say any number of utterances that are constructed to determine phonetic context effects. For instance, if the clinician wants to evaluate the effects on /s/ production of a preceding /k/ sound and a following /p/ sound (e.g., /KSP/) a sentence can be constructed such as "The dress had a bla*ck sp*ot." In addition, phrases may be used instead of sentences. The clinician, then, can use knowledge of coarticulation and devise stimuli to probe phonetic context effects on a given client's articulation. Finally, Kent (1982) urges continued experimentation with phonetic context effects in clinical and research settings because there is much we do not yet understand about this phenomenon:

> *The selection of so-called facilitating contexts involves decisions regarding stress, word position, expected or permissible allophonic variation, frequency of occurrence and the influence of neighboring sounds. . . . The final selection of a facilitating context also should recognize as precisely as possible the nature of the articulation error. It should not be assumed, for example, that the same context will facilitate correct production of /s/ in children who distort the sound by dentalization, lateralization and palatalization.* (75)

With a knowledge of the effects of coarticulation, the clinician may construct a variety of utterance types for a particular client and need not rely solely on instruments devised by others. A thorough assessment could provide significant information that could be used at the outset of treatment if more attention were paid to ferreting out sources of error inconsistency attributable to phonetic context. The clinician should also be willing to experiment with a variety of segmental, suprasegmental, and linguistic complexity variables in the search for sources of inconsistency (Shriberg and Kwiatkowski 1980).

The Phonetic and Phonemic Inventories

A most important source of information about a phonologically disordered client is the phonetic inventory. After gathering a representative sample, one of the first operations a clinician should perform is to inventory the client's sound system in several ways. The phonetic inventory is a summary of sounds the client has produced either correctly or incorrectly in the sample and represents the sounds that can be physically produced by the person. That is, if the client produced a glottal stop, this sound is part of the phonetic inventory. If the client produces an θ/s substitution and never produces the [θ] correctly when it is required to be, the [θ] is still included in the phonetic inventory. The phonemic inventory, on the other hand, includes sounds that are used contrastively and that are implemented to make a meaning difference in the client's language. Thus, although an [θ] may be a part of the child's phonetic repertoire, it may not be part of the phonemic system.

As we will mention later, an examination of the phonetic and phonemic inventories is a critical part of assessing a child's possession and use of distinctive features of English phonemes. There are also some other ways to analyze data from a child's phonetic and phonemic inventories. Some authorities (Elbert 1992; Elbert and Gierut 1986; Maxwell and Rockman 1984) have recommended searching for various types of rules that may or may not be operating in a child's system, and the phonetic/phonemic inventories are an important part of these analyses. For instance, static rules called "phonotactic constraints" (Dinnesen 1984) may be operating to restrict the occurrence of certain sounds or phoneme combinations. Three types of phonotactic constraints have been reported. First, *positional constraints* are rules that allow the production of a sound in only certain contexts or word positions. Second, *inventory constraints* reduce the production of particular sounds because the phonemes are not included in the phonetic inventory. Finally, *sequence constraints* are rules that may not permit the child to produce sounds in particular combinations (e.g., the child can produce the phoneme as a singleton, but not in a cluster). One can see that examination of the phonetic and phonemic inventory is an important part of arriving at an appreciation of a client's phonotactic rule system.

There are a variety of systems for reporting a client's phonetic inventory. It would be most important for a phonetic inventory not only to reflect sensorimotor production of a sound but also to provide some indication of appropriate or phonemic use of the element. The phonetic inventory should also indicate failure to sample certain sounds so that the clinician does not assume the client cannot produce the sounds. The phonetic inventory in the Natural Process Analysis (Shriberg and Kwiatkowski 1980) differentiates between a phone that is used correctly, appears in the sample, is glossed in the sample, and is never glossed. This analysis can tell the clinician if the phonetic element is phonemic (correct anywhere), whether it is used as a substitution for another sound (appears anywhere), whether it should have been in a word (glossed) but was not, or whether the sound was never expected to be produced in the sample. Other systems simply list the phones in the phonetic inventory from left to right in terms of place of articulation in the vocal tract (left=front, right=back) (Maxwell and Rockman 1984). Another way to consider a child's phonetic/phonemic inventory might be to array the phonemes on the continuum of phonological knowledge mentioned earlier. Elbert and Gierut (1986) provide an example of such a summary.

Whatever way the clinician decides to examine a child's phonological system, a phonetic/phonemic inventory is a good starting point because it can give significant insights into phonotactic rules (e.g., inventory constraints) and the child's overall knowledge of the sound system.

Distinctive Feature Analysis

As we mentioned previously, neither traditional analyses or appraisals of phonetic context effects examine all pertinent aspects of a child's articulatory system. Researchers indicate that the most basic unit that speech can be reduced to is the distinctive feature, and the "reality" of features has been demonstrated both acoustically and physiologically (Singh 1976). That is, as humans, we seem to pay attention to certain aspects of the speech signal both in perception and production. Phonemes are evidently made up of "bundles" of distinctive features that combine to produce a variety of different consonant and vowel sounds in a language. Singh (1976) states: "Children do not acquire phonemes one by one; rather, they acquire a feature that provides them with a basis for manifesting a number of phonemes distinctively in speech production and discrimination tasks" (229). Features, then, are a "prerequisite" to phonemes, because without the knowledge of and ability to produce a given feature of language, certain sounds containing that feature will not be produced. For instance, if a child does not learn that the feature of "voicelessness" is important in differentiating certain sounds from each other, the phonemes with the – voice feature will not be produced (/s, f, p, k/ etc.). Distinctive feature theory attempts to specify the characteristics of phonemes—according to the presence (+) or absence (–) of each feature that distinguishes or contrasts one speech sound from another. Table 6.1 depicts a distinctive feature system frequently referred to in the clinical literature.

One difficulty that is immediately apparent to a student studying distinctive features is the number of "systems" available (Singh 1976) and the fact that no single system has received universal acceptance (Fey 1992). Furthermore, these systems have been derived by different procedures and thus have disparate bases (acoustic, articulatory, perceptual). The feature systems also differ in the phonemes included in the scheme, the notation (binary, ternary, quarternary), and the number of features thought to be important. One source of solace to the clinician is the fact that most systems have some things in common. There are certain features that appear to be so significant and strong that they are included in the majority of systems. Specifically, the features of voice, nasality, some feature denoting duration, and a place feature are the most common. Many authorities simply use the traditional place, manner, and voicing features for assessment purposes (Stoel-Gammon 1996)

Several investigations have suggested that there are at least two different types of feature problems exhibited by children: phonetic and phonemic (Elbert 1992; McReynolds and Huston 1971; Pollack and Rees 1972; Ruder and Bunce 1981). One type of distinctive feature difficulty is exemplified by a child who has not acquired

TABLE 6.1   Example of Distinctive Feature Approach to Analyzing Articulation Errors*

Error	Features Used Correctly	Features in Error	
Substitution/Target		Target Phoneme	Substitution
d/s	vocalic, consonantal, high, back, low, nasal	– voice + continuant + strident	+ voice – continuant – strident
d/z	vocalic, consonantal, high, back, low, nasal	+ continuant + strident	– continuant – strident
d/sh	vocalic, consonantal, high, back, low, nasal	– voice + continuant + strident	+ voice – continuant – strident
b/f	vocalic, consonantal, high, back, low, nasal	– voice + continuant + strident	+ voice – continuant – strident
b/v	vocalic, consonantal, high, back, low, nasal	+ continuant + strident	– continuant – strident
d/th (*th*ink)	vocalic, consonantal, high, back, low, nasal	– voice + continuant	+ voice – continuant
d/th (*th*at)	vocalic, consonantal, high, back, low, nasal	+ continuant	– continuant

*The features associated with phonemes are from Chomsky and Halle (1968). Compare the feature bundles of the target and error phonemes to determine features misused. One can easily see the most misused features are the voicing, continuancy, and stridency elements.

the use of a feature at all. The child is not aware of the importance of the feature to differentiate English sounds and has difficulty producing the feature. The child might have one "aspect" or one half of the feature (+ voicing), but does not have the other half (– voicing). Features are rather like light switches; they are only useful when you know about both turning them on and turning them off. Thus, a child has not really acquired the feature of "voice" until both voiced and voiceless sounds can be produced appropriately and contrastively (Grunwell 1988). If a child's phonetic inventory does not include voiceless phonemes used correctly or incorrectly, the child does not have contrastive use of the voice feature. A second type of feature error is shown in a child who has acquired the feature, but does not use it appropriately. Control of features, as with many things, is on a continuum. A child may be aware of the importance of a feature and be capable of producing both aspects (+ and −) of it, yet there are specific contexts in which the feature is not used appropriately. On the other hand, a child may not be able to produce the feature aspects without great difficulty in any context. Several authorities mentioned above have suggested that these two cases represent slightly different diagnostic groups. One child does not "have" the feature, and the other "has" it but is a feature misuser in certain contexts.

Several approaches have been suggested for distinctive feature analysis. McReynolds and Engmann (1975) have prepared a manual featuring detailed clinical worksheets to guide the diagnostician in performing a distinctive feature analysis. This approach is quite time consuming and has been criticized for procedural as well as theoretical shortcomings (Carney 1979; Grunwell 1988). Currently, most authorities recommend the examination of distinctive features as part of the larger process of phonological analysis. That is, when we write phonological rules for a disordered child's system, we can use distinctive features to make our descriptions more specific and look for commonalities across different sound errors. Table 6.1 gives an example of how six individual sound errors can be construed as basically a problem with one distinctive feature (+ continuant). A phonological process analysis of the same errors would reveal a "stopping" rule, which is essentially a misuse of + continuant. It would be important to determine if the child in the example ever produced the + continuant feature in the speech sample. One can easily see that using distinctive features is just another way to look at a client's misarticulations and can add some specificity to our descriptions as well as allow us to see relationships among individual sound errors. Elbert (1992) points out the importance of considering that a child can exhibit *both* phonetic and phonemic problems within the same disordered phonological system.

It was mentioned earlier that a major decision we must make in a distinctive feature analysis is whether a child has not acquired a feature or whether he is a feature misuser. This decision is typically quite easy for a clinician to make after looking at the child's phonetic inventory to see if whole classes of sounds and features are missing. An experienced clinician can examine a child's speech sample and accurately predict which features are the most in error without resorting to the lengthy procedure provided by McReynolds and Engmann (1975). In many cases this may be enough to help the clinician to decide whether the treatment should be directed toward establishing a feature in a child's repertoire or altering the use of a feature that has already been acquired but is being used inconsistently in a child's system.

What are the advantages of considering distinctive features in our analysis of misarticulations? We see four advantages. First, considering distinctive features provides a model for understanding errors in many clients; an error on a given feature (e.g., voicing) that is shared by more than one phoneme accounts for the misarticulation of many phonemes by reducing the seemingly random errors to a simpler pattern. Second, considering distinctive features may provide one gauge of severity of sound substitution, in that the more feature differences between a target sound and its substitution, the more severe the problem may be. Third, it provides a basis for the selection of a target sound for therapy; the clinician can select the phoneme which shares features with many other misarticulated sounds. And fourth, it may provide a basis for more efficient therapy (Costello and Onstine 1976; Ritterman and Freeman 1974) by facilitating generalization to sounds not being directly treated. Therapy directed toward one sound often improves others that are phonetically similar. Considered within the framework of distinctive features, it makes sense that training in features common to many sounds would result in greater improvement in misarticulation than would specific training for each sound error.

Despite the many advantages, however, there are a number of factors that may limit the application of distinctive feature theory to clinical problems. First of all, some procedures for assessment (e.g., McReynolds and Engmann 1975) are quite time consuming; the clinician has to weigh this factor against the purported increase in efficiency. Sommers (1983) has suggested a less formal "short-cut" method of analyzing distinctive features from a sample of speech. Sommers indicates that the briefer method yields similar results at a considerable savings of analysis time. Developments in computer software have included feature analyses that may make the procedure less tedious for clinicians. The second limiting factor is the obvious complexity of the system of analysis. Another drawback is that, on a phonetic level, the distinctive features advocated by Chomsky and Halle may have no conceptual reality (LaRiviere 1974). By that we mean that there may be no one-to-one relationship between distinctive features (an acoustic classification) and articulatory production (a physiological level) (Parker 1976). The physical act of articulation clearly is not a binary function that is either present (+) or absent (–) but is multivaried—a matter of varying degrees. According to Walsh (1974), the categories employed in distinctive feature analysis are overgeneralized and may encompass too great a phonetic space to be of clinical value. Leonard (1973) points out that "articulation therapy involves giving phonetic instructions. Therefore, the features we deal with must have a specific physical interpretation" (141–142). Where it is necessary to use a subphonemic system of analysis, we advocate with others (Eisenson and Ogilvie 1977; Fisher and Logemann 1971; Leonard 1973; McClean 1976; Sommers 1983; Walsh 1974) the selection of one based on a model of speech production rather than on a system limited to an abstract classificatory function. A formal distinctive feature analysis may not be necessary, as indicated by Grunwell (1988):

> The last few paragraphs have seriously thrown into question the clinical value of a formalised distinctive feature analysis procedure. This implication is intentional. None the less, the CONCEPTS of distinctive feature contrasts and natural classes are of major importance and considerable clinical applicability. The concept that phonemes are differentiated by their 'content' of contrastive features enables the clinician to focus on the contrastive/distinctive feature that is in "error" and also to recognise similar "errors" in different phonemes, that is patterns in disordered speech. (157)

We believe that whatever method the clinician uses to analyze distinctive features in a given client, the following are important:

1. The diagnostician should "think features" at some point in the analysis of a child with multiple articulation errors. In other words, one should at least be able to make the judgment as to whether or not all features are present or if error patterns reflect consistent, repeated misuse of specific features in certain contexts.

2. The clinician should determine if a child (a) has not acquired a feature or (b) is a feature misuser. If the child does not evidence a particular feature in his phonetic inventory, then treatment may best be directed toward basic introduction of the feature into the child's repertoire (McReynolds and Engmann 1975; McReynolds and Huston 1971; Pollack and Rees 1972). If the child is a feature misuser, then further phonological analysis (which implies feature use) is indicated, and the clinician must determine the extent and loci of feature misuse. Typical feature analysis techniques (McReynolds and Engmann 1975) do not allow for determining specific contexts in which features are in error. Phonological analysis techniques are more equipped to do this. More-recent nonlinear phonological analyses include a feature level in their hierarchy.

3. Substitution errors especially should undergo a distinctive feature "substitution analysis" in which the feature bundles of the target and substituted sounds are compared and features that are misused are noted by the examiner, as in Table 6.1.

Phonological Analysis

Another approach to analyzing a child's articulatory behavior is to perform a phonological analysis. In 1976, a landmark book by David Ingram entitled *Phonological Disability in Children* was published and sparked an interest in a more linguistic approach to misarticulation analysis. Ingram cited many sources who reported that there were common patterns of articulatory simplification in children's speech (Compton 1970, 1976; Oller et al. 1972; Smith 1973; Stampe 1969). That is, most children develop the ability to articulate gradually and prior to perfecting an adult production, they reduce the complexity of words in characteristic ways. Space in the present chapter does not permit us to provide examples of each phonological pattern reported in the existing literature, and most training programs now include extensive exposure to phonological processes in course work. Readers are referred to any of the above sources for myriad examples of phonological processes.

A phonological approach rests on certain assumptions. First, phonologists assume that there is a structure to every child's sound system and that even in the most unintelligible child there is a pattern of phonemic production. Sounds do not occur in random combinations. Second, a phonological approach assumes an underlying system that gives rise to the observable sound combinations that we hear from children. The implication is that a phonological error may be a product of the underlying system that organizes the overt sound combinations.

Earlier in the present chapter, we indicated that there can be both linguistically based and sensorimotor-based misarticulations. The linguistically generated errors could be construed as products of rules generated by the child's underlying phonological system. Rules, to a certain degree, imply patterns of performance, and phonological "rules" can be written to simply describe these patterns. Phonological rules, then, are descriptive of the way in which a child uses classes of phonemes. Many investigators have reported that, in development, it is commonly observed that children tend to simplify their word productions in comparison to the adult model. The simplifications are typically in the direction of producing physiologically easier sounds for more difficult ones. For reasons not presently known, some children appear to persist in using these simplification strategies; and if enough of these strategies are retained, the child is likely to be quite unintelligible. Most authorities report that many of the patterns of error found in disordered children are those observed in normally developing youngsters at earlier ages (Ingram 1976; Shriberg and Kwiatkowski 1980). Ingram (1976), however, also points out that deviant rules not typically found in normally developing children may appear in phonologically disordered youngsters. Phonological rules can describe these simplification techniques, and each rule implies a change in the use of distinctive features. That is, a child who substitutes stops for continuants is altering an important distinctive feature of the target phonemes.

```
+ continuant      – continuant
     s                 t
     ∫                 t
     f ───────────▶ p
     θ                 t
```

The clinician wishing to gain insight into phonological processes has at least two levels of analysis to choose from. First, there are instruments available that are targeted toward discovering phonological processes in children (Bankson and Bernthal 1990; Compton and Hutton 1978; Hodson 1986; Kahn and Lewis 1986; Lowe 1986; Webb and Duckett 1990; Weiner 1979). These measures provide picture or object stimuli and ask the child to give a single word or connected speech response. These responses are analyzed by the clinician for particular phonological simplifications. Table 6.2 summarizes some of the specific phonological processes examined by the instruments discussed. The reader should consult these references for examples and guidelines in defining the processes.

The Phonological Process Analysis (PPA) (Weiner 1979) is a descriptive procedure that is not sound specific and focuses on patterns. The Phonological Process Analysis uses delayed imitation and is directed toward children between the ages of two and five. It uses action pictures that sample single words and sentence phrases. The stimulus items are organized by phonological process rather than the traditional grouping of phoneme or age of development of sounds.

Another measure is the Compton-Hutton Phonological Assessment (Compton and Hutton 1978) that uses fifty picture stimuli to elicit consonants in initial and final positions of words. The test is aimed at children between the ages of three and seven, and each word is elicited two times to evaluate "consistency" of productions.

TABLE 6.2 Phonological Processes Examined by Selected Evaluation Procedures

Category	Process	PPA	APP	C-H	K-L	NPA	PPACL	PACS	ALPHA
Syllable Structure	Glottal Replacement	×	×		×			×	×
Syllable Structure	Final Consonant Deletion	×	×	×	×	×	×	×	×
Syllable Structure	Unstressed Syllable Deletion	×	×		×	×	×	×	×
Syllable Structure	Consonant Cluster Red	×	×	×	×	×	×	×	×
Syllable Structure	Reduplication	×					×	×	
Syllable Structure	Initial Consonant Deletion		×		×		×		×
Syllable Structure	Epenthesis		×						
Harmony	Labial Assimilation	×	×		×	×	×	×	
Harmony	Alveolar Assimilation	×	×		×	×		×	
Harmony	Velar Assimilation	×	×		×	×	×	×	
Harmony	Nasal Assimilation		×		×	×	×	×	
Harmony	Prevocalic Voicing	×	×		×		×	×	×
Harmony	Devoicing	×	×	×	×			×	×
Harmony	Coalescence		×						
Harmony	Metathesis		×						
Feature Contrast	Stopping	×	×	×	×	×	×	×	×
Feature Contrast	Affrication	×	×	×					×
Feature Contrast	Velar Fronting	×	×	×	×	×	×	×	×
Feature Contrast	Fricative Voicing	×	×	×	×	×	×	×	×
Feature Contrast	Gliding	×	×	×	×		×	×	×
Feature Contrast	Vocalization	×		×			×	×	×
Feature Contrast	Denasalization	×	×				×		
Feature Contrast	Neutralization	×	×						
Feature Contrast	Backing		×		×				×
Feature Contrast	Deaffrication		×	×	×		×		×
Feature Contrast	Palatalization		×						
Feature Contrast	Depalitalization		×				×		
Feature Contrast	Apicalization						×	×	×
Feature Contrast	Labialization						×		×
Feature Contrast	Stridency Deletion								×

Two phonemes are examined in each word sampled. Phonological rules are provided on the scoring sheet to assist the clinician in defining common error patterns.

The Assessment of Phonological Processes (APP-R) (Hodson 1986) elicits and requires transcription of fifty-five utterances. Toys are used instead of pictures and the child spontaneously names each object while the examiner transcribes the responses. All consonants are assessed at a minimum of two times pre- and post-vocalically. Thirty-one consonant clusters are assessed. The test assesses forty-two phonological processes and "articulatory shifts."

The Assessment Link between Phonology and Articulation (ALPHA) (Lowe 1986) is a delayed imitation procedure that also provides a traditional as well as phonological process analysis of a child's responses to fifty target words embedded in sentences. Sixteen processes are specifically targeted, and the test was standardized on over 1300 normal subjects between the ages of three and nine years.

The Kahn-Lewis Phonological Analysis (Kahn and Lewis 1986) utilizes the forty-four words from the Goldman-Fristoe Test of Articulation (Goldman and Fristoe 1986) to examine fifteen phonological processes. Norms for process occurrence are provided for children between the ages of two and six years. Several other authors have advocated using all available phonemes found in single-word items on traditional articulation tests as Kahn and Lewis did above. Preliminary research suggests that traditional test stimuli can be used to aid the clinician in a gross analysis of phonological process use (Garber 1986; Garn-Nunn 1986; Klein 1984; Lowe 1986).

The measures mentioned above can be administered in a reasonable time period (under one hour), and the scoring time will vary with the clinician's experience in using the test and the severity of the phonological disorder under evaluation. The measures, however, do not evaluate spontaneous connected speech, and therefore the phonological rules obtained may only approximate those typically used by the child in conversation (Klein 1984). Some research, however, suggests more similarities than differences between single-word and connected speech productions. Andrews and Fey (1986) evoked the words from the Assessment of Phonological Processes in single-word and connected speech contexts and found that most phonological errors, severity ratings, and clinical recommendations would be similar for either response mode. Table 6.3 illustrates stimulus and task variables in both traditionally oriented and phonological evaluation procedures.

A second level of phonological analysis is to gather a spontaneous speech sample, transcribe it in the International Phonetic Alphabet, and attempt to discern patterns of error (processes) in the data. This is obviously more time consuming than the measures mentioned above, but it is also more valid because the clinician is examining actual utterances that were generated by the client's cognitive-linguistic system. The analysis of a spontaneous speech sample is recommended by Shriberg and Kwiatkowski (1980) in the Natural Process Analysis (NPA). This procedure specifically targets eight processes for analysis and provides a unique and useful phonetic inventory. The Natural Process Analysis can provide valuable information for the practitioner and represents a well-planned procedure.

TABLE 6.3 Stimulus and Task Variables in Tradition (T) and Phonologically (P) Oriented Evaluation Procedures

Procedure	Type	Sample Type		Task		Materials		Norms
		Word	Connected Speech	Spontaneous	Imitation	Picture/Object	L. Sample	
TDTA	T	X		X		X		Y
GFTA	T	X	X	X		X		Y
FLTAC	T	X		X		X	X	N
ARIZONA	T	X	X	X		X		Y
PAT	T	X	X	X		X		Y
APP	P	X		X		X		N
PPA	P	X	X		X	X		N
NPA	P		X	X			X	N
K-L	P	X		X		X		Y
C-H	P	X		X		X		N
PPACL	P	X	X	X			X	N
PACS	TP	X	X	X			X	N
TAP-D	T	X	X	X	X	X		N
ALPHA	TP		X		X	X		Y

Ingram (1981) developed the Procedures for the Phonological Analysis of Children's Language (PPACL), which includes a phonetic analysis, homonym analysis, substitution analysis, and phonological process analysis. Twenty-seven specific processes are targeted. However, Ingram stated that the analysis is "open ended" and can continue "until all the substitutions in a child's speech have been explained" (7).

Grunwell (1985) developed the Phonological Assessment of Child Speech (PACS), which provides a description of analysis procedures for a preferably spontaneous connected speech sample of over 200 words. The procedure results in phonetic analysis, contrastive analysis to determine which phones are used to make meaning differences, and a phonological process analysis. The Phonological Assessment of Child Speech also provides a developmental framework that is missing in many phonological analysis techniques.

There appears to be some agreement that certain processes are "high risk" in phonologically disordered children. Different authorities implicate specific phonological processes as being more "important" than others, at least in terms of focusing on them for assessment targets. Table 6.2 includes the processes thought to be significant enough to test in formal evaluation procedures. Some preliminary evidence exists that suggests that similar phonological processes are detected whether one uses more involved, lengthy procedures (NPA, PPACL) or shorter tasks (APP) (Paden and Moss 1986). This evidence, of course, does not indicate that in-depth phonological analyses and shorter procedures are equivalent, only that they both can identify basic phonological processes. Although there is considerable variation among the assessment techniques in the number of processes examined, there is also a high degree of agreement regarding processes that seem to be most at risk in unintelligible children. The actual number of processes targeted in an evaluation would seem to be related to the clinician's goals in the analysis (Ingram 1981). If the clinician wanted to write a relatively complete generative phonology for a client, it would obviously focus on a larger number of rules than if the clinician's goal were to determine which major processes interfered most with intelligibility. In the latter case, the clinician may find that six phonological processes account for over 80% of the child's misarticulations, and treatment targets might be selected from the processes having the most impact on intelligibility. For instance, if a child is exhibiting unstressed syllable deletion, final consonant deletion and stopping, these will be initial treatment targets; and rules such as epenthesis, vocalization, gliding, and so forth, which may have less effect on intelligibility, will not be of immediate concern. It should be noted that most of the evaluation techniques discussed above allow for the assessment of other processes as discovered by the examiner, even though the processes may not be specifically evaluated.

Recent work in the area of nonlinear phonology (Bernhardt and Stoel-Gammon 1994; Schwartz 1992; Stoel-Gammon 1996) has pointed out the importance and utility of considering hierarchial relationships in child utterances. These relationships among words, syllables, segments, and features are illustrated in Figure 6.3. The initial consonant(s) in a syllable is/are called *onsets* while *rhymes* are a vowel and any consonants following the onset. All English syllables require a rhyme, but the onset is optional as in a vowel-initiated word such as "outside." Segments in

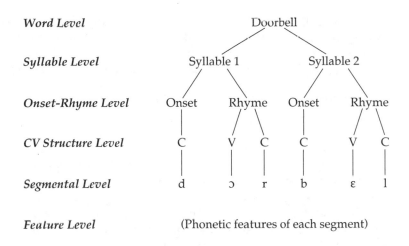

Word Level .... Doorbell

Syllable Level .... Syllable 1 .... Syllable 2

Onset-Rhyme Level ... Onset .. Rhyme .. Onset .. Rhyme

CV Structure Level .... C ... V .. C .... C ... V .. C

Segmental Level .... d ... ɔ .. r .... b ... ɛ .. l

Feature Level .... (Phonetic features of each segment)

**FIGURE 6.3   Hierarchial Levels Discussed in Nonlinear
Phonology**

SOURCE: Adapted from Stoel-Gammon (1996).

this model are similar to phonemes, and features can be viewed from a variety of perspectives as simple as place-manner voicing and as complex as other distinctive feature systems mentioned earlier in the present chapter. The elegance of hierarchial models is that they allow analysis of syllable, onset rhyme, CV structure, and segmental and feature levels and may account for misarticulations in a way not readily possible by traditional or phonological process modes of analysis. Stoel-Gammon (1996) provides excellent examples of using nonlinear phonology in the analysis of disordered phonology.

If a clinician wishes to write phonological rules from a child's conversational sample, there are certain basic issues common to most procedures.

1. *Glossing and Segmentation.* The clinician must interpret the child's utterances and provide adult interpretations or "glosses" of what the child was trying to say. One cannot arrive at a phonological rule system unless the intended utterance is known. Several methods of segmenting or arranging the data have been reported. One method is to arrange correct and incorrect child productions and glosses word by word in phonetic transcription:

Child's Production	Adult Gloss
/ki/	/ki/
/bækɪ/	/bæskɪt/
/pæ/	/fæn/
/go/	/go/

This allows the clinician the opportunity to compare productions with the adult model and hypothesize a phonological reduction pattern (e.g., final consonant deletion in the words "basket" and "fan"). Another method of segmentation is to retain spontaneous connected speech intact and divide the sample into utterances:

Child's Production	Adult Gloss
/tidəgɔgi/	/siðədɔgi/

This method of segmentation can sometimes help the clinician account for certain phonological reductions in a word that are influenced by sounds in previous words. Different authors (Ingram 1981; Shriberg and Kwiatkowski 1980) recommend a variety of methods for organizing segments once they have been glossed (alphabetically, by syllable shape, by consonant, etc.). The purpose of these varied organizational schemes is to aid in the retrieval and comparison of individual words and sounds when attempting to prove the existence of a phonological rule.

2. *Hypothesizing a Natural Process.* After arranging the data from a sample, the clinician attempts to account for errors by hypothesizing a phonological reduction pattern. For instance, when comparing a child's production of a word to the adult gloss it may be noted that there is a deletion of the final consonant. The clinician may hypothesize the process of final consonant deletion. The "high-risk" processes listed in Table 6.1 should be ruled out before any "deviant processes" are suspected.

3. *Finding Support for Hypothesized Rules.* It is not enough to simply postulate that final consonant deletion has occurred in a child's sample. Evidence must be obtained from the utterances to determine whether the process has, in fact, occurred. For instance, the child may have deleted the final consonant in a CVC word. The clinician should examine all other words in the sample that end in singleton consonants to determine the frequency of occurrence of the hypothesized phonological reduction. If there is widespread support for the occurrence of final consonant deletion, then the clinician may write the rule. If only certain final consonants are deleted consistently while others are produced normally, then the clinician must change the hypothesis to a rule that specifies particular kinds of final consonant deletion (e.g., stop and nasal deletion). This is where the use of distinctive features is helpful.

4. *Specification of Frequency of Occurrence.* Authorities differ in their methods of specifying the frequency of occurrence of certain phonological rules. Some processes appear to be obligatory (occur virtually all the time), and others seem to be optional. In specifying optionality of a phonological rule, some authors recommend the three-stage system of "always," "sometimes," and "never" (Shriberg and Kwiatkowski 1980). Other authorities (Ingram 1981) recommend the use of percentage ranges such as 0–20, 21–40, 41–60, 61–80, and 81–100. Whatever method is used, the important thing is to indicate how often the process is occurring.

5. *Writing the Rule.* After the clinician has gathered support for a rule from the transcript, the rule is written specifying the target phonemes, how they are changed, what context they are changed in, and how often the rule occurs. A phonological rule for final stop consonant deletion may look like this:

$$
\left.
\begin{array}{l}
p \\
b \\
t \\
d \\
k \\
g
\end{array}
\right\} \longrightarrow \emptyset \ / \ \text{CV-\#} \ 80\text{--}100\%
$$

This rule says that the consonants *p, b, t, d, k,* and *g* are deleted in the context of the CVC word when the target sound is at the end. The slash stands for "in the context of," the blank represents the location of the target sound, and the # refers to a word boundary. Note that the percentage of occurrence is indicated after the rule.

6. *Recycling of 1–4.* As each rule is written and proof is gathered for each phonological reduction, the clinician repeats the process of examining the errors, hypothesizing a phonological process, looking for data to support the rule, and writing the rule. Soon, the clinician can account for the majority of the errors in the child's transcript with the exception of a small residue of words that the rules do not describe. At this point, the clinician may wish to hypothesize a phonological rule that is not normally seen in children's articulatory development. For instance, the child may delete initial consonants of certain types. The procedure, however, is still the same. The clinician must hypothesize the rule and find support for it before it can be written.

The detection of phonological simplificaton patterns can be a powerful tool in the hands of the clinician. A sample of speech that appears to have many unrelated misarticulations can be reduced to only a few phonological reduction patterns. The clinical implication of these processes is that the child does not need to work on a single sound, but may need to focus on the pattern of error. The assumption is that the observable error pattern is generated by an underlying rule; and if the rule is to be altered, then many of the segments that it affects should be targeted (Compton 1976; Ingram 1976; Hodson and Paden 1983). Again, the only way to discover these patterns of misarticulation is to search for them through a phonological analysis technique. Traditional tests are not constructed for this purpose, although they certainly could be suggestive for further analyses and could provide hints for the clinician as to error patterns.

There are several cautions we might offer regarding phonological analysis of child's misarticulations. First, a phonological approach requires that a clinician transcribe words and/or sentences of spontaneous speech. Although most speech clinicians have completed courses in phonetics during their undergraduate education, many of these courses did not offer students the opportunity to transcribe disordered speech from a variety of male, female, adult, and child speakers. Some clinicians may not have adequate experience to reliably transcribe connected speech. One clinician of our acquaintance remarked that "the only thing I have used my phonetics for in the past ten years is to fill in the little blocks on the Goldman-Fristoe score sheet." It may be quite a leap, then, for some clinicians to transcribe words or connected speech in practice. Second, if our reliability is low in scoring phoneme errors, then we can only assume that reliability is even more of an issue in phonological transcription and analysis because we must construct rules from the data (Shriberg and Kwiatkowski 1977). A third concern is the compelling and captivating nature of phonological analysis. It makes an articulatory assessment rather like an interesting puzzle; and when the clinician reaches the "solution" and divines the phonological rules, it is tempting to view the child's problem from a linguistic-phonological perspective only and apply this type of treatment. Locke (1983) and Fey (1992) caution us about the utility of phonological rules. According to Fey (1992),

> Calling a pattern a phonological rule or process is only a descriptive exercise. The existence of the pattern does not necessarily explain anything; the pattern itself is in need of explanation. . . . We must be cautious that we do not stop our search for causal explanations of disorders simply because we have some elegant descriptive principles and terms that can be used to organize and label them. (230)

Children of various etiological groups will demonstrate phonological regularities in their speech. Even if the disorder has a sensorimotor basis, phonological rules can be written and the child perceived as a phonological-linguistic case. Shriberg and Kwiatkowski (1982a) suggest that the clinician must examine linguistic, sensorimotor, and psychosocial aspects of a child's behavior and select appropriate treatment goals. Clinicians should not assume a linguistically oriented treatment simply because the child exhibits a systematic phonology. The treatment of choice for each child may require different emphases, which could include focusing on sensorimotor aspects of articulation. There is no doubt that phonological analyses are useful and constitute a major innovation in articulatory assessment; but the clinician must be careful to check reliability and should not apply a phonological linguistic interpretation to all errors without examining sensorimotor and social aspects as well.

Assessment of Phonological Knowledge

Some researchers have considered the notion of phonological knowledge in misarticulating children (Elbert and Gierut 1986; Gierut, Elbert, and Dinnsen 1987; Maxwell and Rockman 1984). A basic question revolves around whether a child's phonological system is similar or different from a typical adult system. It is possible that a child's underlying representation of a word is either similar or different from an adult representation. Bernthal and Bankson (1988) illustrate this notion with final consonant deletion:

> One explanation for that process might be that the child misperceives the adult word, e.g., perceives [dɔg] as [dɔ]. A second explanation might be that the child's

underlying lexical representation for dog is [dɔ], so the closest match in his store of lexical items is [dɔ]; thus, [dɔg] becomes [dɔ]. A third possible explanation is that the child's perceptual system functions appropriately and the lexical match between what the child perceives and what he or she has stored is consistent with the adult standard, but he or she has a phonological production rule that calls for the deletion of word-final stops. A fourth possibility is that the child has a motor production problem; in this case the child may have the appropriate perception but does not possess the necessary motor skill to make the physiological gesture to produce the sound. (279)

One might wonder how the clinician is to gain insight into a child's phonological knowledge. While we are just beginning to understand this area, some procedures have been used by researchers. Owing to difficulties inherent in assessing and interpreting a child's perceptual abilities (Locke 1980) and the recent suggestion of independence between the perception and production systems (Dinnsen 1985; Straight 1980), most research has concentrated on data generated from a child's productive system. McGregor and Schwartz (1992) remind us that production data alone are not sufficient to describe the complexities of a child's phonological system. One example of a production analysis is provided by Maxwell and Rockman (1984):

Evidence can be adduced that shows that Jamie does know or does represent these words underlyingly with the appropriate postvocalic obstruents, that is, that he represents them the same way we do, but that his pronunciation of these words is governed by a phonological rule of final obstruent deletion. . . . This evidence is available in his pronunciations of these words or morphemes in their inflected forms, that is, in morphophonemically related words. . . . These data reveal that for each morpheme the omitted consonant in question is not omitted when that consonant is in word-medial position. . . . For example, the morpheme meaning "duck" is pronounced [dʌ] without the final k in its uninflected form but as [dʌk] with the k when inflected with the diminutive morpheme [-i] as in [dʌki]. Morphophonemic evidence of this sort (e.g., k alternating with null) provides clear evidence that Jamie knows that the morpheme meaning "duck" must be represented underlyingly with a postvocalic k. (11–12)

Elbert and Gierut (1986) have suggested a procedure for determining a child's productive phonological knowledge on a six-level continuum from least to most knowledge. Gierut, Elbert, and Dinnsen (1987) summarize the six types of knowledge. It is recommended by Elbert and Gierut (1986) that the clinician gather an extensive sample that includes all phonemes of English in all word positions with a variety of canonical shapes that provide multiple opportunities for phonemic contrast. After examining the child's phonetic and phonemic inventories, phonotactic rules, phonological rules, and allophonic and neutralization rules, the clinician can categorize the types of phonological knowledge a child exhibits for individual sounds, sound classes, or the overall sound system. Gierut, Elbert, and

Dinnsen (1987) found that the phonological knowledge continuum may relate to the amount of generalization to be expected in treatment. Basically, training of sounds with least phonological knowledge resulted in generalization across the entire phonological system, whereas training of sounds with most knowledge resulted in generalization to only the specific class of phoneme trained. Thus, the implication is that greater effects may be obtained by training phonemes for which the child has least knowledge. More research needs to be done in this area.

Other Testing

Five additional areas of examination relate significantly to a competent evaluation of an articulation-disordered client, depending on the type of case and its severity. The clinician should be prepared to assess the following areas as appropriate.

1. *Language Assessment.* The clinician examining a child's articulatory system should expect the bulk of these cases to exhibit some language deviations as well. Many authorities report the high co-occurrence of articulation and language disorders. Paul and Shriberg (1982) report that as many as 86% of articulation-disordered children are also likely to exhibit syntactic delays. The clinician should routinely gather a spontaneous language sample and administer standardized language tests for each articulation-disordered client.

2. *Audiometric Screening.* A second diagnostic procedure that should be routinely administered is an audiometric screening. It is critical that the possibility of hearing impairment be eliminated prior to beginning treatment. This becomes especially important if the parents report suspected auditory problems or if the child has a history of ear infections.

3. *The Oral-Peripheral Examination.* This is an integral part of the articulation examination (see Chapter 9 for guidelines in conducting this procedure). Oral-peripheral examination results may be important in distinguishing a sensorimotor from a linguistic disorder of articulation. Fletcher (1972) provides some normative data on diadochokinetic rates for children, and this should also be included as part of the examination for sensorimotor difficulties.

4. *Auditory Discrimination.* This area has been classically explored in articulation evaluation. Historically, many investigations have shown that articulation-disordered children do not perform as well as normal speakers on auditory discrimination tasks (Bernthal and Bankson 1981; Powers 1971; Winitz 1969). Early treatment programs incorporated an obligatory module of auditory discrimination training (Van Riper and Irwin 1958), and many authorities continue to believe that the assessment of auditory discrimination is an important part of an evaluation (Winitz 1975). Within the past ten years, however, criticisms have emerged regarding clinicians' methods of auditory discrimination testing (Beving and Eblen 1973; Schwartz and Goldman 1974) and the efficacy of auditory discrimination training in treatment (Shelton et al. 1978; Williams and McReynolds 1975). Recently, the most defensible position appears to be assessing the auditory discrimination of misarticulated sounds only (Bernthal and Bankson 1993; Locke 1980) rather than all phonemes and to evaluate it in a way that avoids the use of paired comparisons (mass-math). It is presently not clear if auditory discrimination testing needs to be a part of routine articulatory evaluations or if it should be embarked upon only when some suspicion of a discrimination problem is evidenced in trial therapy. The present authors would favor the latter option.

5. *Phonological Awareness.* Many children with phonological disorders have been shown to exhibit decreased levels of phonological awareness that relate to academic and literacy skills (Bird, Bishop, and Freeman 1995). Clinicians can examine these abilities with a variety of techniques (Ball 1993).

Integrating Data from the Assessment

It is reasonable that subsequent to an articulation evaluation, the clinician should, at the very least, be able to make statements on the following areas: (1) biological prerequisites (hearing, structure/function of the speech mechanism); (2) linguistic ability; (3) phonetic and phonemic inventories; (4) distinctive features acquired, used correctly, absent, or misused; (5) response to stimulation by sounds that the child should have acquired according to normative data; (6) phonological processes evident in the sample; (7) an indication of facilitating phonetic contexts, if any, in cases where stimulability is unproductive; (8) a judgment of intelligibility; (9) a judgment of severity/prognosis.

There are a variety of ways to assess articulatory ability; and the broader the view taken by the clinician, the more realistic the picture obtained of the client. For instance, if only the results of a traditional articulation test are considered, the clinician may be able to summarize a phonetic inventory and make some preliminary judgments about distinctive feature acquisition; but perhaps an inventory of phonological processes may not be possible owing to limited sampling. Furthermore, the norms that might be used in comparing the child's phonetic inventory to other children (Sander 1972; Templin 1957) are not applicable to phonological processes. The eight areas mentioned above are simply different ways of looking at the child's articulatory system and should at least be considered in every case to the extent that the clinician can make a statement about each area. Then, further exploration might be undertaken in areas of concern, such as writing a phonology from a spontaneous speech sample if problems are indicated on measures such as the Phonological Process Analysis or the Assessment of Phonological Processes. If a child is noted to be missing entire classes of phonemes, then a more intensive distinctive feature analysis might be indicated. The point is, that results from a variety of areas need to be considered and used as indicators for further analyses.

Shriberg and Kwiatkowski (1982a; 1994a; 1994b; 1994c) have suggested that clinicians should consider possible causal correlates of articulation disorders. They recommended gathering data on each client in the areas of cognition/language, speech mechanism integrity, and psychological/social parameters. Consideration of these areas helps to keep the clinician from becoming too narrowly focused in the conception of articulation assessment and treatment. It also forces the clinician to at least consider the possibility of a variety of single or interactive maintaining factors in the articulation disorder. If a clinician is enamored of phonology and a linguistic interpretation of most articulation problems, such an approach forces the clinician to at least gather some information on psychosocial and speech mechanism variables. Conversely, if a clinician has a sensorimotor orientation, the approach forces the evaluation of more-linguistic aspects. The findings of such a broad-based analysis may provide the clinician with important information on prognosis and treatment goal that would otherwise have not been considered. Gathering this type of information has allowed Shriberg and Kwiatkowski (1994a; 1994b; 1994c) to construct short and long-term outcome data on children with phonological disorders and to begin to define subgroups of this population.

Severity and Intelligibility

While traditional articulation tests can easily identify children with phonological disorders, the tests have difficulty clearly defining different levels of severity (Garn-Nunn and Martin 1992). Several investigators have considered the problem of assigning a severity rating to children's misarticulation problems. We often hear clinicians rate a child's difficulty as "mild" or "moderate"; and when asked how this was determined, the clinicians sometimes have no empirical basis. Shriberg and Kwiatkowski (1982a) suggest the use of the percentage of consonants correct (PCC) in a spontaneous sample as being a most reliable predicter of severity ratings. They had judges rank order variables that were thought to contribute to severity, and intelligibility was ranked first as an influencing factor. They also had clinicians rate tape-recordings of spontaneous speech on severity (mild, mild-moderate, moderate-severe, severe). Statistical analyses showed that the measure most predictive of severity rating was the PCC. Basically, the PCC is a calculation of the number of correct consonants divided by the numbers of correct plus incorrect consonants. The resulting number is multiplied by 100 to arrive at the PCC. Shriberg (1982b) outlines specific procedures and a worksheet for use in computation of the PCC. The point here is that the percentage of consonants correctly articulated relates to severity and severity relates to intelligibility. The number of errors a child has will obviously affect the PCC.

Hodson and Paden (1983) offer the Composite Phonological Deviancy Score (CPDS) as a measure of severity. The system considers age in the calculation as well as a number of phonological processes occurring in the Analysis of Phonological Processes. Edwards (1992) suggests the Process Density Index, which calculates the number of process applications per word, as a measure of severity and reports good reliability with listener judgments of severity. Shriberg (1993) has developed the Articulation Competence Index for use in genetic research. This index takes into account distorted productions that were not included in the original development of the PCC. Although the above methods may be criticized by some, they are at least attempts to objectify severity in cases of articulation disorders and are available for use by practicing clinicians.

Another gauge of severity might be to have independent judges rate the severity of speech samples based on their perceptual judgments. While this is not a quantitative measure, it certainly is an indication of society's reaction to a person's phonological disorder. Garrett and Moran (1992) compared the ratings of experienced (speech-language pathology majors) and inexperienced (elementary education majors) listeners to more-objective measures such as the PCC and CPDS. They found all measures to be highly intercorrelated. The two objective measures appeared to be useful as clinical indicators of severity. This is especially interesting since the CPDS is derived from a single-word sample and the PCC from connected speech.

Of course, the overall severity of a child's problem will also have to consider other variables in addition to phonology. For instance, if a child has a concomitant language disorder or hearing impairment the severity level increases. Reliability is an important issue in making judgments of severity, and SLPs should become familiar with normative data, especially for younger children. Rafaat, Rvachew, and Russell (1995) found that phonological severity judgments by SLPs for preschool children were not adequate (40% agreement) for children under 3.5 years of age, but were adequate for older preschool children.

No matter how a child performs on an articulation test, a major concern of both the clinician and the parent is intelligibility in spontaneous speech. How understandable is the child in his daily interactions? Intelligibility is difficult to measure since it is affected by many variables (Kent, Miolo, and Bloedel 1994; Kwiatkowski and Shriberg 1992; Weston and Shriberg 1992). For instance, variables such as utterance length, fluency, word position, intelligibility of adjacent words, phonological complexity, grammatical form, and syllabic structure may have an effect on intelligibility judgments for a particular word (Weston and Shriberg 1992). Kent, Miolo, and Bloedel (1994) summarized nineteen different intelligibility evaluation procedures and discussed the issues to be considered in testing intelligibility. They concluded that no single method would be adequate for assessing intelligibility and that a clinician should use some combination of assessment devices. Selection of measurement should consider the child's age, language abilities, other disabilities, time available for assessment/analysis, and the purpose of intelligibility testing.

There are few data relating intelligibility to age, although we know that children become more intelligible as they get older. Generally, a child of age three should be generally intelligible to strangers, and inability to understand a child of this age is reason for clinical intervention (Bernthal and Bankson 1993). A child will be more intelligible to those who know him well because the latter have unconsciously decoded the child's "system" of substitutions and omissions. Kwiatkowski and Shriberg (1992), however, found that caregivers evidenced more difficulty than was anticipated in glossing their children's speech and overestimated their children's syntactic development. Another variable affecting intelligibility is the sound that the child misarticulates. Some sounds occur more frequently in the language than others; and if the child's error is on a sound that occurs frequently, intelligibility will be affected to a greater degree than when errors are on infrequently occurring phonemes. An obvious factor that could logically affect intelligibility is the number of phonemes that a child misarticulates, although Shriberg and Kwiat-kowski (1982b) did not find high correlations between total number of errors and intelligibility. Another variable affecting intelligibility may be the consistency of the error in the child's speech. This would also affect the PCC calculation. A final factor that can affect intelligibility could be the type of error (omissions, substitutions) that the child exhibits (Shriberg and Kwiatkowski 1982b).

At the very least, a clinician can rate the client according to a rating scale. Fudala (1970) recommends using a continuum for rating intelligibility similar to the following:

1. Speech is not intelligible.
2. Speech is usually not intelligible.
3. Speech is difficult to understand.
4. Speech is intelligible with careful listening.
5. Speech is intelligible, although noticeably in error.
6. Speech is intelligible with occasional error.
7. Speech is totally intelligible.

Every assessment of articulatory ability should contain some judgment regarding intelligibility. This is a factor that can be an important deciding variable in making treatment recommendations.

Computer-Assisted Analysis of Phonology

Much of the work in phonological analysis is laborious and repetitive. Some of the major difficulties are keeping track of the data on a host of different worksheets, tallying up percentages and frequency counts, and cross-checking a variety of relationships found in different portions of the client's transcript. The nature of these tasks is ideally suited to computer analysis. The computer can take a corpus of language and the gloss of each utterance and produce more information than even the most zealous clinician would even like to know about a child's phonological system. In some cases, computer analyses of human behavior are rather superficial, and the programs available are just in the early stages of development. In the case of phonological analysis, however, the computer programs are detailed, user friendly, and here to stay! Table 6.4 includes a listing of some popular programs available for phonological analysis. An analysis that might take a clinician several hours to accomplish can actually be completed in less than a few minutes by most programs. The software is compatible with the most popular types of micro-comuputers available in the majority of school systems, universities, and even households of prospective users. The cost of the programs varies from under $100.00 to just over $1000.00. The programs differ in their scope, ranging from those designed to analyze the responses from a particular test of phonology to those focusing on the assessment of spontaneous samples of connected speech. Some of the available programs will be mentioned below; however, some words of caution are in order.

TABLE 6.4   Computer-Assisted Analysis of Misarticulations: Selected Programs

Computer Analysis of Phonological Processes. Hodson, B. (1985). Phonocomp, Box 46, Stonington, IL 62567.

Computerized Profiling. Long, S., and Fey, M. (1993). The Psychological Corporation

Computer Managed Articulation Diagnosis. Fitch, J. (1985). Communication Skill Builders, P.O. Box 42050, Tuscon, AZ 85733.

Diagnostic Articulation Analyzer. Parrot Software, P.O. Box 1139, State College, PA 16804.

LINGQUEST 2. Palin, M., and Mordecai, D., Charles E. Merrill Test Division, 1300 Alum Creek Dr., Box 508, Columbus, OH 43216.

Process Analysis. Weiner, F., Parrot Software, P.O. Box 1139, State College, PA 16804.

Programs to Examine Phonetic and Phonologic Evaluation Records (PEPPER). Shriberg, L. (1986). SDCD, University of Wisconsin, 1025 West Johnson St., Madison, WI 53706.

It would be ideal if the client simply talked into a microphone that was plugged into a computer and in a few seconds a miraculous printout appeared that revealed the secrets of the phonological system. Unfortunately, this is not the case. The clinician must still obtain the sample, transcribe the sample, input the sample into the computer through the keyboard, and in many cases do some other work, responding to menus and prompts produced on the screen. The tasks just described constitute a lot of painstaking work on the part of the clinician. Just transcribing a sample of connected speech can take hours of careful listening. The beauty of computer-assisted analysis is that the clinician does not have to spend several *more* hours of organizing data, scanning the transcript over and over again, and performing mathematical operations. The computer also provides elegant summaries of the data, such as phonetic inventories, canonical shape analyses, positional inventories, phonological process analysis, measures of severity (e.g., PCC, CPDS), and even suggested treatment targets on some programs.

Thus, one misconception that some people might have is that computer analysis takes away all tedious work on the part of the clinician. The truth is, it takes away much of this work, but not all. A second misconception some people may have is that the computer will always come up with the "right answer" with regard to a client's phonology. While the algorithms in most phonology programs are quite sophisticated, they have difficulty dealing with idiosyncratic processes and certain types of analyses. The one thing the clinician can expect, however, is output; it may not always be correct, but it *is* output. A clinician should be aware of the limitations of phonological analysis programs and practice by running phonological samples that they have done by hand to see if there is general agreement between the two methods.

Long-Term Impact of Phonological Disorders

Research has confirmed that many individuals with phonological impairments, whether they receive treatment or not, experience academic difficulties. This, of course, could be related to the co-occurrence of phonological and language disorders in the majority of cases. Lewis and Freebairn (1992) found that subjects with a history of preschool phonological disorders performed more poorly than matched controls did on measures of phonology, reading, and spelling for age groups from preschool to adult. Subjects with a history of language disorder, in addition to the phonological problem, performed even lower on the measures. In a twenty-eight-year longitudinal study, Felsenfeld, Broen, and McGue (1994) followed a group of children who had phonological disorders. These children had phonological disorders as preschoolers, and the problems persisted through first grade. When the researchers interviewed these subjects in adulthood, they found, in comparison to matched controls, reports of lower grades throughout school, more academic remedial services required, and less years of formal education completed. The subjects with a history of phonological disorder also tended to choose more semiskilled or unskilled occupations than the controls did. Bird, Bishop, and Freeman (1995) found that children with phonological disorders scored well below controls on measures of phonological awareness and literacy. These researchers felt that children who start school with severe phonological impairments are especially at risk for developing reading and spelling difficulties.

In view of the relation between phonological disorders and academic performance, clinicians should not underestimate the importance of early assessment, intervention, and counseling.

Bibliography

Allen, D., Bliss, L., and Timmons, J. (1981). "Language Evaluation: Science or Art?" *Journal of Speech and Hearing Disorders* 46:66–68.

Amerman, J., Daniloff, R., and Moll, K. (1970). "Lip and Jaw Coarticulation for the Phoneme /æ/." *Journal of Speech and Hearing Research* 13:148–161.

Anderson, V., and Newby, H. (1973). *Improving the Child's Speech*. 2nd ed. New York: Oxford University Press.

Andrews, N., and Fey, M. (1986). "Analysis of the Speech of Phonologically Impaired Children in Two Sampling Conditions." *Language, Speech and Hearing Services in Schools* 17:187–198.

Avant, V., and Hutton, C. (1962). "Passage for Speech Screening in Upper Elementary Grades." *Journal of Speech and Hearing Disorders* 27:40–46.

Ball, E. (1993). "Assessing Phoneme Awareness." *Language, Speech and Hearing Services in Schools* 24:130–139.

Bankson, N., and Bernthal, J. (1990). *Bankson-Bernthal Test of Phonology*, Chicago, IL: Riverside Publishers.

Battle, D., et al. (1983). "Position Paper–Social Dialects." *Journal of the American Speech-Language-Hearing Association* 25:23–24.

Bernhardt, B., and Stoel-Gammon, C. (1994). "Nonlinear Phonology: Introduction and Clinical Applications." *Journal of Speech and Hearing Research* 37:123–143.

Bernthal, J., and Bankson, N. (1988). *Articulation Disorders*. Englewood Cliffs, NJ: Prentice-Hall.

Bernthal, J., and Bankson, N. (1993). *Articulation and Phonological Disorders*. Englewood Cliffs, NJ: Prentice-Hall.

Beving, B., and Eblen, R. (1973). "Same and Different Concepts and Children's Performance on Speech Sound Discrimination." *Journal of Speech and Hearing Research* 16:513–517.

Bird, J., Bishop, D., and Freeman, N. (1995). "Phonological Awareness and Literacy Development in Children with Expressive Phonological Impairments." *Journal of Speech and Hearing Research* 38:446–462.

Blache, S. (1978). *The Acquisition of Distinctive Features.* Baltimore MD: University Park Press.

Bleile, K., and Wallach, H. (1992). "A Sociolinguistic Investigation of the Speech of African American Preschoolers." *American Journal of Speech-Language Pathology* 1:54–61.

Bowman, S., Parsons, C., and Morris, D. (1984). "Inconsistency of Phonological Errors in Developmental Verbal Dyspraxic Children as a Factor of Linguistic Task and Performance Load." *Australian Journal of Human Communication Disorders* 10:109–120.

Bryant, B., and Bryant, D. (1983). *Test of Articulation Performance: Diagnostic,* Austin, TX: Pro-Ed.

Cammarata, S., and Schwartz, L. (1985). "Production of Object Words and Action Words: Evidence for a Relationship between Phonology and Semantics." *Journal of Speech and Hearing Research* 28:323–330.

Campbell, J., and Shriberg, L. (1982). "Associations among Pragmatic Functions, Linguistic Stress and Natural Phonological Processes in Speech Delayed Children." *Journal of Speech and Hearing Research* 25:547–553.

Carney, E. (1979). "Inappropriate Abstraction in Speech Assessment Procedures." *British Journal of Disorders of Communication* 14:123–135.

Carrell, J., and Tiffany, W. (1960). *Phonetics: Theory and Application to Speech Improvement.* New York: McGraw-Hill.

Chomsky, N. (1957). *Syntactic Structures.* The Hague, Neth: Mouton.

Chomsky, N., and Halle, M. (1968). *The Sound Pattern of English.* New York: Harper and Row.

Cole, P., and Taylor, O. (1990). "Performance of Working-Class African American Children on Three Tests of Articulation." *Language, Speech and Hearing Services in Schools* 21:171–176.

Compton, A. (1970). "Generative Studies of Children's Phonological Disorders." *Journal of Speech and Hearing Disorders* 35:315–339.

Compton, A. (1976). "Generative Studies of Children's Phonological Disorders." In *Normal and Deficient Child Language,* ed. D. Morehead and A. Morehead (Baltimore, MD: University Park Press).

Compton, A., and Hutton, S. (1978). *Compton-Hutton Phonological Assessment.* San Francisco, CA: Carousel House.

Costello, J., and Onstine, J. (1976). "The Modification of Multiple Articulation Errors Based on Distinctive Feature Theory." *Journal of Speech and Hearing Disorders* 41:199–215.

Cypreansen, L., Wiley, J., and Laase, L. (1959). *Speech Development, Improvement and Correction.* New York: Ronald Press.

Daniloff, R., and Moll, K. (1968). "Coarticulation of Lip Rounding." *Journal of Speech and Hearing Research* 11:707–721.

Daniloff, R., Schuckers, G., and Feth, L. (1980). *The Physiology of Speech and Hearing: An Introduction.* Englewood Cliffs, NJ: Prentice-Hall.

Darley, F. (1964). *Diagnosis and Appraisal of Communication Disorders.* Englewood Cliffs, NJ: Prentice-Hall.

Davis, B., and MacNeilage, P. (1990). "Acquisition of Correct Vowel Production: A Quantitative Case Study." *Journal of Speech and Hearing Research* 33, no. 1:16–27.

Dickson, D., and Maue-Dickson, W. (1982). *Anatomical and Physiological Bases of Speech.* Boston, MA: Little, Brown.

Diedrich, W. (1983). "Stimulability and Articulation Disorders." In *Assessing and Treating Phonological Disorders: Current Approaches. Seminars in Speech and Language,* Vol. 4, ed. J. Locke (New York: Thieme-Stratton).

Dillard, J. (1972). *Black English: Its History and Usage in the United States.* New York: Random House.

Dinnsen, D. (1984). "Methods of Empirical Issues in Analyzing Functional Misarticulation." *Phonological Theory and the Misarticulating Child,* ASHA Monographs 22:5–17.

Dinnsen, D. (1985). "A Re-Examination of Phonological Neutralization." *Journal of Linguistics* 21:265–279.

Dubois, E., and Bernthal, J. (1978). "A Comparison of Three Methods for Obtaining Articulatory Responses." *Journal of Speech and Hearing Disorders* 43:295–305.

Dyson, A. (1988). "Phonetic Inventories of 2- and 3-Year-Old Children." *Journal of Speech and Hearing Disorders* 53, no. 1:89–93.

Dyson, A., and Robinson, T. (1987). "The Effect of Phonological Analysis Procedure on the Selection of Potential Remediation Targets." *Language, Speech and Hearing Services in Schools* 18:364–377.

Edmonson, W. (1969). *The Laradon Articulation Scale*. Denver, CO: Laradon Hall.

Edwards, M. (1992). "In Support of Phonological Processes." *Language, Speech and Hearing Services in Schools* 23:233–240.

Eisenson, J., and Ogilvie, M. (1977). *Speech Correction in the Schools*. 4th ed. New York: MacMillian.

Elbert, M. (1992). "Consideration of Error Types: A Response to Fey." *Language, Speech and Hearing Services in Schools* 23:241–246.

Elbert, M., and Gierut, J. (1986). *Handbook of Clinical Phonology: Approaches to Assessment and Treatment*, San Diego, CA: College-Hill.

Eveleigh, K., and Warr-Leeper, G. (1983). "Improving Efficiency in Articulation Screening." *Language, Speech and Hearing Services in Schools* 14:223–232.

Fairbanks, G., (1960). *Voice and Articulation Drillbook*. 2nd ed. New York: Harper and Row.

Faircloth, M., and Faircloth, S. (1970). "An Analysis of the Articulatory Behavior of a Speech-Defective Child in Connected Speech and Isolated Word Responses." *Journal of Speech and Hearing Disorders* 35:51–61.

Farquhar, M. (1961). "Prognostic Value of Imitative and Auditory Discrimination Tests." *Journal of Speech and Hearing Disorders* 26:342–347.

Felsenfeld, S., Broen, P., and McGue, M. (1994). A 28-Year Follow-Up of Adults with a History of Moderate Phonological Disorder: Educational and Occupational Results." *Journal of Speech and Hearing Research* 37:1341–1353.

Fey, M. (1992). "Articulation and Phonology: Inextricable Constructs in Speech Pathology." *Language, Speech and Hearing Services in Schools* 23:225–232.

Fisher, H., and Logemann, J. (1971). *The Fisher-Logemann Test of Articulation Competence*. Boston, MA: Houghton-Mifflin.

Fletcher, S. (1972). "Time-by-Count Measurement of Diadochokinetic Syllable Rate." *Journal of Speech and Hearing Research* 15:763–770.

Fluharty, N. (1974). "The Design and Standardization of a Speech and Language Screening Test for Use with Preschool Children." *Journal of Speech and Hearing Disorders* 39:75–88.

Fristoe, M., and Goldman, R. (1968). "Comparisons of Traditional and Condensed Articulation Tests Examining the Same Number of Sounds." *Journal of Speech and Hearing Research* 11:583–589.

Fudala, J. (1970). *The Arizona Articulation Proficiency Scale*. Beverly Hills, CA: Western Psychological Services.

Gallagher, T., and Shriner, T. (1975). "Articulatory Inconsistencies in the Speech of Normal Children." *Journal of Speech and Hearing Research* 18:168–175.

Garber, N. (1986). "A Phonological Analysis Classification for Use with Traditional Articulation Tests." *Language, Speech and Hearing Services in Schools* 17, no. 4:253–261.

Garn-Nunn, P. (1986). "Phonological Processes and Conventional Articulation Tests: Considerations for Analysis." *Language, Speech and Hearing Services in Schools* 17, no. 4:244–252.

Garn-Nunn, P., and Martin, V. (1992). "Using Conventional Articulation Tests with Highly Unintelligible Children: Identification and Programming Concerns." *Language, Speech and Hearing Services in Schools* 23:52–60.

Garrett, K., and Moran, M. (1992). "A Comparison of Phonological Severity Measures." *Language, Speech and Hearing Services in Schools* 23:48–51.

Gierut, J., Elbert, M., and Dinnsen, D. (1987). "A Functional Analysis of Phonological Knowledge and Generalization Learning in Misarticulating Children." *Journal of Speech and Hearing Research* 30, no. 4:462–479.

Goda, S. (1970). *Articulation Therapy and Consonant Drillbook*. New York: Grune and Stratton.

Goldman, R., and Fristoe, M. (1986). *Goldman-Fristoe Test of Articulation*. Circle Pines, MN: American Guidance Service.

Grunwell, P. (1985). *Phonological Assessment of Child Speech (PACS)*. San Diego, CA: NFER-Nelson, Windsor, UK/College-Hill Press.

Grunwell, P. (1988). *Clinical Phonology*. Baltimore, MD: Williams and Wilkins.

Hamayan, E., and Damico, J. (1991). *Limiting Bias in the Assessment of Bilingual Students*, Austin, TX: Pro-Ed.

Haynes, W., Haynes, M., and Jackson, J. (1982). "The Effects of Phonetic Context and Linguistic Complexity on /s/ Misarticulation in Children." *Journal of Communication Disorders* 15:287–297.

Haynes, W., and Moran, M. (1989). "A Cross-Sectional Developmental Study of Final Consonant Production in Southern Black Children from Preschool through Third Grade." *Language Speech and Hearing Services in Schools* 20: 400–406.

Healy, T., and Madison, C. (1987). "Articulation Error Migration: A Comparison of Single-Word and Connected Speech Samples." *Journal of Communication Disorders* 20:129–136.

Hejna, R. (1963). *Developmental Articulation Test.* Ann Arbor, MI: Speech Materials.

Hodson, B. (1986). *The Assessment of Phonological Processes–Revised.* Austin, TX: Pro-Ed.

Hodson, B., and Paden, E. (1983). *Targeting Intelligible Speech: A Phonological Approach to Remediation.* San Diego, CA: College-Hill.

Hoffman, P., Schuckers, G., and Ratusnik, D. (1977). "Contextual-Coarticulatory Inconsistencies of /r/ Misarticulation." *Journal of Speech and Hearing Research* 20:631–643.

Ingram, D. (1971). *Edinburgh Articulation Test.* London: Edward Arnold.

Ingram, D. (1976). *Phonological Disability in Children.* New York: Elsiever.

Ingram, D. (1981). *Procedures for the Phonological Analysis of Children's Language.* Baltimore, MD: University Park Press.

Irwin, J., and Wong, P. (1983). *Phonological Development in Children 18 to 72 Months,* Carbondale: Southern Illinois University Press.

Johnson, J., Whinney, B., and Pederson, O. (1980). "Single-Word versus Connected Speech Articulation Testing." *Language, Speech and Hearing Services in Schools* 11:175–179.

Johnson, W., Darley, F., and Spriestersbach, D. (1963). *Diagnostic Methods in Speech Pathology.* New York: Harper and Row.

Kahane, J., and Folkins, J. (1984). *Atlas of Speech and Hearing Anatomy.* Columbus, OH: Merrill.

Kahn, L., and Lewis, N. (1986). *Kahn-Lewis Phonological Analysis,* American Guidance Service.

Kenney, K., and Prather, E. (1984). *Coarticulation Assessment in Meaningful Language,* Tucson, AZ: Communication Skill Builders.

Kent, R. (1982). "Contextual Facilitation of Correct Sound Production." *Language, Speech and Hearing Services in Schools* 13:66–76.

Kent, R., and Minifie, F. (1977). "Coarticulation in Recent Speech Production Models." *Journal of Phonetics* 5:115–133.

Kent, R., Miolo, G., and Bloedel, S. (1994). "The Intelligibility of Children's Speech: A Review of Evaluation Procedures." *American Journal of Speech-Language Pathology* 3:81–95.

Klein, H. (1984). "Procedure for Maximizing Phonological Information from Single-Word Responses." *Language, Speech and Hearing Services in Schools* 15:267–274.

Kwiatkowski, J., and Shriberg, L. (1992). "Intelligibility Assessment in Developmental Phonological Disorders: Accuracy of Caregiver Gloss." *Journal of Speech and Hearing Research* 35:1095–1104.

Lariviere, C., et al. (1974). "The Conceptual Reality of Selected Distinctive Features." *Journal of Speech and Hearing Research* 17:122–133.

Leonard, L. (1971). "A Preliminary View of Information Theory and Articulatory Omissions." *Journal of Speech and Hearing Disorders* 36: 511–517.

Leonard, L. (1973). "Some Limitations in the Clinical Application of Distinctive Features." *Journal of Speech and Hearing Disorders* 38:141–143.

Lewis, B., and Freebairn, L. (1992). "Residual Effects of Preschool Phonology Disorders in Grade School, Adolescence and Adulthood." *Journal of Speech and Hearing Research* 35:819–831.

Lidz, C., and Pena, E. (1996). "Dynamic Assessment: The Model, Its Relevance as a Nonbiased Approach, and its Application to Latino American Preschool Children." *Language, Speech and Hearing Services in Schools* 27:367–372.

Locke, J. (1980). "The Inference of Speech Perception in the Phonologically Disordered Child. Part I: A Rationale, some Criteria, the Conventional Tests." *Journal of Speech and Hearing Disorders* 45:431–444.

Locke, J. (1983). "Clinical Phonology: The Explanation and Treatment of Speech Sound Disorders." *Journal of Speech and Hearing Disorders* 48:339–341.

Lowe, R. (1986). *Assessment Link between Phonology and Articulation.* Moline, IL: Linguisystems.

Madison, C. (1979). "Articulation Stimulability Reviewed", *Language, Speech and Hearing Services in Schools* 10:185–190.

Matheny, N., and Panagos, J. (1978). "Comparing the Effects of Articulation and Syntax Programs on Syntax and Articulation Improvement." *Language, Speech and Hearing Services in Schools* 9:57–61.

Maxwell, E., and Rockman, B. (1984). "Procedures for Linguistic Analysis of Misarticulated Speech." *Phonological Theory and the Misarticulating Child*, ASHA Monographs 22:69e

Mazza, P., Schuckers, G., and Daniloff, R. (1979). "Contextual-Coarticulatory Inconsistency of /s/ Misarticulation." *Journal of Phonetics* 7:57–69.

McCauley, R., and Skenes, L. (1987). "Contrastive Stress, Phonetic Context and Misarticulation of /r/ in Young Speakers." *Journal of Speech and Hearing Research* 30, no. 1:114–121.

McClean, J. (1976). "Articulation." In *Communication Assessment and Intervention Strategies*, ed. L. Lloyd (Baltimore, MD: University Park Press).

McClean, M. (1973). "Forward Coarticulation of Velar Movement at Marked Junctural Boundaries." *Journal of Speech and Hearing Research* 16:236–246.

McDonald, E. (1964). *Articulation Testing and Treatment*. Pittsburgh, PA: Stanwix House.

McDonald, E. (1968). *A Screening Deep Test of Articulation*. Pittsburgh, PA: Stanwix House.

McGregor, K., and Schwartz, R. (1992). "Converging Evidence for Underlying Phonological Representation in a Child Who Misarticulates." *Journal of Speech and Hearing Research* 35:596–603.

McLeod, S., Hand, L., Rosenthal, J., and Hayes, B. (1994). "The Effect of Sampling Condition on Children's Productions of Consonant Clusters." *Journal of Speech and Hearing Research* 37:868–882.

McReynolds, L., and Engmann, D. (1975). *Distinctive Feature Analysis of Misarticulations*. Baltimore, MD: University Park Press.

McReynolds, L., and Huston, K. (1971). "A Distinctive Feature Analysis of Children's Misarticulation." *Journal of Speech and Hearing Disorders* 36:155–166.

McReynolds, L., and Kearns, K. (1983). *Single-subject Experimental Designs in Communicative Disorders*. Baltimore, MD: University Park Press.

Milisen, R., et al. (1954). "The Disorder of Articulation: A Systematic Clinical and Experimental Approach." *Journal of Speech and Hearing Disorders* Monograph Supplement 4.

Moll, K., and Daniloff, R. (1971). "Investigation of the Timing of Velar Movements during Speech." *Journal of the Acoustical Society of America* 50:678–684.

Monsees, E., and Berman, C. (1968). "Speech and Language Screening in a Summer Headstart Program." *Journal of Speech and Hearing Disorders* 33:121–126.

Moran, M. (1993). "Final Consonant Deletion in African American Children Speaking Black English: A Closer Look." *Language, Speech and Hearing Services in Schools* 24:161–166.

Oller, K., et al. (1972). "Five Studies in Abnormal Phonology." Unpublished paper, University of Washington.

Paden, E., and Moss, S. (1985). "Comparison of Three Phonological Analysis Procedures." *Language, Speech and Hearing Services in Schools* 16, no. 2:103–109.

Palmer, J. (1984). *Anatomy for Speech and Hearing*. New York: Harper and Row.

Panagos, J., Quine, H., and Klich, P. (1979). "Syntactic and Phonological Influences in Children's Articulations." *Journal of Speech and Hearing Research* 22:841–848.

Parker, F. (1976). "Distinctive Features in Speech Pathology: Phonology or Phonemics." *Journal of Speech and Hearing Disorders* 41:23–39.

Paul, R., and Shriberg, L. (1982). "Association between Phonology and Syntax in Speech-Delayed Children." *Journal of Speech and Hearing Research* 25:536–546.

Pendergast, K., Dickey, S., Selmar, T., and Soder, A. (1984). *Photo Articulation Test*. Danville, IL: Interstate.

Pollack, E., and Rees, N. (1972). "Disorders of Articulation: Some Clinical Applications of Distinctive Feature Theory." *Journal of Speech and Hearing Disorders* 37:451–461.

Poole, E. (1934). "Genetic Development of Articulation of Consonant Sounds in Speech." *Elementary English Review* 11:159–161.

Powell, T. (1995). "A Clinical Screening Procedure for Assessing Consonant Cluster Production." *American Journal of Speech Language Pathology* 4:59–65.

Powers, M. (1971). "Functional Disorders of Articulation: Symptomatology and Etiology." In *Handbook of Speech Pathology and Audiology*, ed. L. Travis (Englewood Cliffs, NJ: Prentice-Hall).

Prather, E., Hedrick, D., and Kern, C. (1975). "Articulation Development in Children Aged 2 to 4 Years." *Journal of Speech and Hearing Disorders* 40:179–191.

Rafaat, S., Rvachew, S., and Russell, R. (1995). "Reliability of Clinician Judgments of Severity of Phonological Impairment." *American Journal of Speech Language Pathology* 4:39–46.

Riley, G. (1971). *Riley Articulation and Language Test*. Los Angeles, CA: Western Psychological Services.

Ritterman, S., and Freeman, N. (1974). "Distinctive Phonetic Features as Relevant and Irrelevant Stimulus Dimensions in Speech Sound Discrimination Learning." *Journal of Speech and Hearing Research* 17:417–425.

Ritterman, S., Zook-Herman, S., Carlson, R., and Kinde, S. (1982). "The Pass/Fail Disparity among Three Commonly Employed Articulatory Screening Tests." *Journal of Speech and Hearing Disorders* 47:429–432.

Rogers, W. (1972). *Picture Articulation and Screening Test*. Salt Lake City, UT: Word Making Productions.

Ruder, K., and Bunce, B. (1981). "Articulation Therapy Using Distinctive Feature Analysis to Structure the Training Program: Two Case Studies." *Journal of Speech and Hearing Disorders* 46:59–65.

Sander, E. (1972). "When Are Speech Sounds Learned?" *Journal of Speech and Hearing Disorders* 44:363–372.

Schissel, R., and James, L. (1979). "A Comparison of Children's Performance on Two Tests of Articulation." *Journal of Speech and Hearing Disorders* 44:363–372.

Schmauch, V., Panagos, J., and Klich, P. (1978). "Syntax Influences the Accuracy of Consonant Production in Language-Disordered Children." *Journal of Communication Disorders* 11:315–323.

Schmitt, L., Howard, B., and Schmitt, J. (1983). "Conversation Speech Sampling in the Assessment of Articulatory Proficiency." *Language, Speech and Hearing Services in Schools* 14:210–214.

Schwartz, A., and Goldman, R. (1974). "Variables Influencing Performance on Speech Sound Discrimination Tests." *Journal of Speech and Hearing Research* 17:25–32.

Schwartz, R. (1983). "Diagnosis of Speech Sound Disorders in Children." In *Diagnosis in Speech-Language Pathology*, ed. B. Weinberg and I. Meitus (Baltimore, MD: University Park Press).

Schwartz, R. (1992). "Clinical Applications of Recent Advances in Phonological Theory." *Language, Speech and Hearing Services in Schools* 23:269–276.

Scripture, M., and Jackson, E. (1927). *A Manual of Exercises for the Correction of Speech Disorders*. Philadelphia, PA: F. A. Davis.

Seymour, H., and Seymour, C. (1981). "Black English and Standard American English Contrasts in Consonantal Development for Four- and Five-Year-Old Children." *Journal of Speech and Hearing Disorders* 46:276–280.

Seymour, H., Green, L., and Huntley, R. (1991). "Phonological Patterns in the Conversational Speech of African American Children." Paper presented at the national convention of the American Speech-Language-Hearing Association, Atlanta, GA.

Shelton, R., Johnson, A., Ruscello, D., and Arndt, W. (1978). "Assessment of Parent-Administered Listening Training for Preschool Children with Articulation Deficits." *Journal of Speech and Hearing Disorders* 43:242–254.

Shelton, R., and McReynolds, L. (1979). "Functional Articulation Disorders: Preliminaries to Treatment." In *Speech and Language: Advances in Basic Research and Practice* (2), ed. N. Lass (New York: Academic Press).

Shriberg, L. (1993). "Four New Speech and Prosody Ovice Measures for Genetics Research and Other Studies in Developmental Phonological Disorders." *Journal of Speech and Hearing Research* 36:105–140.

Shriberg, L., and Kent, R. (1982). *Clinical Phonetics*. New York: Wiley.

Shriberg, L., and Kwiatkowski, J. (1977). "Phonological Programming for Unintelligible Children in Early-Childhood Projects." Paper presented to the convention of the American Speech and Hearing Association, Chicago, IL.

Shriberg, L., and Kwiatkowski, J. (1980). *Natural Process Analysis*. New York: Wiley.

Shriberg, L., and Kwiatkowski, J. (1982a). "Phonological Disorders, I: A Diagnostic Classification System." *Journal of Speech and Hearing Disorders* 47:226–241.

Shriberg, L., and Kwiatkowski, J. (1982b). "Phonological Disorders, III: A Procedure for Assessing Severity of Involvement." *Journal of Speech and Hearing Disorders* 47:256–270.

Shriberg, L., and Kwiatkowski, J. (1988). "A Follow-Up Study of Children with Phonologic Disorders of Unknown Origin." *Journal of Speech and Hearing Disorders* 53:144–155.

Shriberg, L., and Kwiatkowski, J. (1994a). "Developmental Phonological Disorders, I: A Clinical Profile." *Journal of Speech and Hearing Research* 17:1100–1126.

Shriberg, L., Kwiatkowski, J., and Gruber, F. (1994b). "Developmental Phonological Disorders, II: Short-Term Speech Sound Normalization." *Journal of Speech and Hearing Research* 37:1127–1150.

Shriberg, L., Gruber, F., and Kwiatkowski, J. (1994c). "Developmental Phonological Disorders, III: Long-Term Speech Sound Normalization." *Journal of Speech and Hearing Research* 37:1151–1177.

Shriberg, L., Kwiatkowski, J., Best, S., Hengst, J., and Terselic-Weber, B. (1986). "Characteristics of Children with Phonologic Disorders of Unknown Origin." *Journal of Speech and Hearing Disorders* 51:140–161.

Simmons, J. (1988). "Fluharty Preschool and Language Screening Test: Analysis of Construct Validity." *Journal of Speech and Hearing Disorders* 53:168–174.

Singh, S. (1976). *Distinctive Features: Theory and Validation.* Baltimore, MD: University Park Press.

Smit, A. (1986). "Ages of Speech Sound Acquisition: Comparisons and Critiques of Several Normative Studies. *Language, Speech and Hearing Services in Schools* 17:175–186.

Smit, A. (1993a). "Phonologic Error Distributions in the Iowa Nebraska Articulation Norms Project: Consonant Singletons." *Journal of Speech and Hearing Research* 36:533–547.

Smit, A. (1993b). "Phonologic Error Distributions in the Iowa Nebraska Articulation Norms Project: Word Initial Consonant Clusters." *Journal of Speech and Hearing Research* 36:931–947.

Smit, A., Hand, L., Frellinger, J., Bernthal, J., and Bird, A. (1990). "The Iowa Articulation Norms Project and Its Nebraska Replication." *Journal of Speech and Hearing Disorders* 55:779–798.

Smith, N. (1973). *The Acquisition of Phonology.* Cambridge, UK: Cambridge University Press.

Sommers, R. (1983). *Articulation Disorders.* Englewood Cliffs, NJ: Prentice-Hall.

Stampe, D. (1969). "A Dissertation on Natural Phonology." Unpublished dissertation, University of Chicago.

Stockman, I. (1993). "Variable Word Initial and Medial Consonant Relationships in Children's Speech Sound Articulation." *Perceptual and Motor Skills* 76:675–689.

Stockman, I. (1996a). "Phonological Development and Disorders in African American Children." In *Communication Development and Disorders in African American Children,* ed. A. Kamhi, K. Pollock, and J. Harris (Baltimore, MD: Brookes).

Stockman, I. (1996b). "The Promises and Pitfalls of Language Sample Analysis as an Assessment Tool for Linguistic Minority Children." *Language, Speech and Hearing Services in Schools* 27:355–366.

Stockman, I., and Stephenson, L. (1981). "Children's Articulation of Medial Consonant Clusters: Implications for Syllabification." *Language and Speech* 24:185–204.

Stoel-Gammon, C. (1987). "Phonological Skills in 2-Year-Olds." *Language, Speech and Hearing Services in Schools* 18:323–329.

Stoel-Gammon, C. (1996). "Phonological Assessment Using a Hierarchial Framework." In *Assessment of Communication and Language,* Vol. 6, eds. K. Cole, P. Dale, and D. Thal (Baltimore, MD: Paul H. Brookes).

Stoel-Gammon, C., and Dunn, C. (1985). *Normal and Disordered Phonology in Children.* Baltimore, MD: University Park Press.

Stoller, P. (1975). *Black American English.* New York: Delta.

Straight, H. (1980). "Auditory versus Articulatory Phonological Processes and Their Development in Children. In *Child Phonology: Perception, Vol. 2,* ed. G. Yeni-Komshian, C. Kavanagh, and C. Ferguson (New York: Academic Press).

Taylor, O. (1986). "Language Differences." In *Human Communication Disorders: An Introduction*, ed. G. Shames and E. Wiig (Columbus, OH: Merrill).

Templin, M. (1957). *Certain Language Skills in Children: Their Development and Interrelationships.* Institute of Child Welfare, Monograph 26, Minneapolis: University of Minnesota Press.

Templin, M., and Darley, F. (1969). *The Templin-Darley Tests of Articulation.* Iowa City: University of Iowa Bureau of Educational Research and Service.

Van Riper, C. (1963). *Speech Correction: Principles and Methods.* Englewood Cliffs, NJ: Prentice-Hall.

Van Riper, C., and Erickson, R. (1969). "A Predictive Screening Test of Articulation." *Journal of Speech and Hearing Disorders* 34:214–219.

Van Riper, C., and Irwin, J. (1958). *Voice and Articulation.* Englewood Cliffs, NJ: Prentice-Hall.

Van Riper, C., and Smith, D. (1979). *An Introduction to General American Phonetics.* New York: Harper and Row.

Vaughn-Cooke, F. (1976). "The Implementation of a Phonological Change: The Case for Resyllabification in Black English." *Dissertation Abstracts International* 38:234A.

Walsh, H. (1974). "On Certain Practical Inadequacies of Distinctive Feature Systems." *Journal of Speech and Hearing Disorders* 39:32–43.

Washington, J., and Craig, H. (1992). "Articulation Test Performances of Low Income, African American Preschoolers with Communication Impairments." *Language, Speech and Hearing Services in Schools* 23:203–207.

Webb, J., and Duckett, B. (1990). *The Rules Phonological Analysis.* Vero Beach, FL: The Speech Bin.

Weiner, F. (1979). *Phonological Process Analysis.* Baltimore, MD: University Park Press.

Weiner, F. (1981). "Treatment of Phonological Disability Using the Method of Meaningful Minimal Contrast: Two Case Studies." *Journal of Speech and Hearing Disorders* 46:97–103.

Weiner, F., and Ostrowski, A. (1979). "Effects of Listener Uncertainty on Articulatory Inconsistency." *Journal of Speech and Hearing Disorders* 44:487–493.

Wellman, B., Case, M., Mengert, E., and Bradbury, D. (1931). *Speech Sounds of Young Children.* Iowa City: University of Iowa Studies in Child Welfare, no. 5.

Westman, M., and Browen, P. (1989). "Preschool Screening for Predictive Language Errors." *Language, Speech and Hearing Services in Schools* 20:139–148.

Weston, A., and Shriberg, L. (1992). "Contextual and Linguistic Correlates of Intelligibility in Children with Developmental Phonological Disorders." *Journal of Speech and Hearing Research* 35:1316–1332.

Williams, R., and Wolfram, W. (1977). *A Linguistic Description of Social Dialects: Differences vs. Disorders.* Rockville, MD: American Speech-Language-Hearing Association.

Williams, G., and McReynolds, L. (1975). "The Relationship between Discrimination and Articulation Training in Children with Misarticulations." *Journal of Speech and Hearing Research* 18:401–412.

Winitz, H. (1969). *Articulatory Acquisition and Behavior.* New York: Appleton-Century-Crofts.

Winitz, H. (1975). *From Syllable to Conversation.* Baltimore, MD: University Park Press.

Wolfram, W. (1989). "Structural Variability in Phonological Development: Final Nasals in Vernacular Black English." In *Current Issues in Linguistic Theory: Language Change and Variation,* ed. R. Fasold and D. Schiffren (Amsterdam, Neth: John Benjamins).

Wolfram, W. (1991). *Dialects and American English.* Englewood Cliffs, NJ: Prentice-Hall.

Wolfram, W. (1994). "The Phonology of a Sociocultural Variety: The Case of African American Vernacular English." In *Child Phonology: Characteristics, Assessment and Intervention with Special Populations,* ed. J. Bernthal and N. Bankson (New York: Thieme).

Zemlin, W. (1993). *Speech and Hearing Science.* Englewood Cliffs, NJ: Prentice-Hall.

Chapter 7

Disorders of Fluency

Stuttering is a curious, sometimes astonishing, and certainly a difficult way to talk. Why is the flow of speech, seemingly so easy and automatic for others, marred by tense interruptions? Unfortunately, the answer to that question still eludes clinicians and researchers—stuttering remains an enigma.

The puzzling nature of stuttering creates a dilemma for students. Confronted with a voluminous literature and a large number of treatment possibilities—each with its advocates—it is easy to give up in despair. Perhaps the negative attitude toward stutterers held by so many clinicians stems, in part, from overwhelming confusion about the disorder (Ragsdale and Ashby 1982; St. Louis and Lass 1981; Turnbaugh, Guitar, and Hoffman 1979, 1981). Yet, for some beginning clinicians, the dramatic nature of the disorder and even the confusion among experts have a fascinating appeal; they present a challenge.

We will assume in this chapter that the reader has a good foundation concerning the nature of stuttering. Books by Bloodstein (1995), Culatta and Goldberg (1995), Peters and Guitar (1991), and Van Riper (1982) provide excellent discussions of the many aspects of stuttering. We present the following list of "facts" about stuttering that have diagnostic implications and have been gleaned from the literature. For purposes of exposition, we have eschewed lengthy lists of references. Each item can be documented, however, even though some might disagree with our particular selection or interpretation.

1. The basic speech characteristics of stuttering consist of relatively brief part-word (phonemic, syllabic) repetitions and prolongations. These oscillations and fixations may be audible or silent and tend to occur more frequently at the beginning of an utterance and on words and phrases more complex motorically (such as long words and less frequently used words).
2. Stuttering is a disorder of childhood, generally having its onset before the age of six; rarely does it begin in older persons, and when it does it may be a distinct subtype of the disorder (such as neurotic stuttering).

3. Stuttering is found more frequently among males.
4. Stuttering tends to run in families.
5. Stuttering may be precipitated (and perpetuated) by certain environmental events, particularly the critical, demanding behaviors of significant others, usually parents.
6. Stuttering tends to appear more frequently in children described as "sensitive," who may be vulnerable or susceptible to stress. Stutterers may have a low threshold for autonomic arousal.
7. Stuttering tends to appear more frequently in children who were slow in acquiring speech or who manifest certain inadequacies of oral communication (articulation errors, language disturbances) other than fluency breakdowns.
8. Stuttering tends to exhibit cycles of frequency and severity in a given individual.
9. Stuttering is apparently "outgrown" by a significant number of individuals.
10. Stuttering tends to change in form and severity as the individual matures.
11. Stuttering is eliminated or markedly reduced in a variety of conditions: speaking while alone, choral speaking, singing, prolonged or slow speaking, talking in time to rhythm, or under masking conditions.
12. Stuttering, in its developed form, consists largely of escape and avoidance behavior; that is, much of the overt abnormality results from the individual's attempt to cope with the emission of the basic speech disfluency.
13. Stuttering is also characterized by speech and voice abnormalities other than disfluency (such as narrow pitch range, vocal tension, lack of vocal expression, muscular lags, and asynchronies) that can be detected in nonstuttered speech. These anomalies *may* reflect a basic impairment of phonation (difficulty in initiating phonation, making consonant-vowel transitions), respiration (abnormal reflex activity), neuromotor coordination, or cortical integration; they *may*, however, simply be effects of stuttering.
14. Stuttering, in its developed form, is often associated with an expectancy or anticipation of its occurrence.
15. Stuttering is a personal problem; individuals who stutter report fear, frustration, social penalties, dissatisfaction with themselves, lower level of aspiration, and felt loss of social esteem. There is a tendency for problems common to all human beings to become associated with the speech disturbance. However, there is no particular "stuttering personality," nor is the disorder a manifestation of psychoneurosis.

Even though the fluency disorder of stuttering remains a tantalizing mystery, there is much that we can do to help persons who seek our services.

Differential Diagnosis

Speech is fluent when words are produced easily, effortlessly, smoothly, quickly, and in a forward flow. Speech is disfluent when one word does not flow smoothly and quickly into the next. Obviously, then, all speakers are, at times, disfluent and these so-called normal disfluencies should be of no consequence. The SLP needs to be able to differentiate normal from abnormal disfluencies; often this proves to be no easy feat with young children. If the clinician does identify a speaker's disfluencies as abnormal or clinically significant, the next decision is to distinguish the problem of stuttering from other conditions in which speech fluency is disrupted. A final aspect of the differential diagnosis process may be to identify subtypes within the stuttering population, so as to select the most appropriate form of treatment. Let us discuss these three aspects of differential diagnosis, but we will do so in a different order.

Sorting Out the Types of Fluency Disorders

Assuming that the clinician has already identified a speaker as having abnormal amounts and/or types of disfluencies, the diagnostic task is one of deciding *which* disorder of fluency is exhibited. Along with a behavioral analysis of the disfluencies, the case history information will go far in suggesting the disorder type. We will provide an overview of some of the fluency breakdowns that can be confused with the common variety of stuttering, called developmental stuttering (or simply stuttering).

Episodic Stress Reaction

It is well known that most speakers exhibit some degree of disfluency—revisions, interjections, word and phrase repetitions, and occasionally even part-word repetitions and prolongations (Leeper et al. 1990; Pindzola 1991; Yairi 1981; Yairi and Clifton 1972). Speech fluency is often considered a sensitive barometer of a person's psychological state. Stress, particularly communicative stress, tends to increase a speaker's disfluency. If minor stress can affect fluency, then more-intense forms of psychological stress can certainly have a detrimental effect. Examples of conditions that can precipitate a fluency breakdown include battle conditions, intense excitement, emotional upheaval, and stage fright (Gavis 1946; Grinker and Spiegal 1945).

Fluency breakdowns owing to episodic stress show a number of consistent identifying features: an acknowledged source of intense or prolonged stimulation; tension overflow throughout the body (including the oral area), which may also produce a tremulous voice; an exacerbation of "normal" disfluency, including broken words, incomplete phrases, interjections, and repetitions of whole- and part-words; and no avoidance but feelings of fear. Finally, the most crucial characteristic is that the disfluency decreases markedly or stops when (or shortly after) the stress terminates. These acute, or episodic, periods of disfluency are usually not clinically significant.

Psychogenic Stuttering

Most persons who stutter, particularly confirmed adult cases, acquire a negative feeling about their problem. One of our clients summarized it succinctly when he said, "Stutterers are bugged because they are plugged." A few stutterers, however, show symptoms of a primary neurosis—they are "plugged because they are bugged." For these individuals, stuttering is a maladaptive solution to an acute psychological problem.

Psychogenic stuttering has also been known as neurotic or hysterical stuttering. Van Riper (1982) termed the onset and development of this form of disfluency as Track III stuttering.

> Case Example. *Colleen, an eigth-grade parochial school pupil, began to stutter suddenly following the death of her parents in an automobile accident. She collapsed upon hearing the tragic news and remained mute, almost transfixed and catatonic, for several hours. During the planning for the funeral and extended period of the wake, she started to stutter—a monotonous repetition of the initial syllable of words. She showed no struggle, no avoidance behavior. She looked directly at the listener when she spoke and smiled bravely. We followed this case closely until the remission of stuttering two months later, and her disfluency was always the same; it never varied in form or severity from situation to situation. When she read a passage several times, she did not show the typical reduction (adaptation) in stuttering. School documents, as well as interviews with several relatives, indicated that Colleen had no prior speech difficulty. One maternal aunt whom we interviewed did recall, however, that the girl had several "spells" of uncontrolled weeping and laughing during her first menses the year before. The child had received an incredible amount of attention and solace after her parents' death, perhaps even more so because of her "stuttering," from sympathetic adults.*

Psychogenic stuttering is a rare fluency disorder that is characterized by a sudden onset of rather severe stuttering. The onset may occur at any age, including adulthood, yet usually happens in an older child. Some severe (and lasting rather than episodic) psychological trauma, emotional upheaval, or stress seems to precipitate the occurrence of stuttering (Deal 1982; Tippett and Siebens 1991; Van Riper 1982; Weiner 1981). In contrast to the exacerbation of "normal" disfluencies seen in episodic stress, the neurotic stuttering pattern is severe from the beginning, with unvoiced prolongations, laryngeal blocks, tension, and/or lengthy repetitions typical. Although highly aware of these sudden and severe disfluencies, the person may or may not be frustrated by them. The level of concern and motivation to change are important elements for the SLP to assess as they may shape the prognosis for change and the direction of intervention.

Neurogenic Stuttering

Stuttering, or a stutteringlike problem, may occur following nervous system damage, as from stroke, trauma, infection, or tumor. The designation establishes this as a fluency disorder that results from neurological damage. We have observed disfluency in clients suffering from Parkinson's disease, some types of cerebral palsy, apraxia, and other neurological impairments (Helms, Butler, and Canter 1980; Koller 1983; LeBrun, Retif, and Kaiser 1983). There are also reports of fluency disruptions in alcoholics, drug addicts, and patients afflicted with AIDS (Fantry

1990) and with dialysis dementia (Madison et al. 1977). Palilalia, perhaps a sub-type of neurogenic stuttering may be caused by bilateral subcortical brain dam-age. Individuals with palilalia repeat words and entire phrases, typically not sounds or syllables, and they do so with increasing speed and diminishing loud-ness (Kent and LaPointe 1982; LaPointe and Horner 1981). Canter (1971) classified neurogenic stuttering into subtypes, such as dysnomic stuttering, dysarthric stut-tering, apraxic stuttering, and so forth.

Several patients with aphasia with whom we have worked, particularly those clients who show good progress in word finding but who have residual syntactic difficulty, exhibited fluency breakdowns superficially similar to stuttering.

> Case Example. *Mrs. Horn had suffered an aneurysm in the Circle of Willis, leaving her hemiplegic, apraxic, and with mild expressive aphasia. When we ex-amined her, almost a year after the cerebral vascular episode, her speech pattern resembled clonic stuttering. She would begin a word, repeat a phoneme or sylla-ble several times, back up, and try again; if blocked once more, a repetition might reverberate almost endlessly. She frequently pounded on the table as if to time her utterances. We could discern no evidence of fear or avoidance, just severe frus-tration. Interestingly, when she spoke or read swiftly her fluency increased dra-matically; she also talked freely when distracted from closely monitoring the acts of speaking. Here is a sample of her speech taken from a tape recording during a group session: "I can't-I can't (sigh) . . . I-I-I-I have tr-trouble with my, ah, with my speech . . . and, ah, my leg is, is, you know is, stiff."*

The disfluencies noted are rather typical: whole-word repetitions, revisions, inter-jections, broken words, and gaps in the flow of speech. This client had difficulty formulating messages and then programming the proper motor sequences to utter the thought. Unlike stuttering where the difficulty is getting started, Mrs. Horn's fluency breakdowns occurred at any point in a sentence (Brown and Cullinan 1981; Donnan 1979; Rosenbek et al. 1978).

Cluttering

Cluttering is sometimes confused with stuttering, but it encompasses more than just a disorder of fluency. Cluttering has varied symptomatology and co-occurs with other speech, language, and behavioral disorders. According to Weiss (1964, 1968), cluttering symptoms may include: part- and whole-word repetitions, lack of awareness of the disorder, short attention span, perceptual weakness, poorly or-ganized thinking, excessive speech rate (tachylalia), interjections, articulatory and motor disabilities, and grammatical difficulties. Other academic difficulties, noted by clinicians, teachers, and researchers, include reading and writing disorders, dif-ficulty with many language-dependent skills (owing to subtle language disorders), lack of rhythm and musical ability, and restlessness and hyperactivity (Daly 1986; DeFusco and Menken 1979; Irvine and Reis 1980; Weiss 1968).

> Case Example. *Ralph was referred to us as a stutterer by his industrial educa-tion supervisor during his semester of student teaching. When we examined him,*

he revealed no fears or avoidances, exhibited only a few short part-word repetitions, and had no fixations; he said that he enjoyed talking, did a lot of it, and that he was asked frequently to repeat himself, "especially when I talk fast." Ralph's difficulty seemed to take place on the phrase or sentence level; his interruptions broke the integrity of a thought rather than a word. In addition, he frequently omitted syllables and transposed words and phrases; he said "plobably," "posed," and "pacific" for "probably," "supposed," and "specific." Ralph's speech was sprinkled with spoonerisms (he said "beta dase" for "data base") and malapropisms (he described getting lost while hunting because the road he was following "dissipated" and told us he had a good "dialect" going with his roommate). His speech was swift and jumbled; it emerged in rapid torrents until he jammed up, and then he surged on again in another staccato outburst. In spontaneous talking, his message was characterized by disorganized sentences and poor phrasing. He gave the overall impression of being in great haste. When we asked him to slow down and speak carefully, there was a drastic improvement, but he soon forgot our admonishment and reverted to his hurried, disorganized style. By and large, Ralph was unaware and indifferent to his fluency problem. He was an impatient, impulsive young man, always on the go. His course work was characteristically done in a great, almost compulsive rush; he had difficulty reading, and his handwriting was a scrawl.

Distinguishing among Subtypes of Stuttering

Are there different kinds of (developmental) stuttering? Although there is no conclusive answer to that question, clinical opinion is that there must be—if only to explain the wide variety of clients, symptomatologies, and responses to intervention programs. Possibilities that come to mind include interiorized and exteriorized stutterers (Douglass and Quarrington 1952); predominantly clonic (repetitive disfluencies) and predominantly tonic stutterers (with tension, prolongations, and blockages); clients who feature escape techniques; those who are addicted to avoidance; and those who can predict an occurrence of stuttering and those who cannot (Silverman and Williams 1972). Perhaps there are even variations in stuttering that stem from cultural influences (Leith and Mims 1975; Satcher 1986; Shames 1989). These distinctions may be useful in planning treatment.

Ours is an ethnically diverse society and we are only beginning to appreciate how cultural values might affect the incidence, development, and ultimate treatment of communication disorders such as stuttering. Likewise, multicultural sensitivity on the part of the SLP is necessary, but unfortunately not sufficient (Culatta and Goldberg 1995). Early examinations of stuttering within cultures and across nations were motivated by theorists espousing environmental etiologies of stuttering. Table 7.1 cites issues regarding culture and stuttering as presently understood (Bloodstein 1995; Culatta and Goldberg 1995; Dykes 1995). Table 7.2 summarizes differences in the normal disfluencies of Black and White children, adults, and aged persons, whereas Table 7.3 provides an overview of stuttering differences among these same groups. The reader is cautioned that much research is needed in these areas.

TABLE 7.1   Cultural Variables and Stuttering

Gender/Sex. There is unequivocal evidence that more males than females stutter, regardless of the society or national origin.

Parent Variables/Child-Rearing Practices. Glasner (1949) identified harsh discipline, humiliation, and indulgence as directly affecting the occurrence of stuttering.

Demographics. Stuttering is more prevalent in urban, rather than rural areas, according to Brady and Hall (1976). Yet, Dykes (1995) found that rural areas had a greater prevalence of stuttering (.49%) than urban areas did (.34%).

Bilingualism. Bilingual children are more likely to stutter than monolingual speakers, according to Bloodstein (1995) who cites a prevalence rate of 2.8% among bilinguals versus the nearly 1% in the general population. In contrast, Montes and Erickson (1990) found no significant differences in the occurrence of stuttered speech behaviors in English and Spanish bilingual children. They also noted that the types of disfluencies associated with second language learning are often misidentified as stuttering.

Socioeconomic Class. Morgenstern (1956) found more stuttering in the middle and upper-middle classes than in the lower classes.

Race/Ethnicity. Dated studies examined stuttering among the Eskimos and native Americans (see review in Van Riper 1982); however no current research is available on these groups nor on Asian Americans. Leavitt (1974) found the prevalence of stuttering among Puerto Ricans living in New York City to be 0.84%, a value similar to that of Whites; by comparison the prevalence among Puerto Ricans living in San Juan was 1.5%. African American research is presented in separate tables.

TABLE 7.2   Some Studies of Black and White Speakers of Various Age Groups during Normal Disfluencies

Children.

- Preschool Black and White children of low and of middle socioeconomic levels did not show different types of disfluency (Ratusnik, Kirilluk, and Ratusnik 1979).
- Disfluencies of preschool Black children did not differ between males and females; amounts of disfluencies, especially revisions, declined with age (3.5 through 5.5 years) (Anderson 1976).
- No significant differences were found between disfluencies of Black and White first-grade children; both groups exhibited 7–8% disfluency (Brutten and Miller 1988).
- Black preschool children had more repetitions, prolongations, and revisions during narrative discourse than in conversational speech (Robinson and Davis 1992).

Young and Aged Adults.

- Black college football players displayed greater amounts of word and phrase repetitions than did White athletes (Robinson and Crowe 1987).
- Black males and females, aged 61–91, had slower speech rates and greater disfluency rates (especially revisions and repetitions) than White speakers did (Walker et al. 1981).
- Black and White males, aged 65–85, of matched socioeconomic levels were compared; no significant differences were found for race or socioecomomic level with regard to speaking rates, articulatory rates, or frequencies of interjections (approximately 4.75%), revisions (1.22%), and whole-word repetitions (.83%) (Pindzola 1990).

TABLE 7.3

Some Studies Comparing Stuttered Speech among Blacks and Whites of Various Age Groups

Children.

- Analysis of matriarchial families in Tennessee suggests more females stutter among Blacks than among Whites; male-to-female sex ratios were reported as 2.4:1 among Blacks and 5:1 among Whites (Goldman 1967).
- Patriarchial Black families had sex ratios of stuttering similar to sex ratios for Whites (Goldman 1967).
- The male-to-female ratio of stuttering prevalence in African Americans is similar to that of Whites; both were 3.5:1 (Dykes 1995).
- Black male nonstuttering children had closer relationships with their mothers and received more consistent discipline than did Black male stuttering children (Powell 1967).
- The high prevalence of stuttering among Alabama school children (2.1% prevalence) was attributed to the large population of Blacks in the schools (78% Black, 22% White) (Gillespie and Cooper 1973).
- African American male and female students have prevalence rates twice that of White males and females (Dykes 1995).

Young and Aged Adults.

- In a Chicago community college, the prevalence of stuttering was 2.7% for Blacks and .8% for Whites (Conrad 1992).
- Among young adults, racial patterns of disfluency may exist: Whites tend to display overt repetitions and prolongations, while Blacks tend to be more covert and severe. This may be a cultural response to conceal lack of verbal prowess among Blacks (Leith and Mims 1975).
- No known studies of aged adults exist beyond speculations posed by Manning and Monte (1981).

Differentiating Normal Disfluencies from Stuttering

We saved this aspect of the differential diagnosis for last, although the clinician must determine it first. It is a vast topic. The literature shows good agreement regarding the general principles for distinguishing between normal and abnormal but often differs on the specifics. Where to draw the line segmenting normal types and amounts of disfluency from the abnormal is still a matter of clinical judgment; our data is not that precise. Van Riper (1982), however, composed a useful list of distinguishing characteristics. Others have adapted this information for use on various clinical scales (Cooper 1973; Cooper and Cooper 1985; Pindzola 1988).

Gordon and Luper (1992) reviewed six often-used protocols for identifying beginning stuttering. Two of these will be mentioned here. Adams (1977) provides a clinical strategy for differentiating the normal-speaking child from one beginning to stutter; his criteria and guidelines for clinical interpretation are summarized in Table 7.4. Also useful is the Protocol for Differentiating the Incipient Stutterer (Pindzola 1988; Pindzola and White 1986).

TABLE 7.4   Adams' Guidelines for Distinguishing Between the Normally Disfluent Child and the Incipient Stutterer

	Guidelines for Interpretation	
Criterion	Normally Disfluent	Incipient Stutterer
Total frequency (all types)	9 or fewer disfluencies per 100 words	10 or more disfluencies per 100 words
Predominate type	Whole-word and phrase repetitions, interjections, and revisions	Part-word repetitions, audible and silent prolongations, and broken words
Unit repetitions	No more than 2 unit repetitions ("b-b-ball")	At least 3 repetitions ("b-b-b-ball")
Voicing and air flow	Little or no difficulty starting or sustaining voicing or air flow; continuous phonation during part-word repetitions	Frequent difficulty in starting or sustaining voicing or air flow; heard in association with part-word repetitions, prolongations, and broken words; more-effortful disfluencies
Intrusion of the schwa	Schwa not perceived ("ba-ba-baby")	Schwa often perceived ("buh-buh-buh-baby")

In making decisions about normal versus abnormal fluency (stuttering), the clinician should be guided by information available in the literature. The clinician then pulls together a vast array of information collected on and about the client to arrive at a diagnosis. We admit this is a judgment call on the part of the clinician, but if the evaluation is done thoroughly, it is an "informed" judgment call. Here are some guidelines borrowed from the Protocol for Differentiating the Incipient Stutterer (Pindzola 1988; Pindzola and White 1986).

The type of disfluency that predominates in a client's speech and the size of the speech unit affected by the breakdown influence society's judgment of normalcy. For example, repetitions of whole phrases are quite normal; whole-word repetitions are disfluencies typical of both stutterers and nonstutterers. Yet the predominance of part-word repetitions distinguishes stuttering from nonstuttering speakers of all ages, including preschoolers (Yairi and Lewis 1984). Hesitations or pauses before phrases or before words may, likewise, be less innocuous than such gaps within words (i.e., preceding syllables or sounds). The rule of thumb suggested by Perkins (1971) is that the smaller the speech unit affected, the more abnormal the disfluency.

The frequency with which disfluent behaviors occur has long been recognized as important in the diagnosis of stuttering. Some authorities advocate the use of rate of stuttering (calculated as total stuttered words per minute of talking, SW/M) as a frequency measure of choice (Ryan 1974; Shine 1980); others use percentage of stuttered syllables or percentage of stuttered words. There are various norms in the literature; for example, frequencies in excess of 2 percent, 5 percent, or 10 percent may suggest a true stuttering disorder, depending on the strictness of the criterion selected by the clinician (Adams 1977; Metraux 1950; Van Riper 1982; Yairi and Lewis 1984). Being disfluent less than the cutoff percentage presumably indicates normalcy. Ryan (1974) suggests that disfluencies occuring an average of less than one word per two minutes of talking (0.5 SW/M) is within normal limits. Intervention is warranted, he says, if the rate of stuttering is 3 SW/M or more.

As part of the assessment, the clinician will gauge the duration of the client's disfluency. This is often expressed as an average number of reiterations of the repetition or as an average amount of time stuck in an audible or silent prolongation. If the typical duration of prolongations exceeds one second, or if repetitions involve numerous reiterations—say, three to five or more—then these behaviors may be interpreted as signs of stuttering (Adams 1977; Van Riper 1982).

Audible signs of effort while speaking are generally not noted among normal speakers and therefore are indicative of abnormality (Pindzola 1988; Pindzola and White 1986). There are many signs of audible effort; some examples that are typically heard in stutterers include disrupted airflow, hard contacts (explosive, crisp articulation), effort or tension heard in the voice, and a pitch rise during a moment of stuttering.

Van Riper (1982) provides clinical reports that normal disfluencies and perhaps very early stutterings are characterized by repetitions that preserve the normal rhythm and rate of speech. Not until the tempo of the reiterations speeds up or the rhythm becomes irregular and choppy is there substantial reason for concern. The SLP, then, should subjectively judge the client's rhythm, tempo, and speed of disfluencies when trying to make a differential diagnosis.

The presence of learned behaviors, or secondary behaviors, is strongly suggestive of stuttering, rather than normal fluency. The clinician therefore should determine whether the client uses concealment devices (such as word substitutions or circumlocutions), postponement devices, starting tricks, and so forth. Visually, the clinician may note physical involvement of the facial, head, and body regions. Frequently observed contortions are eye blinks, wrinkling of the forehead, distortions of the mouth, overt mandibular tension, head jerks, and the more subtle head turnings to divert eye contact.

Once the SLP has made a differential diagnosis and determined that the client is stuttering, the next issue to be resolved is the developmental progression or severity of the disorder. In actuality, the information gathered to differentiate normal from abnormal speech is part of the same kind of information needed to determine the level of severity. On a continuum between normal and abnormal, the decision is now how far down the abnormal end of the continuum the client is placed. Just as data (e.g., percentage of stuttering, duration of the disfluencies) were used to segment normal from abnormal, so can they be used to categorize the problem as mild, moderate, and severe. Following that, the next decision that confronts the clinician is the recommended course of action. Is treatment warranted? If so, along what lines shall it be devised?

The Appraisal of Stuttering

In our discussion of making a differential diagnosis, we glossed over the details of how to obtain the information necessary to make such a decision. What information is necessary? What published appraisal instruments are available to help collect and make sense of this information? (An annotated listing of some instruments can be found in Pindzola 1986.) What less tangible factors need to be judged, albeit subjectively, by the clinician? We will now try to answer these questions. Bear in mind, however, that the "answers" may differ for different clients, depending on their age, intelligence, reading abilities, and so forth.

Case History Information and Parent Materials

We will discuss two forms of the case history intake: one done with the parents of a child who stutters or is beginning to stutter and one done with a teenager or adult who stutters.

Initial Interview with the Parents

The initial interview with the parents of a child beginning to stutter is of critical importance. We must establish our professional competence, demonstrate our genuine interest, and convince the parents that we can be trusted. In short, our primary task in this initial contact is to build a relationship for subsequent counseling sessions. We also listen carefully to the parents' presenting story: How do they see the child's problem? In their view, what might have caused it? What do they identify as their role in the onset of the child's stuttering? What expectations and apprehensions do they have regarding the nature and the outcome of treatment?

We like to regard the initial interaction between parents and clinician as a time for information gathering and information sharing. As we said, we first want to hear the presenting complaint—and encourage the telling of their child's speech story. We may opt to be more or less directive in our style with the parents; it does not matter, so long as the information we need unfolds. A parent's careful review of the many factors involved in the child's problem tends to foster objectivity. It also shifts the focus away from a general impression of "trouble" to the observation of specific behaviors. Here are some questions we use as guides in assembling information from parents:

1. When did the child begin exhibiting disfluencies?
2. What were the circumstances under which the disfluencies were noted?
3. How long has the child been exhibiting the disfluencies?
4. What changes have been noted in the frequency or form of the disfluencies?
5. What factors seem to increase or decrease the child's disfluency?
6. In what ways has the family tried to help the child?
7. What is the child's reaction to the family's efforts to help?

Additional items to assess in obtaining a case history include (1) a specific review of the familial incidence of stuttering; (2) the impact, if any, of siblings, relatives, teachers, or babysitters upon the child; (3) a description of how the child spends a typical day; and (4) a description of any prior professional treatment.

Case history collection forms, complete with specific questions and answer blanks for recording information, can be found in a number of books and intervention programs (Cooper 1976; Culatta and Goldberg 1995; Goldberg 1981; Luper and Mulder 1966; Peins, McGough, and Lee 1984; Peters and Guitar 1991; Pindzola 1988; Shine 1980; Weiner 1984; Wells 1987; Wingate 1976). The clinician may wish to adopt one or more of these styles.

The case history interview can be done either before or after the child has been seen and evaluated by the clinician. Consequently, this initial meeting may, in fact, involve several points of interaction or separate sessions. We try to refrain from being influenced by the parent's push for us to provide too much information prematurely; naturally they want to know what caused their child's problem and what can be done (quickly) about it. We, however, do enlist the parent's help in collecting observations of the child's behavior in the home environment.

What things at home seem to promote fluency and what seems to promote disfluency? Is it all right for the parents to remind the child to "slow down" (as advocated by Shine 1980 and Cooper 1985) or is that counterproductive and something to be considered taboo (owing to the Wendell Johnson philosophy)? We do not know the answers to these questions for a *particular* child; the parents must find out. Parents' recordings of home behaviors have been advocated by many (Emerick 1983; Pindzola 1988; Shine 1980; Zwitman 1978).

We often find that simply asking parents to monitor the antecedents and consequences of their child's speech disfluencies is sufficiently motivating to engender change. Enviromental events that disrupt a child's flow of speech typically become obvious when parents begin to chart.

Even though there is much information that we simply cannot give the parents early on (often because we do not yet know the information), clincians have a responsiblity to help educate the parents. That is to say, clinicians need to provide a good understanding of stuttering and its many ramifications. In addition to what clinicians say, they like to provide the parents with reading materials; some are of their own preparation, while others are brochures and booklets from published sources. The interested reader might consider the materials by Cooper (1979), Emerick (1983), Johnson (1961), and Robinson (1966). The Stuttering Foundation of America (P.O. Box 11749, Memphis, TN 38111), the Stuttering Resource Foundation (123 Oxford Road, New Rochelle, NY 10804), the National Stuttering Project (4601 Irving Street, San Francisco, CA 94122), and the American Speech-Language-Hearing Association (10801 Rockville Pike, Rockville, MD 20852) have pamphlets or booklets available for parents. We find these materials more useful and up-to-date than the sources previously mentioned. Other tools that clinicians use in helping parents are two excellent films: *Family Counseling* (Walle 1975) and *Is It Me? Is It You?* (Walle 1977). Both films are invaluable in helping parents understand how they can help children overcome the broken and hesitant speech often displayed between two and six years of age.

The clinician may wish to have one or both parents complete a checklist or questionnaire that may prove useful in identifying parental perceptions, attitudes, and topics in need of exploration at subsequent counseling sessions. Table 7.5 lists some of the available instruments for a clinician to consider in working with parents.

It is important that parents obtain some closure from these initial interviews. Let us demonstrate a typical conversation, showing how we relate our diagnostic findings to the parents of a client named Stephen.

Stephen does indeed have some breaks in speech, more than normal for a child of his age. He is doing some stuttering, but it is still the "good kind": He is not strug-gling or avoiding and, most important, he doesn't seem to be very aware that talk-ing is tough (we drew a rough sketch of the stuttering gauge depicted in Figure 7.1 and showed them that Stephen exhibited only the first three early danger signs of stuttering, based on the 1974 film by Walle). We want to prevent the disorder from developing further and cannot do anything without your help. We need to find out why he is having speech breaks; we need to know when he does it, under what circumstances. In short, we have to start looking at behaviors, at what he does, not a condition he has. In many cases like this, if we identify and alter cer-tain enviromental situations, the child stops stuttering. You were very wise to bring him in now, before the fear and frustration have a chance to develop. Let's plan on meeting again tomorrow, and together we can begin to review Stephen's background and then decide how to gather information on what is happening now.

Case History Interview with Older Clients

The case history and initial interview with an older client who stutters are obvi-ously different from those we just described. Prior to undertaking formal obser-vation and testing, clinicians like to perform an intake interview. This brief preliminary discussion is designed to accomplish four objectives: (1) to inform the client what to expect in the diagnostic session, (2) to determine why the client is coming for treatment at this particular time, (3) to assemble historical information, and (4) to establish a working relationship.

Because the clinician wants the client to be a partner in the exploration of the problem, it is important for the client to know *what* the clinician intends to do and *why* the clinician proposes to do it. By structuring the clinical transaction so the clients know what role they are to play in their own recovery, the clinician is es-

---

TABLE 7.5   Some Assessment Instruments for Use with Parents of Young Stutterers

Parent Attitudes Toward Stuttering Checklist
  Cooper (1976), Cooper and Cooper (1985)

The Child Fluency Assessment Instrument
  Goldberg (1981) (contains parental questionnaire)

Parental Diagnostic Questionnaire
  Tanner (1987)

Assessment of Stuttering Behaviors
  Tanner (1990)

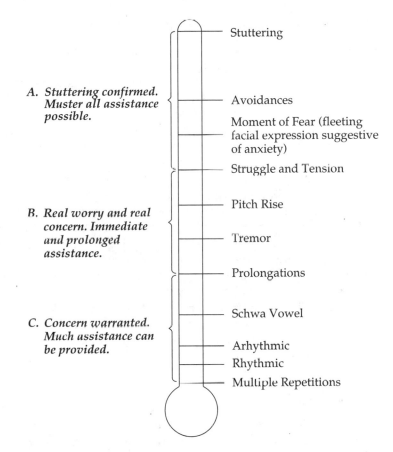

A. Stuttering confirmed.
Muster all assistance
possible.

Stuttering

Avoidances

Moment of Fear (fleeting
facial expression suggestive
of anxiety)

Struggle and Tension

B. Real worry and real
concern. Immediate
and prolonged
assistance.

Pitch Rise

Tremor

Prolongations

C. Concern warranted.
Much assistance can
be provided.

Schwa Vowel

Arhythmic

Rhythmic

Multiple Repetitions

FIGURE 7.1　The Danger Signs of Developing Stuttering

tablishing a therapeutic contract. The reader may also wish to consult Silverman (1980) who discusses the role of the client in defining treatment goals through the use of the Stuttering Problem Profile.

Case history questionnaires are readily available in many books and intervention programs. Examples include those by Culatta and Goldberg (1995), Goldberg (1981), Peters and Guitar (1991), Wells (1987), and Wingate (1976). Naturally, the clinician asks about the duration of the problem, what professional help has been sought, recent changes in the speech, and a description of the current speaking difficulties.

The clinician also likes to determine why the client is coming (or being sent) to an SLP at this particular point in time. Has the individual undergone a "bottoming-out" experience, a severe crisis in his/her social, occupational, or educational life? What does he/she expect from treatment? What do others expect? Answers to these questions are useful in determining the client's motivation and in making a prognosis. All in all, the initial contact with a client is of inestimable importance in establishing a working relationship.

Differentiating and Predictive Scales

As we discussed earlier in this chapter, one of the clinician's major responsibilities is differentiating normal speakers having usual disfluencies from persons who are stuttering. This may be obvious in the evaluation of some clients, but it may be quite difficult with others—particularly young children.

Complicating the issue further with young children is the notion of spontaneous recovery. Estimates are that as many as 80 percent of the children who begin to stutter spontaneously recover or "outgrow" the problem (Andrews and Harris 1964). We should also report that Young (1975) and Martin and Lindamood (1986) concluded, after a critical review of the literature, that the 80 percent recovery figure is too high; spontaneous recovery rates may be as low as 30 percent. Still, the clinician needs to know which disfluent children will likely outgrow the problem and which seem destined for chronic difficulties and therefore need clinical intervention. Although clinicians are far from being able to precisely differentiate these two types of children, they do have assessment instruments that help them in their predictions. We cite the Stuttering Chronicity Prediction Checklist (Cooper 1973; Cooper and Cooper 1985) and the Stuttering Prediction Instrument for Young Children (Riley 1981) as examples. In the hands of an experienced clinician, all assessment indices provide information useful in "guessing" who will and who will not outgrow stuttering without help. Table 7.6 lists many of the available assessments instruments, useful for a variety of purposes.

Severity Scales

The clinician's primary mission in the evaluation of a person who stutters is to perform a careful analysis of the individual's speech disfluency behavior. Not only is this necessary for differential diagnosis, but also for the appraisal of the severity of the disorder. With regard to treatment, the disfluency assessment also accomplishes two basic purposes: It delineates the behaviors to be altered, and it provides a base measure to which the clinician can refer when monitoring the impact of treatment. The majority of published assessment instruments help the clinician determine the extent of the speech problem. We will call these instruments *severity scales,* whether or not the "score" from the test yields a severity modifier, such as mild to very severe.

Table 7.6 listed some of the available instruments that assess the overt features of stuttering. Many aspects of the stuttering problem can be tapped by using a variety of these instruments, including the frequency of disfluency, the duration of the disfluency, the physical behaviors that accompany speech attempts, and so forth. Judging from the length of this (nonexhaustive) list, there are many severity scales from which to choose. We will highlight one of these scales and will recommend Chapter 3 of Culatta and Goldberg (1995) for an overview of many published instruments.

In wide use is the Stuttering Severity Instrument (Riley 1972, 1994). This SSI, as it is often known, is useful with both children and adults and has provisions for testing those who can and cannot read. The number of syllables (previous editions

TABLE 7.6   Some Available Instruments for the Assessment of Overt Features of Stuttering, including Diagnostic, Severity, and Predictive Scales

Southern Illinois Behavior Checklist
   (Brutten and Shoemaker 1974)

Syracuse University Fluency Diagnostic Summary Sheet
   (Conture 1990)

A Stuttering Chronicity Prediction Checklist
   (Cooper 1973) Cooper and Cooper (1985)

Concomitant Stuttering Behavior Checklist
   (Cooper 1976) Cooper and Cooper (1985)

Stuttering Frequency and Duration Estimate Record
   (Cooper 1976) Cooper and Cooper (1985)

Client and Clinician Perceptions of Stuttering Severity Ratings
   (Cooper 1976) Cooper and Cooper (1985)

The Preschool Fluency Baseline Record
   (Culp 1984)

Severity Scale (S-Scale)
   (Erickson 1969)

The Child, Adolescent, Adult Fluency Assessment Instrument
   (Goldberg 1981, three multifaceted assessment systems)

Scale for Rating the Severity of Stuttering
   (Johnson, Darley, and Spriestersbach 1963)

The Stuttering Severity Scale (SS Scale)
   (Lanyon 1967)

Stuttering Diagnostic and Evaluative Checklist
   (Luper and Mulder 1966)

Checklist of Physical Behaviors Accompanying Stuttering
   (Peins, McGough, and Lee 1984)

A Protocol for Differentiating the Incipient Stutterer
   (Pindzola 1988; Pindzola and White 1986)

Stuttering Severity Instrument for Children and Adults
   (Riley 1972, 1994)

Stuttering Prediction Instrument for Young Children
   (Riley 1981)

Stuttering Interview (Forms A and B)
   (Ryan 1974)

Assessment Form: Systematic Fluency Training for Young Children
   (Shine 1980)

The Stocker Probe Technique for Diagnosis and Treatment of Stuttering in Young Children
   (Stocker 1980)

Assessment of Fluency in School-Age Children
   (Thompson 1983)

Profile of Stuttering Severity: A Revised Scale
   (Van Riper 1982)

Stutterers' Physiological Assessment
   (Wells 1987)

Severity Rating Guide
   (Wingate 1976)

used words) stuttered and the number of total syllables (or words) spoken are computed by the SLP as the client reads and/or is engaged in conversation. Frequency, expressed as percentage of stuttered syllables, is then computed. The clinician also monitors the duration of the longest stuttering events and rates the presence and conspicuousness of physical behaviors concomitant with the speech attempts. Frequency, duration, and physical concomitant task scores are then combined for a total score. The severity of the client's stuttering can be ascertained by comparing the total score to the normative data provided in the test manual. Stuttering severity may be described as very mild, mild, moderate, severe, or very severe in this manner.

Recently, Bakker and Riley (1997) made available a software program, the Computerized Scoring of Stuttering Severity, that provides the clinical measures required in the SSI. It obtains the percentage of stuttered syllables, mean duration of the three longest stuttering events, mean duration of all stuttering events, fluent speaking rate, and length of periods of fluent speech.

At this point we would like to mention that the Individualized Education Program (IEP) format adopted by most school districts requires a statement regarding the educational and psychological severity of a student's handicapping condition. The SLP who works in the public schools, then, must categorize the severity of the student's stuttering along the continuum of very mild to very severe. The ease of administration and the usefulness of the results may account for the popularity of the SSI among clinicians, especially those employed by the schools (e.g., Howard County, MD 1985). (Treatment approaches with built-in IEP formats include those by Cooper and Cooper 1985 and Pindzola 1988.)

The appraisal of the overt symptoms of stuttering need not require administration of a published test. The clinician's analysis, whether using a formal published test or an informal look at a speech sample, should include a thorough description of the stuttering pattern (topography) and measures of the relative frequency with which various features of the pattern occur. Descriptions of the process can be found in the writings of Conture (1990), Starkweather, Gottwald, and Halfond (1990), and Peters and Guitar (1991).

The Assessment Process

We will now walk the reader through our assessment process. The first step in the disfluency analysis is to obtain a representative sample of the client's speech. The operative word here is *representative;* stuttering is an intermittent disorder, and the amount of difficulty an individual has is contingent on the speaking task, the situation, and other variables. If it is possible, there are obvious advantages to collecting samples of the client's "real" communication in naturalistic settings—the playground, informal group situations, the family dinner table. Generally, however, clinicians rely on data obtained from speaking tasks, such as reading aloud a standard passage, giving a monologue, or conversing. Be sure to tape-record, or, even better, videotape, the session and note the time elapsed for each segment of the total sample: It will then be easier to specify rather precise frequency and severity values. We always ask the stutterer to discuss both neutral topics (hobbies, sports, vacations) and threatening topics (family, school, dating) to ensure that we obtain a range of speaking difficulty. It is important to know what produces stress and how the individual responds to it; we experiment in the session with things like hurrying the client, feigning listener loss, and asking the client to repeat. .

An Overall Description

We begin the analysis with a global description of the individual's speech behavior. What is his/her normal speech like in terms of rate, rhythm, degree of tension, articulation, and voice? What are the salient features of the stuttering pattern?

Core Behaviors

The lowest common denominators of the problem of stuttering seem to be repetitions (oscillative phenomena) and prolongations (fixative phenomena). Although most individuals have either predominately repetitive or predominately tense disfluency patterns, all stutterers exhibit a variety of forms of the speech interruption. A key feature of the disfluency analysis, therefore, is a precise description of these core behaviors.

With respect to *repetitions,* the clinician wants to identify the size of the unit (phrase, whole-word, syllable), the number of oscillations per unit (e.g., b-boy vs. b-b-b-b-boy), their tempo and degree of tension involved, and how they are terminated. Are there silent oscillations of articulatory postures? Does the client have difficulty finding the proper vowel during the course of the repetitions?

In terms of *prolongations,* the clinician is interested in the anatomical site of the fixations, whether they are silent or audible, how long they last, the degree of tension involved, and how they are terminated.

Struggle-Tension Features

Very rarely does a client exhibit *only* repetitions and prolongations. Anyone who has observed persons who stutter knows that they appear tense and often make irrelevant sounds and movements while attempting to speak. Persons who stutter which display a wide variety of these mannerisms, may vary in frequency of occurrence and degree of involvement in particular clients; some individuals manifest an astounding array of eye blinking, head jerking, postponement rituals, and other behaviors, whereas others appear relatively quiescent, at least overtly. The clinician should take note of these "accessory features." Several scales listed in Table 7.6 can be used as well. For example, the Southern Illinois Behavior Checklist (Brutten and Shoemaker 1974) lists ninety-seven different behaviors and is designed so that both the client and the clinician can record the presence of various mannerisms.

Covert Measures

In developed stuttering, the overt symptoms may be only the tip of the problem. After years of difficulty in speaking, especially since the amount of difficulty varies with the speaking situation, it is only natural that the person would develop hidden feelings and attitudes about speech. The negative feelings may be generalized

but are often directed toward particular speaking situations, conversational partners, and even particular word and phoneme combinations. Following on the
heels of apprehension, dislike, and fear of these events comes the avoidance of
them. Therefore, measuring the covert side of a client's stuttering problem is often
part of the diagnostic process. Early on, perhaps in the initial session, we attempt
to discuss with the client his/her feelings, attitudes, fears, and experiences. This
helps us "get to know" the client and better understand the depth of the problem.
Counseling may need to be part of the treatment program for some clients. In addition to discussions of feelings, the clinician can utilize published instruments.
Sentence completion tasks and adjective checklists help to identify attitudes and
personality traits. Several of these tasks and checklists are listed in Table 7.7.

We would be remiss if we did not acknowledge that some behavioral clinicians opt not to measure, or clinically deal with, covert feelings and attitudes. The

**TABLE 7.7   Some Available Instruments for the Assessment of Covert
Features of Stuttering, including Perception/Attitude
Scales and Situation/Avoidance Checklists**

Iowa Scale of Attitude Toward Stuttering
  (Ammons and Johnson 1944)

Modified Erickson Scale of Communication Attitudes
  (Andrews and Cutler 1974)

Communication Attitude Test
  (Brutten and Dunham 1989)

Fear Survey Schedule
  (Brutten and Shoemaker 1974)

Speech Situation Checklist
  (Brutten and Shoemaker 1974)

Stuttering Attitudes Checklist
  (Cooper 1976, 1985)

Situation Avoidance Behavior Checklist
  (Cooper 1976, 1985)

Adjective Checklist
  (Erickson 1969)

Role Construct Repertory Test
  (Fransella 1972)

A-19 Scale for Children Who Stutter
  (Guitar and Grims 1977)

Stutterer's Self-Ratings of Reactions to Speech Situations (ARSF Scale)
  (Shumak 1955)

Perceptions of Stuttering Inventory (PSI)
  (Woolf 1967)

Hierarchy Ranking
  (Wells 1987, several versions)

focus of intervention may, indeed, be to train fluency and let the covert aspects drop out of the client's repertoire on their own, in due time. Likewise, the clinician may use an attitude scale as a baseline measure, proceed with a behavioral approach that focuses only on the overt side of stuttering, and then probe for attitudinal change as a consequence of successful fluency.

The clinician *is* interested in avoidance behaviors that the client exhibits. We feel that, clinically, avoidance behavior is an important feature to deal with because it tends to reinforce and compound the stutterer's difficulty. Rather than diminish, fears tend to incubate and grow when a person recoils from them; avoidances cause apprehension to increase and the problem to expand.

Avoidance is characterized by reduction or cessation of communication: The stutterer retreats from the act of talking. The clinician can discern the types of speaking situations and listeners who increase or decrease the client's stuttering. This evaluation can be accomplished by interviewing or by having the client fill out a checklist. The clinician can devise a form for recording data (simply listing different speaking situations, topics of conversation, and so forth) or use a published inventory. Table 7.7 lists assessment instruments useful with the covert side of stuttering. We will highlight a few.

The Speech Situation Checklist (Brutten and Shoemaker 1974) has the client rate his/her degree of emotional response and severity of speech disruption in fifty-one life situations. Although no formal instrument is supplied, Shames and Egolf (1976) list various circumstances (audience size, specific people, different talking situations) and suggests tactics for sampling actual speech behavior under those conditions. In addition to listing the conditions under which stuttering is increased or reduced, the clinician may ask the client to rank-order the items in terms of speech difficulty and emotional impact, as done by Wells (1987).

In addition to situation fears, many who stutter report that they have particular difficulty with certain words and speech sounds. We make a list of these items and then examine the speech sample to determine if in fact there is more stuttering on some sounds or words. During attempts at trial treatment, we like to show the client ways of ameliorating the stuttering and often use his/her most feared words as stimuli.

Any assessment of stuttering should also include the client's own perceptions of the magnitude of the problem. The clinician can obtain the stutterer's self-rating of severity in many of the instruments listed in Tables 7.6 and 7.7. In particular, we like to administer the Perceptions of Stuttering Inventory (Woolf 1967). The PSI, as it can be called, is an instrument devised to assess three dimensions of stuttering behavior: struggle, avoidance, and expectancy, as perceived by the person who stutters. It yields a profile that the clinician can then compare to scores obtained by a reference group of stutterers.

Having now discussed the predictive instruments, severity scales, and covert measures typically used in the evaluation of stuttering, let us turn our attention to some general evaluation principles and special considerations for clients of various ages.

Evaluation at the Onset of Stuttering

Experienced clinicians agree that the problem of stuttering is much easier to prevent or manage in children than to treat in chronic adult clients. Indeed, the early detection and management of children's beginning to stutter is one of the most significant contributions a speech clinician can make. The SLP must seek answers for a great many questions: Is the child stuttering? If so, how far has the disturbance progressed? When did it begin? What factors were associated with the onset of the problem? How aware is the child of the speech disturbance? How do listeners attempt to help, and how does this affect the child's efforts? How can the SLP alter the child's environment to prevent the problem from getting worse?

Throughout this book, we have repeatedly suggested that diagnosis and treatment are not separate undertakings. The careful assessment of a client's problem is often therapeutic; only by working with an individual (and his/her parents) for a period of time does the clinician truly come to know the dimensions of the problem. This is particularly true in the management of children beginning to stutter.

In many cases, a physician is the first professional to be consulted by parents. The clinician is wise to enlist the support of local pediatricians in the early identification of children beginning to stutter.

We agree with Wyatt (1969) that the onset of stuttering is a crisis situation in which swift intervention is absolutely essential. In planning for the evaluation, we delineate several objectives that will guide the clinician's efforts:

1. Determine if the child is stuttering (problem–no problem determination).
2. If so, identify to what stage or level of development the disorder has progressed (severity determination).
3. Obtain the parent's perception of the onset and current status of the problem.
4. Sample the child's general level of functioning in regard to auditory, motor, social, articulatory, and cognitive-linguistic abilities.
5. Commence the development of a counseling relationship with the parents.

We have already discussed most of these objectives. Various assessment instruments are available to help the clinician make a differential diagnosis, determine the severity of the speech difficulties, appraise the home situation and parental attitudes, and begin a healthy dialogue with the parents of the child who is beginning to stutter. What remains to be discussed are the ancillary areas that need to be assessed in the young child.

Several authorities recommend assessing the child's rate of speech, as well as the parents' rates (Peters and Guitar 1991; Starkweather, Gottwald, and Halfond 1990). Normative data for children can be found in Pindzola, Jenkins, and Lokken (1989). Speech rate is a basic element of fluency and therefore warrants assessment. The rate at which parents talk may be demanding of fluency in the child.

Speed and coordination of repetitive oral movements may be tested using Fletcher's (1972) norms for diadochokinesis. Also, Riley and Riley (1986) have published the Oral Motor Assessment Scale.

Phonological disorders seem to co-occur frequently with stuttering, as do language delays or disorders (Conture 1990). Various articulation and language tests should be used as part of a thorough fluency evaluation. Information contained in Chapters 4, 5, and 6 certainly pertains. The presence of speech and language disorders concomitant with stuttering will affect the planning of an appropriate treatment program.

Along with these areas of assessment, we routinely screen the oral mechanism, voice, and hearing. We advocate referral for additional testing of cognitive, motoric, and psychological status, as needed, with particular clients.

A Direction for Treatment

Even though it is beyond the scope of this chapter to discuss the myriad of treatment programs available, we do wish to point out to the reader that different philosophies exist regarding the treatment of young persons who stutter, such as those between the ages of two and nine years. In addition, although many preschoolers continue to receive intervention services in clinics and through private practitioners, with the implementation of PL 94–457 more and more are being treated by the public school SLP. School systems serve children ages three to five, and many are responsible for the birth-through-age-two population. Four treatment options may be considered.

In the first option, environmental treatment, the SLP determines that the most prudent course of action is to work through the significant others in the child's life—parents and teachers—to modify the daily environment. The goal is to structure the child's environment to make it more conducive to fluency. The child is not seen for treatment; typically, parents and teachers meet regularly with the clinician to discuss environmental modifications and results. Opting for only environmental treatment is commonly done for the child "at risk" for developing stuttering or for the child beginning to stutter who displays early developed symptoms. Modifying parental and teacher reactions to disfluencies; altering the pace and organization of home and school; and generally educating significant others about fluency, disfluency, and the modeling of good speech habits are beneficial. Reduction in communicative pressures that the child is vulnerable to are a necessary and important aspect of treatment.

A second treatment option is to combine the environmental treatment with direct, but modified, therapy for the child. Sessions may be individual but are often in groups. The treatment is considered modified as it does not focus on specific symptoms of stuttering. Rather, treatment may emphasize the concept of rhythm by having children sing, speak to a rhythm, practice rhymes, use choral speaking, and just generally experience much success in easy, fluent speech. Modified treatment often involves language treatment. The language skills of a child who stutters may be somewhat delayed. The length and complexity of utterances affect the likelihood of even normal speakers' having a disfluency. By shoring up weak language skills, and by systematically controlling the linguistic output of young clients (e.g., sentence length and syntactic complexity), SLPs are able to reduce or eliminate stuttering. Additionally, some SLPs may include in the modified program mention of "smooth" and "bumpy" speech and train the children to identify samples of each. Altering the "bumpy" speech, however, is not done in this form of treatment.

A third option of treatment for the young child who stutters is to combine the environmental approach with direct intervention. The child attends individual or group treatment sessions (depending upon the severity of the problem) with the purpose of modifying specific stuttering symptoms. A variety of therapeutic emphases are possible. The student may be taught a new, fluent way of talking by learning patterns such as "slow speech," "breathy speech," "stretchy speech," the "easy speaking voice," "slow, easy speech," and other similar strategies for fluency. Discussions of feelings and attitudes are often a component of the treatment program for children ready to address personal issues surrounding their speech difficulties.

The fourth option of direct stuttering modification alone expands the details involved in mastering strategies, techniques, or targets for fluency. The absence of co-occurring environmental treatment may be a function of (1) the setting in which services are provided (parents may not be available to participate fully in the intervention program); or (2) the child's stuttering symptoms may have progressed beyond the level where environmental manipulations would be expected to have much effect. In such cases, efforts need to be focused on direct treatments using greater specificity.

Prognosis with Young Children

We are very impressed with the efficacy of treatment for young children who are beginning to stutter. When the clinician can intervene before the child develops fear and avoidance reactions, and if the parents are amenable to counseling, the prognosis for recovery is excellent. There are several factors that the clinician must consider when estimating a client's prospects for recovery:

1. How long has the child been stuttering? The older the child is and the longer his/her exposure to adverse enviromental reactions, the poorer the prognosis.
2. What type and intensity of enviromental reactions has the child been exposed to? In our experience, children who have been slapped or have suffered other forms of physical abuse have the worst problems.
3. Is the child aware of speaking difficulties? The more heedful the child is of speech interruptions, the less positive the prognosis. (This may be argued as evidence of the progression of the disorder; hence the less favorable prognosis.)
4. What type of speech disfluency characteristics are present? The more danger signs present—in particular, cessation of phonation, stoppage of airflow, dysrhythmia, tension, and fear—the poorer the prognosis.
5. How amenable are the parents to counseling? An all-out concerted effort at the home front is ideal, perhaps essential, for amelioration.
6. What is the child's level of intelligence? We have had more limited success with "slow" children.
7. Are there organic or neurotic factors that figure in the onset of stuttering? Chances for recovery are more limited if either is present.

Our clinical success or failure with children who are beginning to stutter is also related to the characteristic pattern of factors present at the onset of stuttering. Apparently, there are several ways of becoming a stutterer (Van Riper 1982; Yairi 1983). We find the model developed by Myers and Wall (1982) useful for synthesizing diagnostic information and making a prognosis about a young disfluent child. The many variables that may be involved in the onset of stuttering are organized into three major categories: physiological, psycholinguistic, and psychosocial (Figure 7.2). Note how the three categories overlap. For example, a child delayed in language development and deficient in motor skills could be particularly suceptible to high parental standards or communication competition with siblings. These same thoughts are amplified by Starkweather, Gottwald, and Halfond (1990) and by Wells (1987).

One question continues to nag clinicians who work with young children. Would the children have gotten better without the clinicians' help, owing simply to the passage of time and some internal recovery potential in the child? Although we cannot answer that question with any authority, we do see that in most instances, the child's recovery from stuttering occurred too swiftly after the initiation of treatment (two weeks to several months) to be attributed to spontaneous

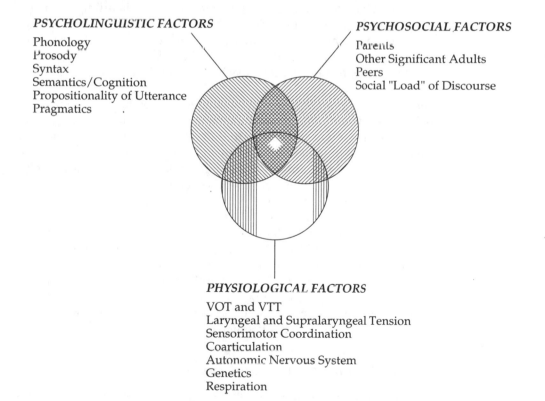

PSYCHOLINGUISTIC FACTORS

Phonology
Prosody
Syntax
Semantics/Cognition
Propositionality of Utterance
Pragmatics

PSYCHOSOCIAL FACTORS

Parents
Other Significant Adults
Peers
Social "Load" of Discourse

PHYSIOLOGICAL FACTORS

VOT and VTT
Laryngeal and Supralaryngeal Tension
Sensorimotor Coordination
Coarticulation
Autonomic Nervous System
Genetics
Respiration

FIGURE 7.2   Factors Influencing Early Childhood Stuttering

recovery. The interested reader may consult the work of Wyatt (1969) for a list of variables contributing to and inhibiting progress and that of Yairi et al. (1996) for insights into unassisted recovery from stuttering.

Evaluation of the School-Aged Student

Elementary Students

Appraising and treating elementary school students who stutter is particularly challenging. This group of children, approximately seven- to twelve-years-old, is no longer beginning to stutter; they are not simply repeating and hesitating. They struggle noticeably when speaking and attempt to avoid or disguise their difficulty; they are frustrated and it is now necessary to deal directly with the stuttering.

The clinician is faced with several thorny problems when planning an examination of a young person who stutters: (1) Young children frequently lack the insight and cooperation necessary to analyze their problem objectively and rationally. (2) Children are reluctant or unable to verbalize their internal feelings freely. (3) The speech clinician is associated in the child's mind with the teaching personnel, who may in some cases be penalizing or disturbing listeners. In addition, the clinician may be identified with authority figures; this tends to undermine a trusting relationship. (4) Last, and perhaps most significant, the child usually has no choice about entering treatment; most likely the student is brought for evaluation by the parents, referred by a teacher, or identified in a screening by a speech clinician.

The clinician may find that these students respond to an honest, straightforward clinical approach. With early elementary school children, we use descriptive language, such as "tensing" or "getting stuck," to inquire about their speaking difficulty, not out of any fear of the word *stuttering,* but simply because the term either doesn't mean much to the child or, in some cases, is too negatively charged. With older elementary school children, we use a frank, direct style. Establish trust and confidence by showing the client that the clincian is competent and *knows* about the problem of stuttering.

The evaluation of a student does not differ greatly in substance from an assessment of an older individual except that with young children, enviromental, parental, and school factors are more important. In order to reveal the range of information generally sought, Figure 7.3 outlines an assessment plan prepared by a diagnostic team composed of a faculty member and graduate students. The plan was compiled for the evaluation of a ten-year-old child referred to a university speech clinic by a public school clinician.

Junior and Senior High School Students

The assessment and treatment of stuttering in older students is even more challenging than with the youngsters. Denial of the problem, lack of cooperation, and lack of motivation seem typical in the teenagers we have seen.

FIGURE 7.3   Assessment Plan for Alan Schlicher

I. **Identifying Information**
   Obtain all the usual information regarding address, grade level, and so on. This can be obtained from Mrs. Hronkin, the referral source, or in the parent interview. Be sure to inquire about living arrangements: Ms. Hronkin mentioned that a parental grandfather may reside with the family, and apparently he is a dominant force in the family (reportedly, he is against Alan receiving speech therapy and insists he overcame stuttering by eating mashed potatoes!).

II. **Description of Stuttering**
   A. *Global description.* What are the salient descriptive features of Alan's stuttering behavior? Is it basically fixative or oscillative? Are there long silent periods of internal struggle, or does he exhibit a more overt pattern?
   B. *Core behaviors.* Make an analysis of the repetitions and prolongations observed—the number of oscillations per unit, tempo, duration, and so forth.
   C. *Tension-struggle features.* Note the occurence and location of any ancillary behaviors.
   D. *Frequency.* This analysis will serve as our baseline for reevaluation of Alan, so we need to be especially precise. Collect data (count repetitions, prolongations, other salient features of his moments of stuttering) on at least three types of speech samples—reading, paraphrasing, and spontaneous speech. We can compute the relative frequency of stutterings per minute, or per total words uttered, by analyzing the videotape later.
   E. *Severity.* We will use the Stuttering Severity Instrument (Riley 1994); this instrument employs the three dimensions of frequency, duration, and physical concomitants and yields a score that can be converted to a percentile. A severity measure like this (particularly when it allows the examiner to score a client on a common scale of 0 to 100) is useful when communicating the results of the evaluation to the parents, teacher, even the child himself.
   F. *Variations in frequency/severity.* Explore with the child and his parents whether his stuttering comes and goes in cycles, which situations or listeners provoke variations in his problem, and whether there are any words or sounds that are particularly difficult. Determine what impact delayed auditory feedback and masking noise have on his speech.
   G. How does the child try to control his stuttering? What techniques has he devised for coping with speech interruptions? How effective are they? Additionally, we need to identify which speech-altering strategies—slowing, easy onset, and so forth—induce fluency. Use Cooper's (1982) Disfluency Descriptor Digest as a checklist to record observations.
   H. Can the child predict when he is about stutter? Ask him if he can; but also have him underline words he thinks he might stutter on as he reads silently a simple passage. Have him read it aloud and determine the degree to which he can accurately predict his stuttering.
   I. What is the client's poststuttering behavior? Does he continue talking, give up, become angry, or cry? Does he appear indifferent?

III. **Attitude Dimension**
   This is the most difficult and least reliable aspect of the evaluation. Some information can be obtained through observation of Alan and his parents and by what they say about the problem. We can also administer several self-inventory scales such as the A-19 Scale developed by Guitar (1977). What is the child's attitude toward treatment? How much does he know about stuttering? Has he been teased at school or home because of his problem?

Continued

FIGURE 7.3   *Continued*

IV. **Case History**

We will want to obtain background information with respect to four basic areas: history of general development (motor, language, social), onset and development of stuttering, medical history, and family history. These areas can be explored in the parent interview.

V. **Present Functioning**

A. *Personality.* Describe the child's personality in general terms (shy, aggressive, and so on) and identify any special features (fears, tics, nail-biting, and the like) that may apply to him. Ascertain his special interests or hobbies.

B. *School.* Obtain information relevant to his academic and social adjustment in school.

C. *Related testing.* Is a psychological or medical referral indicated? Perform screening evaluations on the child's motor behavior, hearing, and language ability. The latter is particularly important, as there is some evidence that children who stutter may have a language disability. Plan to use the testing format suggested by Riley and Riley (1986). They advocate evaluating the following skills:

1. Attending behavior: Is the child distractible? Does he perseverate?
2. Auditory processing: Does he delay in responding to tasks? Does he request repetitions of instructions?
3. Sentence formulation: Is there any evidence of a breakdown in word order?
4. Oral motor: What is the child's diadochokinetic rates for /p/, /k/, and /t/? Is there any evidence of articulatory imprecision?

D. *Diagnostic session.* How did the child behave during the diagnostic session? What could be discerned about his level of motivation? How did he respond when put under communicative stress? How did he respond to trial therapy?

The assessment outline does not differ much from the example shown for Alan Schlicher. The process, however, is very adultlike; environmental and parental factors are downplayed.

Direction for Treatment

The treatment of stuttering among some older children, adolescents, and adults is of the direct type. Obviously, programs differ in complexities and emphases for these disparate age groups. As negative feelings and attitudes develop late in the evolution of stuttering, treatment for the older student often involves explorations into these psychological topics. The emotional crisis of stuttering escalates during the teenage years when social interactions become so critical. (Students may benefit from reading, *Do You Stutter: A Guide for Teens,* published by the Stuttering Foundation of America.) Physiological modifications of speech are often components in adolescent and adult fluency programs. Physiological targets may include breath, voice onset, and rate, as well as a host of others. Computerized instrumentation may help in the training of these speech targets. Much practice is necessary to habituate new speaking patterns, and support from family, friends, and school personnel can be critical to success.

Prognosis

What factors are crucial for improvement with students? What variables should the clinician consider when making a prognosis? We believe that the most significant improvement in treatment is noted in cases with the following operative factors:

1. No prior record of unsuccessful treatment (An absence of treatment seems more conducive to success than a history of therapeutic failure.)
2. Cooperative parents, willing to participate meaningfully in a program of counseling
3. More severe stuttering pattern (Mild stutterers typically show little improvement.)
4. A predominantly clonic stuttering pattern featuring struggle and escape (Students adept at avoidance generally have more difficulty.)
5. Cooperative teachers and other school personnel
6. No other significant problems (reading difficulty, a scholastic problem independent of stuttering, and so on)
7. Other available resources (expertise in scouting, athletics, music)
8. A schedule of intensive therapy (at least three, preferably four, contacts a week)

Assessment of the Adult Who Stutters

The disorder is fully developed in the adult client: Speech interruptions are more complex and characteristically compulsive; fears and apprehensions become chronic; avoidance, disguise, and negative attitudes hamper and distort the individual's relationships with others. At this stage, a speech breakdown is not simply a response, it is also a stimulus—the problem has become cyclic and self-reinforcing. Clinicians agree that the treatment of stuttering at this advanced stage is complicated—but far from impossible. There is a bewildering array of treatment approaches (and indices of their successes); we, however, will not attempt to summarize them here.

Prognosis

Making a prognosis about success and failure in stuttering is an inexact science. Recent research efforts have tried to delineate some factors that may be involved in determining successful outcomes. The reader is referred to the works of Boberg, Howie, and Woods (1979), Guitar (1976), and Perkins (1983). We present an incomplete and heuristic list of factors that help in making prognoses. The items are presented in random order, for at present we have no data that would allow us to assign weight to them.

1. *Severity.* Paradoxically, persons with more severe stuttering, other factors being equal, seem to make better progress than do milder cases.

2. *Motivation and Attitude.* Motivation to change is, of course, a most significant variable in all intervention programs. The better the client's pretreatment attitude, the more successful the outcome of treatment is likely to be.

3. *Timing.* A client's motivation for treatment is often related to crucial life experiences. Persons who have reached a critical stage and feel blocked by their disordered speech, barred from job advancement, education, or marriage, and who voluntarily seek treatment have a more favorable prognosis.

4. *Age.* Adolescents, particularly between the ages of thirteen and sixteen, are especially resistant to treatment. Similarly, clients over forty tend to do poorly in treatment.

5. *Sex.* Women seem to be more difficult to treat than men.

6. *Nonstuttered Speech.* The more well integrated the client's nonstuttered speech is, in terms of prosody, the better the prognosis.

7. *Type of Stuttering.* Those with predominantly repetitive stuttering make more rapid progress than do those with predominantly fixative disfluencies; clients who feature escape reactions are easier to work with than chronic avoiders. Interiorized stutterers—especially those manifesting laryngeal blocking—are very resistant to treatment.

8. *Concomitant Problems.* Clients presenting with organic complications (e.g., sensory, intellectual, or motor impairments) or psychological symptoms require more prolonged treatment and do less well than clients without concomitant problems.

9. *Prior Treatment and Intensive Treatment.* Clients with a history of therapeutic failure have a poor prognosis. Token treatment may be worse than no treatment at all. When intensive treatment (minimum daily contact of at least one hour) is available and the client can participate in a comprehensive program, the prospects for recovery are more favorable.

Bibliography

Adams, M. (1977). "A Clinical Strategy for Differentiating the Normally Nonfluent Child and the Incipient Stutterer." *Journal of Fluency Disorders* 2:141–148.

Ammons, R., and Johnson, W. (1944). "Studies in the Psychology of Stuttering." *Journal of Speech Disorders* 9:39–49.

Anderson, B. (1976). "An Analysis of the Relationship of Age and Sex to Type and Frequency of Disfluencies in Lower Socioeconomic Preschool Black Children." *Dissertation Abstracts International* 7:75–81.

Andrews, G., and Cutler, J. (1974). "Stuttering Therapy: The Relation between Changes in Symptom Level and Attitudes." *Journal of Speech and Hearing Disorders* 39:312–319.

Andrews, G., and Harris, M. (1964). *The Syndrome of Stuttering.* Clinics in Developmental Medicine No. 17. London: William Heinemann.

Bakker, K., and Riley, G. (1997). *Computerized Scoring of Stuttering Severity.* Austin: TX, Pro-Ed.

Bloodstein, O. (1995). *A Handbook on Stuttering.* Chicago: National Easter Seal Society.

Boberg, E., Howie, P., and Woods, L. (1979). "Maintenance of Fluency: A Review." *Journal of Fluency Disorders* 4:93–116.

Brady, W. A., and Hall, D. E. (1976). "The Prevalence of Stuttering among School-Age Children." *Language Speech Hearing Services in Schools* 7:75–81.

Brown, C., and Cullinan, W. (1981). "Word-Retrieval Difficulty and Disfluent Speech in Adult Anomic Speakers." *Journal of Speech and Hearing Research* 24:358–365.

Brutten, E., and Dunham, S. (1989). "The Communication Attitude Test: A Normative Study of Grade School Children." *Journal of Fluency Disorders* 14:371–377.

Brutten, E. J., and Miller, R. (1988). "The Disfluencies of Normally Fluent Black First Graders." *Journal of Fluency Disorders* 13:291–299.

Brutten, E., and Shoemaker, D. (1974). *The Southern Illinois Behavior Check List.* Carbondale, IL: Southern Illinois University.

Canter, G. J. (1971). "Observations on Neurogenic Stuttering: A Contribution to Differential Diagnosis." *British Journal of Disorders of Communication* 6:139–143.

Conrad, C. (1992). "Fluency in Multicultural Populations." In *Communication Disorders in Multicultural Populations,* ed. L. Cole and V. Deal (Rockville, MD: ASHA).

Conture, E. G. (1990). *Stuttering* (2nd ed.). Englewood Cliffs, NJ: Prentice-Hall.

Cooper, E. B. (1973). "The Development of a Stuttering Chronicity Prediction Checklist: A Preliminary Report." *Journal of Speech and Hearing Disorders* 38:215–223.

Cooper, E. B. (1976). *Personalized Fluency Control Therapy.* Allen, TX: DLM/Teaching Resources.

Cooper, E. B. (1979). *Understanding Stuttering: Information for Parents.* Chicago: National Easter Seal Society.

Cooper, E. B. (1982). "A Disfluency Descriptor for Clinical Use." *Journal of Fluency Disorders* 7: 355–358.

Cooper, E. B. and Cooper, C. (1985). *Personalized Fluency Control Therapy—Revised.* Allen, TX: DLM/Teaching Resources.

Culatta, R., and Goldberg, S. A. (1995). *Stuttering Therapy: An Intergrated Approach to Theory and Practice.* Needham Heights, MA: Allyn and Bacon.

Culp, D. M. (1984). "The Preschool Fluency Development Program: Assessment and Treatment." In *Contemporary Approaches in Stuttering Therapy,* ed. M. Peins (Boston, MA: Little, Brown).

Daly, D. A. (1986). "The Clutterer." In *The Atypical Stutterer: Principles and Practices of Rehabilitation,* ed. K. O. St. Louis (Orlando, FL: Academic Press).

Deal, J. (1982). "Sudden Onset of Stuttering: A Case Report." *Journal of Speech and Hearing Disorders* 47:301–304.

DeFusco, E., and Menken, M. (1979). "Symptomatic Cluttering in Adults." *Brain and Language* 8:25–33.

Donnan, G. A. (1979). "Stuttering as a Manifestation of Stroke." *Medical Journal of Australia* 1: 44–45.

Douglass, E., and Quarrington, B. (1952). "The Differentiation of Interiorized and Exteriorized Secondary Stuttering." *Journal of Speech and Hearing Disorders* 17:377–385.

Dykes, R. L. (1995). "Prevalence of Stuttering among African-American School-Age Children in the South: A Survey of Speech-Language Pathologists' Caseloads." Unpublished master's thesis, Auburn University, AL.

Emerick, L. (1983). *With Slow and Halting Tongue.* Danville, IL: Interstate Printers and Publishers.

Erickson, R. (1969). "Assessing Communication Attitudes among Stutterers." *Journal of Speech and Hearing Research* 12:711–724.

Fantry, L. (1990). "AIDS-Related Acquired Stuttering." *Quo Vadis* 2, no. 2:6.

Fletcher, S. (1972). "Time-by-Count Measurement of Diadochokinetic Syllable Rate." *Journal of Speech and Hearing Research* 15:763–770.

Fransella, F. (1972). *Personal Change and Reconstruction.* London: Academic Press.

Gavis, L. (1946). "Bombing Mission No. 15." *Journal of Abnormal and Social Psychology* 41:189–198.

Gillespie, S. K., and Cooper, E. B. (1973). "Prevalence of Speech Problems in Junior and Senior High School." *Journal of Speech and Hearing Research* 16:739–743.

Glasner, P. J. (1949). "Personality Characteristics and Emotional Problems in Stutterers under Age Five." *Journal of Speech and Hearing Disorders* 14:135–138.

Goldberg, S. A. (1981). *Behavioral Cognitive Stuttering Therapy.* Tigard, OR: C.C. Publications.

Goldman, R. (1967). "Cultural Influences on the Sex Ratio in the Incidence of Stuttering." *American Anthropologist* 69:78–81.

Gordon, P., and Luper, H. (1992). "The Early Identification of Beginning Stuttering, I: Protocols." *American Journal of Speech-Language Pathology* 1:43–53.

Grinker, R., and Spiegal, J. (1945). *War Neuroses.* Philadelphia, PA: Blakiston.

Guitar, B. (1976). "Pretreatment Factors Associated with the Outcome of Stuttering Therapy." *Journal of Speech and Hearing Research* 19:590–600.

Guitar, B., and Grims, S. (1977). "Developing a Scale to Assess Communication Attitudes in Children Who Stutter." Paper presented at the convention of the American Speech-Language-Hearing Association, Atlanta, GA.

Helms, N. A., Butler, R. B., and Canter, G. J. (1980). "Neurogenic Acquired Stuttering." *Journal of Fluency Disorders* 5:269–279.

Howard County (MD) Public School System (1985). "Communication Rating Scales, Service Delivery Model, and Dismissal Criteria for Speech-Language Services." Paper presented at the convention of the American Speech-Language-Hearing Association, Washington, DC.

Irvine, T., and Reis, R. (1980). "Cluttering as a Complex of Learning Disabilities." *Language, Speech and Hearing Services in Schools* 11:3–14.

Johnson, W. (1961). *Stuttering and What You Can Do About It.* Mineapolis: University of Minnesota Press.

Johnson, W., Darley, F., and Spriestersbach, D. (1963). *Diagnostic Methods in Speech Pathology.* New York: Harper and Row.

Kent, R., and LaPointe, L. (1982). "Acoustic Properties of Pathological Reiterative Utterances: A Case Study of Palilalia." *Journal of Speech and Hearing Research* 25:95–99.

Koller, W. (1983). "Disfluency (Stuttering) in Extrapyramidal Disease." *Archives of Neurology* 40:175–177.

Lanyon, R. I. (1967). "The Measurement of Stuttering Severity." *Journal of Speech and Hearing Research* 10:836–843.

LaPoint, L., and Horner, J. (1981). "Palilalia: A Descriptive Study of Pathological Reiterative Utterances." *Journal of Speech and Hearing Disorders* 46:34–38.

Leavitt, R. R. (1974). *The Puerto Ricans: Cultural Change and Language Deviance.* Tucson, AZ: University of Arizona Press.

LeBrun, Y., Retif, J., and Kaiser, G. (1983). "Acquired Stuttering as a Forerunner of Motor Neuron Disease." *Journal of Fluency Disorders* 8:161–167.

Leeper, L., Culatta, R., Pindzola, R., and Duchin-Ceska, S. (1990). "Elderly Speakers' Rate/Fluency: What We Know, What It Means." Paper presented at the convention of the American Speech-Language-Hearing Association, Seattle, WA.

Leith, W., and Mims, H. (1975). "Cultural Influences in the Development and Treatment of Stuttering: A Preliminary Report." *Journal of Speech and Hearing Disorders* 40:459–466.

Luper, H. L., and Mulder, R. L. (1966). *Stuttering Therapy for Children.* Englewood Cliffs, NJ: Prentice-Hall.

Madison, D., Baehr, E. T., Bazell, M., Hartman, R. W., Mahurkas, S. D., and Dunea, G. (1977). "Communicative and Cognitive Deterioration in Dialysis Dementia: Two Case Studies." *Journal of Speech and Hearing Disorders* 42:238–243.

Manning, W. H., and Monte, K. L. (1981). "Fluency Breaks in Older Speakers: Implications for a Model of Stuttering Throughout the Life Cycle." *Journal of Fluency Disorders* 6:35–48.

Martin, R. R., and Lindamood, L. P. (1986). "Stuttering and Spontaneous Recovery: Implications for the Speech-Language Pathologist." *Language, Speech, and Hearing Services in Schools* 17:207–218.

Metraux, R. (1950). "Speech Profiles of the Preschool Child 18 to 54 Months." *Journal of Speech Disorders* 15:37–53.

Montes, J., and Erickson, J. G. (1990). "Bilingual Stuttering: Exploring a Diagnostic Dilemma." *Ethnotes* 1:14–15.

Morgenstern, J. J. (1956). "Socioeconomic Factors in Stuttering." *Journal of Speech and Hearing Disorders* 21:25–33.

Myers, F., and Wall, M. (1982). "Toward an Integrated Approach to Early Childhood Stuttering." *Journal of Fluency Disorders* 7:47–54.

Peins, M., McGough, W. E., and Lee, B. S. (1984). "Double Tape Recorder Therapy for Stutterers." In *Contemporary Approaches in Stuttering Therapy*, ed. M. Peins (Boston: Little, Brown).

Perkins, W. H. (1971). *Speech Pathology: An Applied Behavioral Science.* St. Louis, MO: Mosby.

Perkins, W. H. (1983). "Learning from Negative Outcomes in Stuttering Therapy, II: An Epiphany of Failures." *Journal of Fluency Disorders* 8: 155–160.

Peters, T. J., and Guitar, B. (1991). *Stuttering: An Integrated Approach to Its Nature and Treatment.* Baltimore, MD: Williams and Wilkins.

Pindzola, R. H. (1986). "A Description of Some Selected Stuttering Instruments." *Journal of Childhood Communication Disorders* 9:183–200.

Pindzola, R. H. (1988). *Stuttering Intervention Program: Age 3 to Grade 3.* Austin, TX: Pro-Ed.

Pindzola, R. H. (1990). "Disfluency Characteristics of Aged, Normal-Speaking Black and White Males. *Journal of Fluency Disorders* 15, no. 4: 235–243.

Pindzola, R. H. (1990). "Disfluency Characteristics of Aged, Normal-Speaking Black and White Males." *Journal of Fluency Disorders* 15:235–243.

Pindzola, R. H., Jenkins, M., and Lokken, K. (1989). "Speaking Rates of Young Children." *Language, Speech and Hearing Services in Schools* 20: 133–138.

Pindzola, R. H., and White, D. (1986). "A Protocol for Differentiating the Incipient Stutterer." *Language, Speech and Hearing Services in Schools* 17:2–15.

Powell, H. (1967). "Child-Rearing Practices Reported for Young Male Negro Stutterers and Nonstutterers in Two South Carolina School Districts." *Dissertation Abstracts International* 28, no. 3A:1149–1150.

Ragsdale, J., and Ashby, J. (1982). "Speech-Language Pathologists' Connotation of Stuttering." *Journal of Speech and Hearing Research* 25:78–80.

Ratusnik, D. L., Kirilluk, E., and Ratusnik, C. M. (1979). "Relationship among Race, Social Status, and Sex of Preschoolers' Normal Disfluencies: A Cross-Cultural Investigation." *Language, Speech, and Hearing Services in Schools* 10:171–177.

Riley, G. (1972). "A Stuttering Severity Instrument for Children and Adults." *Journal of Speech and Hearing Disorders* 37:314–322.

Riley, G. (1981). *Stuttering Prediction Instrument for Young Children.* Tigard, OR: C. C. Publications.

Riley, G. (1994). *Stuttering Severity Instrument for Children and Adults.* Tigard, OR: C. C. Publications.

Riley, G., and Riley, J. (1986). *Oral Motor Assessment and Treatment.* Tigard, OR: C. C. Publications.

Robinson, F. B. (1966). *What Parents and Teachers Should Know about Children Who Stutter.* Washington, DC: National Association of Hearing and Speech Agencies.

Robinson, T. L., and Crowe, T. A. (1987). "A Comparative Study of Speech Disfluencies in Nonstuttering Black and White College Athletes." *Journal of Fluency Disorders* 12:147–156.

Robinson, T. L., and Davis, J. G. (1992). "Speech Fluency Skills in African American Preschoolers during Narative Discourse." Paper presented at the annual convention of the American Speech-Language-Hearing Association, San Antonio, TX.

Rosenbek, J., Messert, B., Collins, M., and Wertz, R. (1978). "Stuttering Following Brain Damage." *Brain and Language* 6:82–96.

Ryan, B. (1974). *Programmed Therapy for Stuttering in Children and Adults.* Springfield, IL: Charles C. Thomas.

Satcher, D. (1986). "Research Needs for Minority Populations." In *Concerns for Minority Groups in Communication Disorders,* ed. F. H. Bess, B. S. Clark, and H. R. Mitchell (Rockville, MD: ASHA Reports 16).

Shames, G. H. (1989). "Stuttering: An RFP for a Cultural Perspective." *Journal of Fluency Disorders* 14:67–77.

Shames, G. H., and Egolf, D. (1976). *Operant Conditioning and the Management of Stuttering.* Englewood Cliffs, NJ: Prentice-Hall.

Shine, R. E. (1980). *Systematic Fluency Training for Children.* Austin, TX: Pro-Ed.

Shumak, I. (1955). "A Speech Situation Rating Sheet for Stutterers." In *Stuttering in Children and Adults,* ed. W. Johnson (Mineapolis: University of Minnesota Press).

Silverman, F. (1980). "Stuttering Problem Profile: A Task That Assists Both Client and Clinician in Defining Therapy Goals." *Journal of Speech and Hearing Disorders* 45:119–123.

Silverman, F., and Williams, D. (1972). "Prediction of Stuttering by School-Age Stutterers." *Journal of Speech and Hearing Research* 15:189–193.

Starkweather, C. W., Gottwald, S. R., and Halfond, M. M. (1990). *Stuttering Prevention: A Clinical Method.* Englewood Cliffs, NJ: Prentice Hall.

St. Louis, K., and Lass, N. (1981). "A Survey of Communication Disorder Students' Attitudes toward Stuttering." *Journal of Fluency Disorders* 6:49–79.

Stocker, B. (1980). *The Stocker Probe Technique.* Austin, TX: Pro-Ed.

Tanner, D. (1987). *Parental Diagnostic Questionnaire* (rev.). Austin, TX: Pro-Ed.

Tanner, D. (1990). *Assessment of Stuttering Behaviors.* Oceanside, CA: Academic Communication Associations.

Thompson, J. (1983). *Assessment of Fluency in School-Age Children.* Austin, TX: Pro-Ed.

Tippett, D. C., and Siebens, A. A. (1991). "Distinguishing Psychogenic from Neurogenic Dysfluency When Neurologic and Psychologic Factors Coexist." *Journal of Fluency Disorders* 16:3–12.

Turnbaugh, K., Guitar, B., and Hoffman, P. (1979). "Speech Clinicians' Attribution of Personality Traits as a Function of Stuttering Severity." *Journal of Speech and Hearing Research* 22:37–45.

Turnbaugh, K., Guitar, B., and Hoffman, P. (1981). "The Attribution of Personality Traits: The Stutterer and Nonstutterer." *Journal of Speech and Hearing Research* 24:288–291.

Van Riper, C. (1982). *The Nature of Stuttering* (2nd ed.). Englewood Cliffs, NJ: Prentice Hall.

Walker, V. G., Hardiman, C. J., Hedrick, D. L., and Holbrook, A. (1981). "Speech and Language Characteristics of an Aging Population." In *Speech and Language: Advances in Basic Research and Practice*, ed. N. Lass (New York: Academic Press).

Walle, E. (1974). *The Prevention of Stuttering, I: Identifying Danger Signs* (a film). Memphis, TN: Speech Foundation of America.

Walle, E. (1975). *The Prevention of Stuttering, II: Parent Counseling and Elimination of the Problem* (a film). Memphis, TN: Speech Foundation of America.

Walle, E. (1977). *The Prevention of Stuttering, III: SSStuttering and Your Child. Is It Me? Is It You?* (a film). Memphis, TN: Speech Foundation of America.

Weiner, A. (1981). "A Case of Adult Onset of Stuttering." *Journal of Fluency Disorders* 6:181–186.

Weiner, A. (1984). "Vocal Control Therapy for Stutterers." In *Contemporary Approaches in Stuttering Therapy*, ed. M. Peins (Boston, MA: Little, Brown).

Weiss, D. A. (1964). *Cluttering.* Englewood Cliffs, NJ: Prentice Hall.

Weiss, D. A. (1968). "Cluttering: Central Language Imbalance." *Pediatric Clinics of North America* 15:705–720.

Wells, G. B. (1987). *Stuttering Treatment: A Comprehensive Clinical Guide.* Englewood Cliffs, NJ: Prentice Hall.

Wingate, M. E. (1976). *Stuttering Theory and Treatment.* New York: Irvington.

Woolf, G. (1967). "The Assessment of Stuttering as Struggle, Avoidance, and Expectancy." *British Journal of Disorders of Communication* 2: 158–171.

Wyatt, E. (1969). *Language Learning and Disorders of Communication in Children.* New York: Free Press.

Yairi, E. (1981). "Disfluencies of Normally Speaking Two-Year-Old Children." *Journal of Speech and Hearing Research* 24:490–495.

Yairi, E. (1983). "The Onset of Stuttering in Two- and Three-Year-Old Children: A Preliminary Report." *Journal of Speech and Hearing Disorders* 48:171–177.

Yairi, E., Ambrose, N., Paden, E., and Throneburg, R. (1996). "Predictive Factors of Persistence and Recovery: Pathways of Childhood Stuttering." *Journal of Communication Disorders* 29:51–77.

Yairi, E., and Clifton, N. F. (1972). "Disfluent Speech Behavior of Preschool Children, High School Seniors, and Geriatric Persons." *Journal of Speech and Hearing Research* 15:714–719.

Yairi, E., and Lewis, B. (1984). "Disfluencies at the Onset of Stuttering." *Journal of Speech and Hearing Research* 27:155–159.

Young, M. (1975). "Onset, Prevalence, and Recovery from Stuttering." *Journal of Speech and Hearing Disorders* 40, no. 1:49–58.

Zwitman, D. (1978). *The Disfluent Child.* Baltimore, MD: University Park Press.

Chapter 8

Assessment of Aphasia and Adult Language Disorders

When an adult suddenly loses the easy use of language, it is a devastating experience for the individual and for the family. Aphasia, and other adult language disorders, affect that which makes us uniquely human—our ability to communicate with each other by a system of language symbols.

The Nature of Aphasia

Aphasia is the most common disorder of communication resulting from brain injury. Damage occurs in the hemisphere of the brain that is dominant for language; for most of us, this is the left hemisphere. An adult with aphasia has a basic interference with *comprehension* and *use* of language in its many forms. More specifically, aphasia is a syndrome of language deficits resulting from destruction of cortical tissue and is characterized by one or more of the following symptoms:

1. Disturbance in receiving and decoding symbolic materials via auditory, visual, or tactile channels (Although the individual can still hear and see, there is difficulty deciphering the learned associations of messages.)
2. Disturbance in central processes of meaning, word selection, and message formulation
3. Disturbance in expressing symbolic materials by means of speech, writing, or gesture

Aphasia may result from trauma, brain tumors, certain inflammatory processes, and degenerative diseases. The vast majority of aphasias, however, are the consequence of a cerebrovascular accident (CVA), commonly called stroke or brain attack.

The cerebrovascular accident is a relatively common illness that affects approximately a half million persons each year. In the United States, CVA now stands as the third leading cause of death (outdistanced only by heart disease and cancer). No one knows precisely how many surviving stroke victims are left with language impairment; estimates suggest at least a quarter of the victims present some degree of aphasia that warrants treatment.

Neurological disease and accident can affect anyone, regardless of ethnicity. Public health demographics, however, show that neurological impairments affect individuals from the multicultural community to a disproportionate extent (Reyes 1995; Wallace 1993). Cerebrovascular accident is the leading cause of neurological impairment among African Americans, Hispanics and certain Asian/Pacific Americans. Primary risk factors for CVA in these groups include hypertension (excerbated by underutilization of health care services and high cholesterol diets), arteriosclerosis (accentuated by diets high in fats and salt), sickle cell anemia (reduced red blood cells affects oxygen-carrying capacity, and sickle-shaped cells fail to pass through smallest blood vessels in the brain), and substance abuse (e.g., crack causes vasoconstriction that may lead to stroke).

Etiology can influence the onset, progress, and type of aphasia symptoms. According to Rosenbek, LaPointe, and Wertz (1989), the onset of symptoms is likely to be insidious when caused by tumor, and abrupt when due to CVA. They go on to state that improvement is more likely if the aphasia is caused by a CVA than by a tumor, and patients with tumors may have wide differences in abilities across modalities (reading, writing, listening, speaking). Such large differences are less likely from a CVA. Aphasia resulting from trauma is often accompanied by a greater variety of cognitive deficits, but it shows a faster recovery than does aphasia resulting from CVA.

There are a host of other disorders that may resemble aphasia and have brain damage as their basis. These include the language of confusion, language of intellectual deterioration (dementia), communication deficit subsequent to a nondominant lesion (usually right hemisphere damage), language associated with psychosis, and motor speech disorders. These disorders will be discussed later in this chapter as part of the differential diagnosis process.

The severity of aphasia can vary greatly, from minimal, temporary language dysfunction to almost total and permanent inability to use and comprehend language. It is important to remember that the impoverishment of language observed in aphasia is *not* due to loss of mental capacity, impairment of sensory organs, or paralysis of the speech apparatus. These problems, however, can co-occur with aphasia, making differential diagnosis important.

Classifying a patient as to the *type* of aphasia displayed can be an important feature of diagnosis and treatment planning. Many labels and classification systems have been put forth through the years for this purpose. Three methods are currently in wide use: (1) fluent-nonfluent dichotomy, which is based on the patient's length of utterance; (2) the "Boston" classification system by Goodglass and Kaplan (1983); and (3) the Western Aphasia Battery (WAB) taxonomy by Kertesz (1979, 1980). The Boston and WAB systems are quite similar and use fluency, auditory comprehension, repetition, and naming abilities for arriving at a diagnostic label. Table 8.1 lists characteristics of each of the major types of aphasia (Fitch-West 1984; Goodglass and Kaplan 1983).

Although there is some controversy as to our ability to localize language functions in the brain, there is fairly good agreement with site of lesion information

TABLE 8.1   Neurolinguistic Features of the Major Types of Aphasia

Broca's Aphasia

Impaired fluency; limited verbal output
Relatively good auditory comprehension
Impaired articulatory agility
Stereotyped grammar
Telegraphic and agrammatic (especially reduced use of articles, prepositions, auxiliaries, copulas, and derivational endings)
Prosodic alterations

Transcortical Motor Aphasia

Preserved ability to repeat
Nonfluent
Some auditory comprehension impairment, similar to Broca's aphasia
Superior naming ability compared to spontaneous speech

Global Aphasia

Severe loss of all receptive modalities
Severe loss of all expressive modalities
Almost totally absent speech
Stereotypic utterances (perhaps with normal melody and intonation)

Wernicke's Aphasia

Fluent; copious verbal output
Impaired auditory comprehension (often severe)
Frequent paraphasias (especially semantic types)
Neologisms and jargon, if severe
Normal articulatory agility
Normal prosody
Normal or supranormal phrase length
Full range of grammatical forms
Preserved syntax
Impaired naming and repetition abilities

Transcortical Sensory Aphasia

Preserved ability to repeat
Conversation resembles symptoms of Wernicke's aphasia
Extreme difficulty with nouns
Excessive paraphasias
Impaired auditory comprehension, resembling Wernicke's

Continued

TABLE 8.1   *Continued*

Conduction Aphasia

Poor repetition ability
Fluent speech; good articulation and phrase length
Frequent paraphasias (especially literal types)
Some auditory comprehension impairment
Acute awareness of errors

Anomic Aphasia

Severe word-finding deficits
Frequent circumlocutions
Minimal paraphasic errors
Fluent speech; good articulation and phrase length
Appropriate grammatical forms
Good auditory comprehension

and the language characteristics seen in individual patients. Primary language areas of the left hemisphere and associated aphasias are shown in Figure 8.1. As can be seen, anterior lesions generally produce nonfluent aphasia, such as Broca's and transcortical motor aphasias. Posterior lesions are associated with the fluent aphasias, such as Wernicke's, conduction, and transcortical sensory aphasias.

Site of lesion (anatomical areas affected) and type of lesion (tumor, CVA, and so forth) can usually be determined by modern methods of brain imaging such as computerized tomography (CT), positron emission tomography (PET), and magnetic resonance imaging (MRI). An example of a CT scan is shown in Figure 8.2. These methods have contributed greatly to aphasiology and are reviewed by Metter and Hanson (1985). Although such anatomical evidence supplied by the neuro-

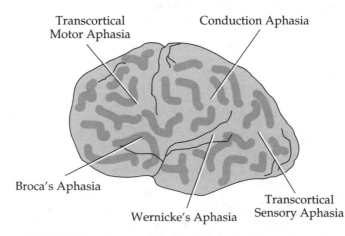

FIGURE 8.1   Areas of the Left Hemisphere Associated with Some of the Types of Aphasia

FIGURE 8.2   **Computed Tomographic (CT) Scan (with x-ray pictures taken from many angles and computerized) of a Patient with Broca's Aphasia Showing a Lesion in the Left Hemisphere)**

(Photograph courtesy of D. Shah, M.D., Hines V.A. Hospital.)

radiologist is diagnostically valuable, the speech-language pathologist may be wise to focus on carefully describing what the individual can and cannot do with respect to language. The clinician must first and foremost delineate the patient's ability to talk, listen, read, and write.

In our zeal to identify the neurolinguistic dimensions of aphasia, it is possible to forget that brain injury is a grave health problem. The individual has suffered a major life crisis that has profound medical, psychological, and social consequences. In addition to the language impairment, the patient may present paralysis or paresis of the extremities (generally the right side, sometimes including the face), sensory abnormalities, and behavioral disturbances. There seems to be little,

if any, relationship between these difficulties and the extent of the language impairment. Above all, the clinician must remember that aphasia is both a personal
catastrophe and a family crisis, as Buck (1968) so eloquently points out.

Case History

It is wise for SLPs to remember that they work with *persons* who have aphasia, not
aphasia. Language treatment for an adult with aphasia has to be very personalized. Therefore, SLPs need to know as much as possible about their clients when
planning a rehabilitation program. What sort of people were the clients before the
strokes? How did they meet their problems? What educational levels were achieved?
What were their occupations? Their avocations? What changes in behaviors, if any,
have occurred following the brain injuries? The style, pace, and content of treatment will be based on the answers to these and many other questions.

Unfortunately, the aphasic patient is often in no position to provide the kind of
detailed information we seek. In some instances, official records (educational tests,
military records) and personal documents (diaries, letters) are helpful. Usually, however, we must rely on the accuracy and veracity of informants who are familiar
with the patient. The most common method of assembling information about the
language-impaired individual is a case history form that is filled out by a spouse or
other close relative. Sample questions from a typical case history form are listed in
Table 8.2. Ideally, the clinician also interviews the respondent to clarify any ambi-
guities in the written information and to permit additional questioning. Keep in
mind, however, that a long-term marriage partner typically sees the patient as less
impaired than objective language testing may show (Helmick, Watamori, and
Palmer 1976). On the contrary, Holland (1977) points out that acontextual tests of
language do not measure communication and that the client may, in fact, perform
better in a "real" setting.

In discussing neurogenic communication disorders in Hispanic-Americans,
Reyes (1995) notes that the case history must be expanded to include information regarding each of the patient's languages. Reyes recommends collecting the following
additional case history information for optimal case planning and management:

1. Languages spoken in the home, community, and in school during childhood
   and premorbidly
2. Degree of speaking, reading, and writing proficiency in each language premorbidly
3. Frequency and type of code switching premorbidly (i.e., alternating use of two
   languages at the word, phrase, clause, or sentence level)
4. Language in which television, movies, radio, and newspapers were most often
   received premorbidly
5. Proficiency of significant others in each language (spouse, children, parents,
   siblings)
6. Attitudes of self and of significant family members toward bilingualism

TABLE 8.2   Sample Questionnaire Topics for a Case History

Personal

Marital status
Name and occupation of spouse
Names and locations of children
Information about grandchildren
Amount of education
Occupation
Current employment status (retired?)
Hobbies and special interests
Preferences in reading material, television entertainment, and use
   of writing
Preferred hand
Native language, knowledge of others
Description of personality
Description of involvement in group activities (e.g. bowling leagues,
   church fellowships)
Description of any changes in mood, personality, ability to care for
   self, and the like, since the injury

Medical

Date of injury
Cause of injury (accident, stroke, disease)
Length of unconsciousness, if any
Description of paralysis, if any
Complaints of dizziness, faintness, headaches if any
Description of any visual or hearing problems
Description of any other problems, illnesses, or injuries

Communicative

Description of the patient's speech at the onset of the problem
Description of how the speech has changed
Check the appropriate column as it applies to the patient *now:*

Can	Cannot	
___	___	indicate meaning by gesture.
___	___	repeat words spoken by others.
___	___	use one or a few words over and over.
___	___	use swear words (often).
___	___	use some words spontaneously.
___	___	say short phrases.
___	___	say short sentences.
___	___	follow requests and understand directions.
___	___	follow radio or television speech.
___	___	read signs with understanding.
___	___	read newspapers, magazines.
___	___	tell time.
___	___	write name without assistance.
___	___	write sentences, letters.
___	___	do simple arithmetic.
___	___	handle money, make change.

The interview of a family member also allows the SLP to learn something of the family dynamics that may impact on treatment outcome. There are many difficulties with which the family must cope—often, unfortunately, without professional guidance (Derman and Manaster 1967; Porter and Dabul 1977). We may want to consider the following: In terms of life cycle, at what stage is the family? Are there young or adolescent children? Is it a middle-aged couple, now alone and with leisure and peak earning power? What premorbid marital problems existed? Will they be exacerbated or will the family unit draw more closely together to meet the threat? Does the spouse have health problems? How does the family handle the fear of recurring strokes? Are there financial difficulties? Is there any guilt? How are they coping with the communication impairment? What are their impressions of the physical changes?

As we conduct the interview, it is wise to remember that relatives need information, reassurance, and an outlet for frustration (Derman and Manaster 1967). Thus, there is only an imaginary line between case history interviewing and the start of family counseling.

In addition to the case history, the SLP may wish to prepare an index that reflects the severity of the patient's total disability. The SLP can choose from several published scales, among them the Maryland Disability Index, the Communication Status Chart (Wisconsin Division of Health 1966), the Pulses Profile and Barthel Index (Granger and Albrecht 1979), the Functional Performance Assessment (Harvey and Jellinek 1983), and the Functional Life Scale (Sarno and Sarno 1973). We prefer the latter device because it provides a quantitative measure of the individual's ability to participate in all phases of daily activity—in the home, outside the home, and in social interaction. It should also be mentioned that other ways to assess the psychosocial impact of adult language impairment have been put forth by Evans and Northwood (1983) and by Muller, Code, and Mugford (1983).

Health history of the patient is ascertained, in part, during the case history interview (recall Table 8.2), but medical records provide greater specificity. Information concerning the current medical episode is particularly useful in differential diagnosis and treatment planning. Rosenbek, LaPointe, and Wertz (1989) suggest that the following medical data be collected:

1. Major and secondary medical diagnoses (e.g., thrombosis of left middle cerebral artery, organic brain syndrome, diabetes, CVA with right hemiparesis, and the like)
2. Date of onset as regards etiology of communication disorder
3. Localization of brain damage (hemisphere and lobes affected) and source of data (e.g., CT, MRI, and other techniques)
4. Previous CNS involvement (type and date of onset)
5. Brain stem signs (e.g., facial weakness, extraocular movement, dysphagia, other bulbar signs)
6. Limb involvement
7. Vision (acuity, corrective lens, visual field deficits, etc.)
8. Hearing (acuity, discrimination, amplification, etc.)

Access to the patient's medical chart is therefore essential to the SLP. In addition to the physician/neurologist report, entries by the neuroradiologist, social worker, nurse, and other health care professionals are enlightening. Important information can be gained from this telegraphic chart note entered by a neurologist:

This alert, oriented adult male suffered a CVA on 3-19-96. Expressive-receptive aphasia. Right hemiplegia. Babinski sign on the right. Gross motor functioning of involved leg is returning; arm and hand are doubtful. CT scan revealed a focal lesion in the left parietal-temporal region. Right side astereognosis. Right homonomous hemianopsia.

This brief report told us several important things about the patient: The neurologist observed that the brain damage was apparently localized and was not widespread; he also observed that the aphasia was probably not transitory, as lesions in the region cited generally result in more persistent language impairment; the patient could not identify objects by touch when they were placed in his right hand; and he could not see in the right field of vision. This last anomaly would require that we present testing materials from the patient's left side. Information assembled by the neurologist is, of course, very useful to the SLP. In addition to the size and locale of the lesion, the nature of the injury may be pertinent diagnostically. (For example, patients incurring traumatic brain injury often experience a different course of recovery from persons suffering vascular episodes.) The chart note also underscores the importance of being familar with pertinent medical terminology.

After garnering case history information, the SLP should have a rather detailed description of the salient aspects of the patient's premorbid personality, health history and current status, and social orientation. But what impact would this sudden illness have? How much change could be expected, and in what areas? Would the patient's responses to the language impairment and physical disabilities merely be an exaggeration of earlier behavior patterns?

There are only limited answers to these questions. We suspect, however, that the nature of the illness, the treatment the patient receives, and premorbid factors are all crucial in determining the impact of the problem upon the individual. In summary, any and all information about the individual that can be pulled together is important and may shape our course of assessment and treatment.

Diagnosis and Formal Testing

A comprehensive evaluation of an adult aphasic includes several clinical tasks: (1) a review of pertinent medical information and the sequence of events leading up to the referral; (2) a preliminary interview with the patient's spouse or other close relatives; (3) a case history, including information about the impact of brain injury on the patient and how much natural or spontaneous recovery has taken place; (4) an inventory of the client's language/communication performance; (5) observation and related testing (including informal assessments, oral peripheral examination, hearing test, and the like); and (6) a diagnostic determination with recommendations as to the nature of treatment and a judgment about the individual's prospects for recovery. In arriving at a diagnosis, the clinician first determines whether or not a communication problem exists and, if it does, what kind of problem. This involves sorting out among various possible conditions and among subtypes within specific conditions. This decision-making process is shown schematically in Figure 8.3.

Having discussed the first three tasks in the list, let us now turn our attention to the fourth and see how the evaluation process leads to a diagnosis. The SLP may need a quick idea of the client's language abilities and disabilities in order to determine the need for further testing and to better choose the most appropriate standardized tests to employ. A screening test, therefore, may be administered.

Screening for Aphasia

A screening instrument is designed to swiftly evaluate a patient's language abilities before the administration of a more thorough (and lengthy) examination. One reason for using a screening instrument is that it allows the SLP to quickly advise relatives and health care professionals about the best means of communicating with the patient. Additionally, patients' symptoms change rapidly during the first days and months following brain injury; screenings allow for frequent reassessments to document the patient's progress (or lack of progress) and to modify sug-

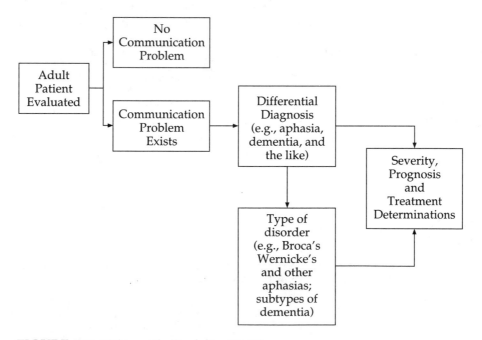

FIGURE 8.3 Diagnosis Decision Matrix

gestions as to how best to communicate with the patient. Frequent readministrations of formal, standardized tests—many lasting one to six hours—would not be practical.

Some screening tests were designed as screening devices per se; others are merely shortened versions of published language examinations for aphasia. Table 8.3 lists some of the available screening tests for aphasia.

Many experienced clinicians design their own screening device—usually one that is more cursory than published tests. In some work settings, for example, the SLP must quickly (in five minutes or so) interview and screen all newly admitted patients to determine if a communication problem exists and to decide whether to suggest that the physician order a speech-language consult. This is done because third-party reimbursement agencies require that evaluations be medically necessary and physician ordered. Typically, the SLP will elicit spontaneous conversation and judge it for contextual accuracy, topic maintenance, length of utterance, syntactic variety, facility with word selection, and fluency. Limited or absent conversation may lead the SLP to quickly assess more-basic skills, such as naming and pointing to objects in the room, repeating, following commands (nonverbally), and responding to yes/no questions (verbally or gesturally). Such a quick, albeit

---

TABLE 8.3   Some Screening Tests for Aphasia

Halstead-Wepman Aphasia Screening Test
   (Halstead and Wepman 1949)

Short Examination for Aphasia
   (Schuell 1957)

Sklar Aphasia Scale (SAS)
   (Sklar 1966)

A Short Form of the Token Test
   (Spellacy and Spreen 1969)

Screening Test of Aphasia
   (Emerick and Coyne 1972)

Aphasia Language Performance Scales (ALPS)
   (Keenan and Brassell 1975)

Shortened Version of the PICA (4 subtests)
   (DiSimoni et al. 1975)

Shortened Version of the PICA (2 of the objects in 17 subtests)
   (DiSimoni, Keith, and Darley 1980)

Very Short Form of the Minnesota Aphasia Test
   (Powell, Bailey, and Clark 1980)

Whurr Aphasia Screening Test
   (Whurr 1983)

Bedside Evaluation and Screening Test of Aphasia (BEST)
   (Fitch-West and Sands 1987)

Acute Aphasia Screening Protocol
   (Crary, Haak and Malinsky 1989)

incomplete, screening permits the clinician to judge (1) whether or not a communication problem exists on a gross level, (2) the need for further testing (and hence the need for a physician-ordered consult), and (3) which formal tests would be best suited to the patient's level of functioning.

No matter which form of screening is done, the SLP should enter a summary note in the patient's medical chart. An example follows:

> *The results of the screening test are encouraging. Mr. Tenhave has good auditory recognition (pointing to objects and pictures when named), and his comprehension for auditory materials is good within his limited auditory memory span. His listening is accurate for simple, short messages. He seems to understand more than he really does because he is alert and well oriented, and he picks out a crucial word in a sentence. He has a good supply of automatic (counting, emotional language) and reactive speech. He frequently gives associations when asked to name objects or pictures; for example, he said "pedal" for "brake." His gestures are not more complex than his verbal output. I did not ask him to write at this time, but it is my impression that his language deficit cuts across all modalities. No dysarthria was observed, although he did simplify complex words such as "Methodist." He is making a great many attempts at self-correction. On balance, then, I would say that he has a good prognosis for functional use of language.*

We offer a final word of caution: Screening tests were not designed to replace longer, more comprehensive evaluations. As Schuell (1966) points out, screening tests fail to sample behaviors in all communicative modalities, and they do not provide a sufficient sample in the modalities that are tested to make a confident differential diagnosis or to plan treatment.

Standardized Testing

In order to devise a plan of treatment, as well as to predict the probable course and outcome of treatment, the SLP needs a comprehensive appraisal of the patient's present language abilities. Where is the patient having difficulty? Which modalities are working best? How are errors made and are there discernable patterns to the errors? To answer these and other questions, we inventory the patient's language.

The SLP has many published tests from which to choose; Table 8.4 lists some of the more commonly used tests of aphasia. Many of these instruments have been reviewed in detail elsewhere (Buros 1978; Darley 1979; Davis 1993; Kertesz 1979; Rosenbek, LaPointe, and Wertz 1989; Tikofsky 1984). Only a cursory discussion of the more popular—and different—tests will be presented here.

Beginning clinicians often ask which aphasia test they should select for examining patients. We prefer not to advocate any particular instrument but instead ask the clinicians to specify their purposes in testing. What do they want the test to show? If prediction of the course of the patient's recovery is important, the PICA (Porch, 1981) or the Western Aphasia Battery (WAB) (Kertesz 1980) are the instruments of choice; if the clinician is more interested in the site of lesion, the Boston Diagnostic Aphasia Examination (Goodglass and Kaplan 1983) or the WAB are in-

TABLE 8.4   Commonly Used Tests for Aphasia

Aphasia Language Performance Scales (ALPS)
  (Keenan and Brassell 1975)

Examining for Aphasia
  (Eisenson 1994)

Boston Diagnostic Aphasia Examination (BDAE)
  (Goodglass and Kaplan 1983)

Boston Assessment of Severe Aphasia
  (Helm-Estabrooks et al. 1989)

Communicative Abilities in Daily Living
  (Holland 1980)

Communicative Effectiveness Index
  (Lomas et al. 1989)

Functional Communication Profile
  (Sarno 1969)

Minnesota Test for Differential Diagnosis of Aphasia (MTDDA)
  (Schuell 1973)

Multilingual Aphasia Examination (MAE)
  (Benton and Hamsher 1989)

Neurosensory Center Comprehensive Examination for Aphasia
  (Spreen and Benton 1977)

Porch Index of Communicative Ability (PICA)
  (Porch 1981)

Western Aphasia Battery
  (Kertesz 1980)

dicated; if the clinician wants to know how the patient performs on basic-to-complicated language functions, then the Minnesota Test for Differential Diagnosis of Aphasia (Schuell 1973) is a good choice. To sample a patient's communication ability in natural settings, the checklist called the Functional Communication Profile (Taylor 1963) or the more extensive Communicative Abilities in Daily Living (Holland 1980) would be the instruments of choice.

In the hands of a skilled and perceptive clinician who is thoroughly familiar with the materials, *any* of the published tests will provide a detailed description of an aphasic patient's language disturbance. As we pointed out earlier in this book, a test is only a tool, a way to help the clinician make relatively precise observations of a particular individual. Nation and Aram (1977) state the issue succinctly: "A good diagnostician relies on the feelings that have resulted as much as on the tools that were administered" (258). None of the published aphasia tests are pure, and none are sacrosanct. With this in mind, let us discuss four popular tests that are very different in philosophy and content.

The Porch Index of Communicative Ability
Better known as the PICA (Porch 1981), this is a psychometrically well-constructed test that assesses verbal, gestural, and graphic responses to common objects. The

test features a multidimensional scoring system, using one to sixteen categories, that allows the clinician to make precise observations of the patient's responses. Scores with percentile norms, performance plots, and recovery curves are generated through data manipulation. Speech-language pathologists have found the overall score (as a single index of communication ability) and the recovery predictions extremely useful information to share with physicians.

In mild criticism of the PICA, we dislike the rigidity of the test and feel that the standard procedure breaks down the patient-clinician relationship. As Keenan and Brassell (1975) state, "A badly presented item is a minor error, far less important than an impersonal or mechanical response to the patient" (36). Additionally, we find that test administration is time comsuming and that starting the examination with the most difficult task often overwhelms the aphasic and disturbs his/her subsequent performance. The PICA offers only limited information about a patient's verbal ability: Only four of the eighteen subtests elicit verbal behavior; only one of the four, "describing how objects are used," affords any insight into how the patient talks. Finally, we do not feel that a clinician should abrogate his/her personal clinical responsibility for judgment by deferring to a test or the numerical scores it generates. A combination of clinical intuition, patient observations, lesion information, *and* test scores/performances should shape our diagnoses and predictions.

The Boston Diagnostic Aphasia Examination
The BDAE (Goodglass and Kaplan 1983) operates on the localization premise that test scores and profiles correspond to specific types of aphasia. We particularly recognize as a strength the conversational and expository speech section that rates six features: melodic line, phrase length, articulatory agility, grammatical form, paraphasia, and word finding. Subtests cover a wide variety of skills and modalities, making it a well-rounded examination. Supplementary tests are included for use with related disorders. We, however, do find that the BDAE is a lengthy test and one that may frustrate low-level patients. The Computerized Boston (Code, Heer, and Schofield 1989) is a computerized scoring program for the BDAE.

Communicative Abilities in Daily Living
Holland (1980) designed the CADL to sample the patient's functional communication skills in naturalistic situations. It is to supplement traditional tests of aphasia, not replace them. As such, it does not lend itself to differential diagnosis. The content of the CADL is unique; it includes categories such as role-playing, utilizing nonverbal context, and analyzing speech acts. All in all, it is a test that measures what it purports—communication in daily activities.

Aphasia Language Performance Scales
The ALPS, by Keenan and Brassell (1975), is a quick-to-administer test that emphasizes an informal conversational approach. It contains four 10-item scales: listening, talking, reading, writing. Items are presented in an increasingly complex order and may be omitted if judged too difficult or too easy for a patient. We find

the ALPS a useful test for low-level patients but also consider it rather cursory for differential diagnosing and treatment planning.

Regardless of the test used, the evaluation process permits the clinician to identify islands of communication ability the patient retains. In many instances, however, the SLP will want to do additional, more extensive testing in particular areas. Some specialized tests follow.

1. *Auditory Comprehension.* Almost every comprehensive aphasia battery has at least one section that evaluates auditory comprehension. Since the integrity of the auditory modality is so crucial in predicting recovery, several specialized tests have been published. The most notable of them include the Token Test (DeRenzi and Vignolo 1962) and its many versions, the most popular of which is the Revised Token Test (McNeil and Prescott 1978); the Auditory Comprehension Test for Sentences (ACTS) (Shewan 1980); and the Functional Auditory Comprehension Task (FACT) (LaPointe and Horner 1978).

2. *Expressive Abilities.* Early aphasia batteries have been criticized for not evaluating the spontaneous speech of patients. The Boston Diagnostic Aphasia Examination (Goodglass and Kaplan 1983), in contrast, does elicit conversational and expository speech. The test's "Cookie Theft" picture description task and ratings based on the patient's verbal output are well known. Recently, *discourse analysis* has become refined and the work of Ulatowska and colleagues shows clinical promise (Ulatowska, North, and Macaluso-Haynes 1981; Ulatowska and Bond 1983; Ulatowska et al. 1983). On a syntactic level, the Sentence Completion Test (Goodglass et al. 1972) is useful in assessing sentence construction abilities and the patient's use of derivations.

3. *Reading Ability.* The Reading Comprehension Battery for Aphasia (LaPointe and Horner 1979) and the Battery of Adult Reading Function (Gonzales-Rothi, Costett, and Heilman 1984) are useful in-depth measures of reading ability.

4. *Intelligence.* The Coloured Progressive Matrices (Raven 1963) is useful in assessing nonverbal skills, while the Wechsler Adult Intelligence Scale (Wechsler 1955) is a traditional battery with many useful subtests.

5. *Others.* Additional special testing almost surely includes an oral-peripheral and motor examination and a test of hearing acuity, as well as others deemed necessary for particular patients.

Differential Diagnosis

The SLP must often distinguish between aphasia and a number of other conditions involving abnormality in language and/or speech. A variety of special tests may be needed to supplement standard aphasia batteries in order to facilitate differential diagnosing. Table 8.5 lists some tests useful in differentiating aphasia from other adult language disorders, as gathered from the literature (Bayles 1984; Hagen 1984; Marquardt 1982; Myers 1984). Special tests delineate patient's strengths and

TABLE 8.5   Useful Tests for Cognitive-Communicative Assessments

Assessment of Cognitive Abilities
(Adamovich and Henderson, 1985)

Benton Revised Visual Retention Test (BVRT-R)
(Benton, 1974)

Blessed Orientation and Memory Examination
(Blessed, Tomlinson, Roth, 1968)

Boston Naming Test
(Kaplan, Goodglass, and Weintraub, 1983)

Cognitive Assessment of Minnesota
(Rustad, et al., 1993)

Coloured Progressive Matrices
(Raven, 1963)

Detroit Test of Learning Aptitude (DTLA) (selected subtests)
(Baker and Leland, 1959)

Developmental Test of Visual Perception
(Frostig, 1963)

F-A-S Word Fluency Measure
(Borkowski, Benton, and Spreen, 1967)

Galveston Orientation and Amnesia Test (GOAT)
(Levin, O'Donnell, and Grossman, 1979)

Geriatric Mental Status Interview (GMS)
(Gurland, Copeland, Sharpe, and Kelleher, 1976)

Geriatric Rating Scale (GRS)
(Plutchik and Conte, 1972)

Global Deterioration Scale of Primary Degenerative Dementia (GDS)
(Reisberg, Ferris and Crook, 1982)

Halstead-Reitan Battery
(revised frequently; consult Lezak, 1983 for description)

Hooper Visual Organization Test
(Hooper, 1958)

Illinois Tests of Psycholinguistic Abilities (ITPA) (selected subtests)
(Kirk, McCarthy, and Kirk, 1968)

Luria-Nebraska Neuropsychological Battery
(consult Lezak, 1983 for description)

Mattis Dementia Rating Scale (MDRS)
(Mattis, 1976)

Mental Status Questionnaire (MSQ)
(Goldfarb and Antin, 1975)

Mini-Mental State Examination (MMS)
(Folstein, Folstein, and McHugh, 1975)

Nonsense Syllable Learning Task
(Alexander, 1973)

Nonverbal Test of Cognitive Skills
(Johnson and Boyd, 1981)

TABLE 8.5   *Continued*

Peabody Picture Vocabulary Test-Revised
(Dunn and Dunn, 1981)

Reading Comprehension Battery for Aphasia
(LaPointe and Horner, 1979)

Revised Token Test
(McNeil and Prescott, 1978)

Ross Information Processing Assessment-Geriatric
(Ross-Swain and Fogle, 1996)

Ross Test of Higher Cognitive Processes
(Ross and Ross, 1976)

Wechsler Adult Intelligence Scale (WAIS) (selected subtests)
(Wechsler, 1955)

Wechsler Memory Scale
(Wechsler and Stone, 1948)

weaknesses beyond the realm of language; areas such as intelligence, cognition, perception, mood, and behavior need to be tapped.

We present the following brief discussion of some disorders that might be confused with aphasia. Keep in mind, however, that impairment of symbolic functioning can coexist with any of these conditions.

Psychosis

Although it is rather easy for the professional to distinguish *aphasia* from *psychosis*, it is understandable why laypersons are often confused. The aphasic may say yes when he/she means no, use obscenities and other antisocial language or gestures freely, laugh or cry often, lapse into euphoria, deny his/her symptoms, or withdraw into severe depression and despair. The distinguishing features of psychosis are, however, rather obvious: severe personality decomposition—not just frustration or emotional overflow when trying to comprehend or speak—and distortion of, or loss of contact with, reality. The vast majority of aphasic patients do not show evidence of mental deterioration or gross disturbances in processing reality. Additionally, the person with aphasia will generally try hard to communicate with others; for the psychotic, interpersonal contact is irrelevant.

Considering all the frustrations that persons with aphasia encounter, we have often wondered why they do not behave in a more abnormal manner than they do. Indeed, their demeanor and social interaction, aside from the language impairment, are remarkably normal. Nevertheless, some individuals with aphasia do experience psychotic episodes and periods of severe depression.

Language of Confusion

According to Darley (1982), the *language of confusion* describes patients with irrelevant and confabulatory language, unclear thinking, reduced recognition of the environment, faulty memory, and disorientation to time and place. Syntax, word retrieval, auditory comprehension, and ability to repeat are usually not impaired. The patient's relatively good language is, therefore, unlike aphasia.

In persons who exhibit the language of confusion, the injury to the brain is widespread—usually bilateral—and often due to trauma. The following case example illustrates the irrelevance and confusion:

> *Tom Snively, a 20-year-old college junior, suffered a closed head injury in a skiing accident. He was in a coma for two weeks. Now, two months post onset, he is an inpatient in the Marquette Rehabilitation Center. When evaluated with a standard test of aphasia, Tom showed no disturbance of vocabulary or syntax; he did have some limited word-finding difficulty. The examiner noted, however, that the young man had trouble attending and staying in touch with the test situation. The patient tended to give responses that, although syntactically correct, were often irrelevant. Additionally, Tom was disoriented and particularly in response to open-ended questions gave rambling, fabricated answers. Here is a portion of an interview conducted by a medical social worker that reveals the patient's disorientation and tendency to confabulate:*
>
> Worker: *Where are you?*
>
> Tom: *Ah, in training camp. Colorado Springs. And tomorrow we do time trials for the giant slalom.*
>
> Worker: *But, what is this place?*
>
> Tom: *A training center. I had a hamstring pull and need whirlpool treatments.*

In addition to language confusion and other cognitive symptoms, patients may show changes in personality as well. Areas to be assessed include orientation, memory, reasoning, story retelling, and verbal explanations, to name but a few. The SLP may wish to select from tests presented in Table 8.5. Regarding prognosis, the confusion may range from mild and temporary, such as in concussion or hypothermia, to profound and chronic, as in head injury or drug overdose.

Language of Generalized Intellectual Deterioration

Dementia refers to a group of disorders that feature generalized intellectual decline. The deterioration of emotional control, cognitive skills, and language use is caused by diffuse, bilateral subcortical and cortical brain injury or atrophy. Dementia is caused by, among other factors, infectious diseases, tumor, multiple strokes, and Parkinson's and Alzheimer's diseases. Unlike language confusion, dementia often has a gradual, insidious onset.

Before a clinical diagnosis of dementia can be confirmed, several key features must be present (Berg et al. 1982):

1. A sustained deterioration of *memory*, plus a disturbance in at least three of the following areas: (a) orientation in time and place; (b) judgment and problem

solving (dealing with everyday situations); (c) community affairs (shopping, handling finances); (d) home and avocations; and (e) personal care
2. A gradual onset and progression
3. A duration of at least six months or longer.

Generalized intellectual decline and cognitive dysfunction are hallmarks of dementia that are evident in the patient's overt language. Table 8.6 highlights differences between dementia and aphasia (Bayles and Kaszniak 1987; Rosenbek, LaPointe, and Wertz 1989).

TABLE 8.6   Cognitive and Communicative Differences between Aphasia and Dementia

Variable	Aphasia	Dementia
Progression	There is rapid onset; improvement is typical.	There is slow onset and progressive deterioration.
Cognition	Cognition is generally intact.	Cognition is mildly to profoundly impaired; it worsens with the condition; problem solving is poor.
Memory	Memory is generally intact.	Memory ranges from mildly forgetful to profoundly impaired or amnesic; it worsens with the condition.
Emotionality	Mood is typically appropriate with occasional periods of depression or frustration.	Person is typically labile; is apathetic and withdrawn; intermittently shows agitation; and can exhibit depression or mania.
Pragmatics	Socially appropriate skills are evident despite some comprehension failures; communication efforts typically show relevance.	Social skills are mildly to severely affected; inappropriate behaviors and irrelevant comments are typical; thought processes are disorganized.
Repetition ability	This ability is slightly to severely impaired.	This ability is generally intact unless the condition is severe.
Semantics	Work retrieval difficulties can be mild to severe; semantic and literal paraphasias may be used.	Impairment ranges from mild word-retrieval difficulties to visual misrecognitions to severe vocabulary reductions.
Syntax	Syntax is affected to varying degrees; it can be classified as fluent or nonfluent based on length of utterance.	Syntax is intact when disorder is mild; there is reduction of syntactic complexity as the disorder progresses.
Phonology	Phonology is impaired in nonfluent aphasia; it may be present as literal paraphasia in fluent aphasia.	Phonology is generally intact unless the condition is severe; dysarthria is possible.

In order to illustrate the salient behavioral and communicative symptoms observed in dementia, we include a portion of a diagnostic report on a patient in the second phase of Alzheimer's disease (Powell and Courtice 1983):

This 64-year-old patient manifested the following behaviors: lowered drive and energy level; memory loss; slow reaction time; and difficulty making decisions. Her personality has changed in the past year so that now she typically is dull, bland, and unresponsive socially.

Mrs. Davis's language abilities are only mildly impaired at this time. She can match objects; point to and name pictures; and repeat words, phrases, and short sentences. Phonologically and syntactically, her speech is within normal limits. She does have limited output, however, and restricted usage. The patient's speech performance is slow and often, after trying to respond to a task, she will say, "I don't know."

The patient's language disturbance was more evident on tasks requiring greater intellectual effort and abstraction. For example, Mrs. Davis was unable to find and correct semantic errors in sentences ("My sister is an only child") or discern the ambiguity in sentences ("Visiting relatives can be a nuisance").

The Arizona Battery for Communication Disorders of Dementia (ABCD) (Bayles and Tomoeda 1991) profiles patient performance along the subtests of mental status, linguistic expression, visuospatial construction, episodic memory, and linguistic comprehension. The ABCD is a popular test and can be used to document disease effects over time, as with Alzheimer's. Dementia scales are also provided by Mattis (1976) and by Reisberg, Ferris and Crook 1982). As so few standardized language tests exist for assessing dementia (and the subtypes of dementia), clinicians often draw from other tests and subtests. Cognitive and communicative areas to assess in patients with suspected dementia might include: memory, orientation, associative thought, intelligence, reasoning (both verbal and nonverbal), story retelling, object descriptions, explanations, and vocabulary. Many of the tests listed in Table 8.5 would be appropriate to use.

Right Hemisphere Impairment

Most individuals are left hemisphere dominant for language; yet, injury to the right hemisphere can cause communication deficits. According to Myers (1984), problems are mostly perceptual and prosodic. Linguistic deficits become apparent only with higher order, complex tasks. The communicative inefficiencies resulting from right hemisphere damage do not resemble aphasic symptoms. Table 8.7 summarizes deficits typically seen in patients with right hemisphere damage (Myers 1984). The interested reader is referred to the book detailing aspects of right hemisphere communication disorders (Tompkins 1995).

Only in recent years have tests of right hemisphere communication impairment been marketed. Typically, SLPs and/or neuropsychologists form a test battery using selected subtests from standard tests of aphasia, learning aptitude tests,

TABLE 8.7   Sequelae of Right Hemisphere Damage

General Symptoms

Neglect of the left half of space
Denial of illness
Impaired judgment
Impaired self-monitoring
Poor motivation

Visuospatial Deficits

Visual memory and imagery problems
Facial recognition difficulties (disorientation to person)
Geographic and spatial disorientation (to place)
Visual field deficits (especially left)
Visual hallucinations
Visuoconstructive deficits (constructional apraxia)

Deficits in Affect and Prosody

Indifference reaction
Reduced sensitivity to emotional tone
Impaired prosodic production and comprehension

Lingusitic Deficits

Problems with figurative language (interprets literally)
Impaired sense of humor
Linguistic deficits, including
    Comprehension of complex auditory material
    Word fluency
    Word recognition and word-picture matching
    Paragraph comprehension
Higher-order communication deficits, including
    Difficulty organizing information
    Tendency to produce impulsive answers with unnecessary detail
    Insensitive to contextual cues and pragmatic aspects of communication

perceptual tests, and others (recall Table 8.5). Informal test items also are often part of the assessment battery. Of particular importance are the patient's abilities/ disabilities with visuospatial perception, prosody, judgment, and high-level communication. Nevertheless, three cohesive tests in clinical use are presented.

The Right Hemisphere Language Battery (RHLB) (Bryan 1989), published in England, consists of seven subtests: metaphor-picture matching, written metaphor choice, inferred meaning comprehension, humor appreciation, lexical semantic recognition, emphatic stress production, and discourse production. Rating scales for scoring the discourse sample along eleven parameters are used.

The Mini Inventory of Right Brain Injury (MIRBI) (Pimental and Kingsbury 1989) is a twenty-seven-item screening tool that assesses visual scanning, integrity of gnosis, body image/body schema and praxis, visuoverbal processing, visuosymbolic processing, affective language, higher-level language skills, emotion and affect processing, and general behavior/psychic integrity.

The Rehabilitation Institute of Chicago Evaluation of Communication Problems in Right Hemisphere Dysfunction (RICE) (Burns, Halper and Mogil 1985) has five sections focusing on general behavioral patterns, visual scanning and tracking, assessment and analysis of writting errors, assessment of pragmatic communication violations, and metaphorical language.

Motor Speech Disorders

Motor speech disorders often coexist with language disorders, particularly aphasia. The presence of a speech disorder certainly affects the language treatment goals and procedures. For example, facilitative articulation techniques must often be incorporated into the total management program. The evaluation of a patient with brain damage, therefore, should include tasks to determine the existence of either *apraxia of speech* or *dysarthria*. We will discuss these disorders, and the process of differential diagnosis, in Chapter 9.

Determining the Type of Aphasia

Once the SLP has narrowed down the diagnostic options and determined that the patient has aphasia, the next step is to decide which *type* of aphasia is exhibited. The characteristics of the various types of aphasia were summarized in Table 8.1. Communicative abilities and disabilities are considered in "fitting" the patient into a diagnostic category. Many of the published tests facilitate this decision-making process by profiling patient scores from the various subtests. Clinical experience and expertise are often invaluable, as well.

Summary

What is aphasia and what is not aphasia remains controversial, even among the experts. Many definitions of aphasia exist—some broad and all-encompassing and others quite specific and limiting. Speech-language pathologists will be wise to keep this in mind as they seek to differentiate aphasia from other speech and language disorders. In the final analysis, labels we use reflect speech-language diagnoses, not medical diagnoses. The evaluation process is likened to taking an inventory of the patient's communicative strengths and weaknesses; this can be done informally as well.

The Art of Informal Assessment

Regardless of which standardized test the clinician administers, for treatment planning it is important to examine *how* the patient made the errors. Did the patient seem to perseverate? At what level of complexity did responses break down? Did the patient give synonyms or associations for words when asked to name pictures or objects? For example, when asked to name a picture of a dollar bill, a patient who says, "Put it . . . pocket . . . wallet . . ." is making a "better error" than a response of "soup" or "don't know." Was the patient attempting to correct the errors? Are responses significantly delayed? How did the patient respond to various cueing techniques? What strategies, if any, were used to assist in word retrieval—using gestures, writing, semantic, or phonetic cues? Answers to these questions are based more on clinician observations during the testing process than on test scores. Informal assessment with activities that probe treatment levels and cueing needs may be most insightful.

In evaluating a patient, it is not *necessary* to use a "test" at all; some SLPs prefer to rely on observation of the patient in the natural environment. The Functional Communication Profile (Taylor 1963) and the informal assessment tasks prepared by Ulatowska, Macaluso-Haynes, and Mendel-Richardson (1976) are useful in providing a structure for observing the patient's communication abilities in real situations. Ideas may also be borrowed from the CADL (Holland 1980), without actually administering the test, for clinical insights of the patient's functional use of language in contrived situations. Functional communication skills exhibited by the patient are relevant to designing treatment. Questions that should come to the mind of the clinician include: Which of the patient's strategies should be capitalized on and reinforced? Which can be made more effective? Which strategies are counterproductive and interfering? Should alternative modes of communication be employed to develop functional responding? The evaluation provides an excellent time to observe *patient-generated facilitation strategies,* such as gesturing an action to aid in word retrieval, finger tapping to pace speech production, requesting repetitions or using a delay to gain extra processing time, and the like. In addition, before designing a management program, the SLP must consider *characteristics of the stimulus* and which *cues and prompts* may be presented to the patient to increase the likelihood of response accuracy. Treatment probes to determine these things may be initiated during the evaluation stage but should continue to be used throughout the management program to maintain efficiency. (Patient progress is often uneven, and "steps" in the program may be skipped from time to time.)

Characteristics of the stimulus affect the patient's ability to respond. The prevailing clinical assumption is that parameters of the stimulus can be hierarchically arranged to produce a level of responding that is not only continual but also correct (appropriate) more than half of the time (Marquardt 1982). The writings of Darley (1976), Duffy (1981), and Marquardt (1982) provide good reviews of stimulus attributes and their therapeutic applications. Some general guidelines can be summarized here; the clinician may want to probe the patient's needs regarding the following stimulus characteristics:

1. Presentation of a stimulus through more than one modality increases the likelihood of a correct response. This also provides more contextual information.
2. Salient and nonambiguous stimuli affect performance positively—for example, large pictures without distracting backgrounds, or intense auditory stimuli with a favorable signal-to-noise ratio.

3. Reduced length and complexity of presentation, such as using short words or short and grammatically simple sentences, improves comprehension and production accuracy.
4. Presentation of stimuli at reduced rates for longer periods of time and with an imposed response delay affects performance favorably.

Various cues and prompts may be presented to increase the likelihood of response accuracy. These may be provided by the clinician initially and later, through training, may be faded from use or become self-generated cues, thus helping the patient become a self-sufficient, functional communicator. McDearmon and Potter (1975) categorized types of cues, and their work should be consulted by the interested reader. "Associational" cues include such things as the use of sentence completion, first sounds, function, or rhyme to trigger word retrieval. "Symbolic" prompts are written, printed, or spoken words, whereas "realistic" prompts show attributes of the stimulus. Examples of realistic prompts include a picture of an object, the object itself, or sensory properties of the stimulus, such as the ticking of a clock to evoke the response "clock" or the feel of water to evoke its name. Cueing characteristics and optimal hierarchies are an often-researched area in aphasiology. Table 8.8 lists a ten-level cueing hierarchy, based on the work of Linebaugh and Lehner (1977), which is useful in assisting patients with word retrieval problems. Cue the patient at the highest step possible to initially aid in word recall and back down the steps, supplying more assistance, as needed. Table 8.9 explains strategies suggested by Whitney (1975) that might prove helpful during the informal assessment and that later can be integrated into treatment. We have often used such stop-and-go strategies to elicit optimal, elaborate, on-target responses from our patients in both assessment and treatment situations.

TABLE 8.8 A Hierarchy for Word Retrieval

Step 1. Ask patient, "Say (<u>word</u>)." (Patient imitates.)

Step 2. Ask patient to complete sentence with first and second phonemes supplied (e.g., "You sleep in a b_____ .").

Step 3. Ask patient to complete sentence with first phoneme supplied (e.g., "You sleep in a b_____ .").

Step 4. Ask patient to complete sentence with first phoneme silently articulated (e.g., "You sleep in a . . . [form /b/ on lips]").

Step 5. Ask patient to complete sentence (e.g., "You sleep in a _____ .").

Step 6. State function, demonstrate function, and supply a carrier phrase (e.g., "You sleep on it . . . motion sleep . . . it's a _____ .").

Step 7. State function and supply a carrier phrase (e.g., "You sleep on it; it's a _____ .").

Step 8. Direct the patient to demonstrate the function (e.g., "Show me what you do with it.").

Step 9. Direct the patient to state the function (e.g., "What do you do with this?").

Step 10. Request the name (e.g., "What's this?").

TABLE 8.9   Compensatory Strategies for Aphasia

Comprehension Strategies

- Repeat the utterance for the patient; later ask the patient to assume the responsiblity of requesting repeats.
- Augment verbal material with the same information in writing; patient eventually should ask for material to be written if this modality aids comprehension.

"Stop" Strategies

These strategies are useful with patients who have fluent aphasia. These strategies assist in controlling fluency and monitoring empty speech or paraphasic errors.

- If desired, model a slow rate of speech and monitor the patient's pace, stopping to correct when needed.
- Encourage the patient to listen to himself/herself. Frequent verbal reminder to "listen" may be employed.
- Actively stop the patient's speech output, if necessary. This can be done by touching the lips, saying "Stop," using a gesture signal (such as hand up) or any combination of these that successfully terminate the jargon. Fading of the stop cue should be incorporated into the treatment plan.
- Encourage self-correction in the patient. Direction to use another strategy, such as a word-retrieval technique, may be helpful.

"Go" Strategies

These strategies are useful with patients who have nonfluent aphasia. "Go" strategies encourage the patient to keep communication going by using telegraphic speech, gestures, or graphics on which to expand.

- Get the patient started; the clinician can suggest a gesture or "key word" to initiate a telegraphic response.
- Keep the patient going; the clinician can replay or feed back to the patient what was initially said and encourage expansion or elaboration.

Summing Up the Findings

Patient abilities and disabilities are determined through the formal and informal evaluation process. Such information permits the SLP to diagnose the type of aphasia (or other communication disorder), if any. The diagnostic label is useful as a "summary statement." The information collected is used in determining the patient's prognosis for recovery. Furthermore, it shapes the direction that treatment will take. Of course, the ultimate goal of evaluation and diagnosis is to ensure that the patient's symptoms are managed appropriately.

Prognosis

Selecting patients for treatment who have the best chance of recovery from aphasia is an unsettling task. Rather than abandon anyone, the clinician's impulse is to attempt to work with every person even though prospects for improvement in cases of severe language impairment are dim (Sarno, Silverman, and Sands 1970). When there is little real progress, the patient's labors are like those of Sisyphus.

How, then, can the SLP identify patients with the best potential? A list of interrelated factors that we have found helpful for making a prognosis is presented here; however, we trust the reader's forecasting will be guided by three important maxims: (1) Do not make a final prognosis on the basis of a single evaluation session—a period of trial therapy is always highly informative; (2) do not make a prognosis solely on the basis of a single measure of behavior (such as one test); and (3) be sure you understand the value of predictors—they can be potent self-fulfilling prophecies.

1. *Initial Severity.* Initial severity of aphasia is the single best predictor of recovery, according to Kertesz (1979). The more severe the patient's language impairment is at the time of assessment, the poorer the prognosis. Three aspects of language functioning are particularly important in predicting recovery:

- *Auditory recognition.* Patients who make errors (even a few errors—two or three out of ten items—are significant) when identifying pictures or common objects named by the examiner have an unfavorable prognosis; an impairment at this level is apparently irreversible (Schuell 1973).
- *Comprehension.* Patients who have marked difficulty in comprehending verbal messages make poor candidates for treatment. In fact, a reliable index of the severity of language impairment in aphasia is the degree of disturbance in comprehension (Schuell 1973).
- *Speech fluency.* Patients who speak more fluently seem to make better recoveries. But the presence of jargon, especially when it is coupled with lack of self-monitoring, euphoria, or denial, is a poor clinical sign.

2. *Time Elapsed since Onset.* Many studies have concluded that patients who receive language treatment before six months has elapsed since the cerebral insult show the most significant gains in treatment. The longer the time elapsed since onset of aphasia and the beginning of treatment, the poorer the prognosis (Fitch-West 1984). Habits of dependence, withdrawal, and possible secondary gains accruing from a nonverbal role tend to defeat therapeutic intervention.

3. *Type of Aphasia.* Recovery of aphasia seems to follow a pattern of evolution (Kertesz 1979). Progress in global aphasia is often poor, but when improvement occurs it is toward the symptoms of Broca's aphasia. Broca's aphasia typically shows fair-to-good recovery; when symptoms diminish, the patient usually retains word-retrieval difficulty and dysfluency. Wernicke's aphasia carries a split prognosis, with some patients doing fairly well and others poorly. Although the symptoms of Wernicke's aphasia often persist, recovery can occur with symptoms evolving toward conduction or anomic types of aphasia. Conduction aphasia improves toward symptoms of anomic aphasia or may recover completely. Anomic aphasia also shows complete recovery or recovery with only the persistence of mild word-retrieval difficulties.

4. *Etiology.* Depending on the location and extent of the lesion, patients who have suffered traumatic brain injury tend to make better recoveries than do individuals who have had thrombotic or other vascular episodes and tumors (Rosenbek, LaPointe, and Wertz 1989).

5. *Age.* The importance of age as a prognostic variable is not clear, as it often overlaps with factors such as etiology. For example, trauma patients tend to be younger than CVA patients. However, it can generally be said that younger patients recover faster and more adequately than do older patients. Presumably this is because younger brains show more plasticity and older patients may have more widespread cerebral damage due to arteriosclerosis. In addition, aphasic patients in or near retirement may lack the energy and motivation to persist in a treatment program.

6. *Presence of Other Health Problems.* In our clinical experience, aphasic patients presenting health problems in addition to the brain injury (such as diabetes, systemic vascular disease, or kidney disease) often do poorly in treatment.

7. *Family Response.* Patients whose families provide supportive understanding and appropriate stimulation and who permit the individual to regain his/her role within the family unit have a more favorable prognosis.

8. *Extent of the Lesion.* The more extensive the brain injury, the poorer the prospects for recovery.

9. *Location of the Lesion.* This variable overlaps with type of aphasia. In general, damage occurring posterior to the fissure of Rolando, especially at the junction of the parietal and temporal lobes, tends to result in more persistent aphasia (Fitch-West 1984).

10. *Premorbid Personality.* The more outgoing, flexible individual generally responds better to treatment than does an inhibited, introverted person. Personality and temperment are often said to have altered as a result of brain damage. Behavior patterns seen in some aphasic patients have been labeled "egocentricity," "catastrophic response," "concretism," and the like. Despite the tremendous frustration and alteration in self-concept that aphasia produces, most of our clients have not exhibited much change in their basic personality traits.

11. *Intelligence and Education.* The more intelligent, better educated patients make better candidates for treatment. Although this is generally true, a few of our most highly educated patients were so vividly aware of the discrepancy between their premorbid abilities and their present condition, they simply withdrew in futility.

12. *Self-Monitoring.* Patients who are aware of their errors and attempt to correct them have a more favorable prognosis than those who do not.

13. *Handedness.* Left-handed patients have better prognoses than right-handed ones (Fitch-West 1984). However, it may be that left-handed individuals are more likely to become aphasic regardless of which hemisphere of the brain is damaged, suggesting that left-handers show bilateral language representation.

The reader may want to consult the following references for further information regarding prognosis in aphasia: Keenan and Brassell (1974), Kertesz and McCabe (1977), Marshall and Phillips (1983), Fitch-West (1984), and Crary and Haak (1988).

Early Intervention

We cannot overemphasize the critical importance of early intervention in the clinical management of persons with aphasia; this position becomes obvious when we consider that aphasia is a personal and family catastrophe (Buck 1968). Early support and counseling for the patient and for the family are greatly needed. Early initiation of language stimulation is also wise. We offer the following five concluding points for consideration in early intervention with acute patients: (1) Nurses and others who work with the patient should receive inservice training on how to deal adequately with aphasic patients. Consult the work of Leutenegger (1975) and Haynes and Greenberg (1976) for useful material for in-service training. (2) There should be information-sharing and planning conferences with professional team members—the physician, physical therapist, occupational therapist, social worker, and others concerned with the rehabilitation of the patient. (3) Supportive interviews with the aphasic patient should be conducted to provide release of feelings and to offer reassurance that a professional clinician is concerned and attempting to do something about the language problem. (4) Family counseling is most important. Families are confronted with a crisis when an adult member is suddenly afflicted with a potentially deadly, often mysterious illness that results in such profound physical and psychological alterations. A serious illness disrupts communication patterns, dissolves or shifts roles, and forces family members to assume unfamiliar responsibilities. The resolution of the crisis situation and the manner in which members reorganize the family structure will have profound implications for the patient's rehabilitation (Kinsella and Duffy 1978). The maintenance of a supportive, nonthreatening environment for the brain-injured patient is crucial to recovery. (5) Last, design a treatment program that is appropriate for the patient and modify it as the patient's abilities and disabilities change. With recovery from brain damage, patient's symptoms will evolve, making dynamic treatment with frequent reassessments a necessity.

A discussion of treatment philosophies and treatment approaches is beyond the scope of this book. The reader is encouraged to consult many of the fine books on the clinical management of adult communication deficits. Among these books are those by Chapey (1994); Davis (1993); Davis and Wilcox (1985); Eisenson (1984); Jenkins et al. (1975); Johns (1978); Rosenbek, LaPointe, and Wertz (1989); Schuell, Jenkins, and Jimenez-Pabon (1989); and Shewan and Bandur (1986).

Bibliography

Adamovich, B. B., and Henderson, J. A. (1985). "Assessment of Cognitive Abilities." In *Cognitive Rehabilitation of Closed Head Injured Patients*, ed. B. B. Adamovich, J. A. Henderson, and S. Auerbach (San Diego, CA: College-Hill).

Alexander, D. A. (1973). "Some Tests of Intelligence and Learning for Elderly Psychiatric

Patients: A Validation Study." *British Journal of Social and Clinical Psychology* 12:188–193.

Baker, H. J., and Leland, B. (1959). *Detroit Test of Learning Aptitude.* Indianapolis, IN: Bobbs-Merrill.

Bayles, K. A. (1984). "Language and Dementia." In *Language Disorders in Adults: Recent Advances,* ed. A. L. Holland (San Diego, CA: College-Hill).

Bayles, K. A., and Kaszniak, A. W. (1987). *Communication and Cognition in Normal Aging and Dementia.* San Diego, CA: College-Hill.

Benton, A. L. (1974). *Revised Visual Retention Test: Clinical and Experimental Application* (4th ed.). New York: Psychological Corporation.

Benton, A. L., and Hamsher, K. (1989). *Multilingual Aphasia Examination.* Palo Alto, CA: Psychological Corporation.

Berg, L., Hughes, C. P., Coben, L. A., Danziger, W. L., and Martin, R. L. (1982). "Mild Senile Dementia of Alzheimer Type: Research Diagnostic Criteria, Recruitment, and Description of a Population Study." *Journal of Neurology, Neurosurgery and Psychiatry* 45:962–968.

Blessed, G., Tomlinson, B. E., and Roth, M. (1968). "The Association between Quantitative Measures of Dementia and of Senile Change in the Cerebral Grey Matter of Elderly Subjects." *Journal of Psychiatry* 114:797–811.

Borkowski, J. G., Benton, A. L., and Spreen, D. (1967). "Word Fluency and Brain Damage." *Neuropsychologia* 5:135–140.

Bryas, K. L. (1989). *The Right-Hemisphere Language Battery.* Kibworth, Eng.: Far Communications.

Buck, M. (1968). *Dysphasia.* Englewood Cliffs, NJ: Prentice Hall.

Burns, M. S., Halper, A. S., and Mogil, S. I. (1985). *Rehabilitation Institute of Chicago Evaluation of Communication Problems in Right-Hemisphere Dysfunction (RICE).* Rockville, MD: Aspen.

Buros, O., ed. (1978). *The Eighth Mental Measurements Yearbook.* Vol. 2. Highland Park, NJ: Gryphon Press.

Chapey, R. (1994). 3rd ed. *Language Intervention Strategies in Adult Aphasia.* Baltimore, MA: Williams and Wilkins.

Code, C., Heer, M., and Schofield, M. (1989). *The Computerized Boston.* Palo Alto, CA: Psychological Corporation.

Crary, M. A., and Haak, N. J. (1988). "One Perspective on Recovery in Aphasia." *NSSLHA Journal* 16, no. 1:76–92.

Crary, M., Haak, N. J., and Malinsky, A. (1989). "Peliminary Psychometric Evaluation of an Acute Aphasia Screening Protocol." *Aphasiology* 3:611–618.

Darley, F. L. (1976). "Maximizing Input to the Aphasic Patient: A Review of Research." In *Clinical Aphasiology Conference Proceedings,* ed. R. Brookshire (Minneapolis, MN: BRK Publishers).

Darley, F. L. (1979). *Evaluation of Appraisal Techniques in Speech and Language Pathology.* Reading, MA: Addison-Wesley.

Darley, F. L. (1982). *Aphasia.* Philadelphia: Saunders.

Davis, G. A. (1993). *A Survey of Adult Aphasia and Related Language Disorders.* 2nd ed. Englewood Cliffs, NJ: Prentice Hall.

Davis, G. A., and Wilcox, M. J. (1985). *Adult Aphasia Rehabilitation: Applied Pragmatics.* San Diego, CA: College-Hill.

DeRenzi, E., and Vignolo, L. A. (1962). "The Token Test: A Sensitive Test to Detect Receptive Disturbances in Aphasics." *Brain* 85:665–678.

Derman, S., and Manaster, A. (1967). "Family Counseling with Relatives of Aphasic Patients." *Journal of American Speech and Hearing Association* 8:175–177.

DiSimoni, F. G., Keith, R. L., and Darley, F. L. (1980). "Prediction of PICA Overall Score by Short Versions of the Test." *Journal of Speech and Hearing Research* 23:511–516.

DiSimoni, F. G., Keith, R. L., Holt, D. L., and Darley, F. L. (1975). "Practicality of Shortening the Porch Index of Communicative Ability." *Journal of Speech and Hearing Research* 18: 491–497.

Duffy, J. (1981). "Schuell's Stimulation Approach to Rehabilitation." In *Language Intervention Strategies in Adult Aphasia,* ed. R. Chapey (Baltimore, MD: Williams and Wilkins).

Dunn, L. M., and Dunn, L. M. (1981). *Peabody Picture Vocabulary Test—Revised.* Circle Pines, MN: American Guidance Service.

Eisenson, J. (1984). *Aphasia in Adults.* Englewood Cliffs, NJ: Prentice Hall.

Eisenson, J. (1994). *Examining for Aphasia.* 3rd ed. Austin, TX: Pro-Ed.

Emerick, L. (1971) *Appraisal of Language Disurbance.* Marquette: Northern Michigan University Press.

Emerick, L., and Coyne, J. (1972). *Screening Test of Aphasia.* Danville, IL: Interstate Printers and Publishers.

Evans, R., and Northwood, L. (1983). "Social Support Needs in Adjustment to Stroke." *Archives of Physical Medicine and Rehabilitation* 64:61–64.

Fitch-West, J. (1984). "Aphasia Rehabilitation." In *Communication Disorders: Remedial Principles and Practices,* ed. S. Dickson (Glenview, IL: Scott Foresman).

Fitch-West, J., and Sands, E. S. (1987). *The Bedside Evaluation Screening Test (BEST).* Frederick, MD: Aspen.

Folstein, M. F., Folstein, S. E., and McHugh, P. R. (1975). "Mini-Mental State: A Practical Method for Grading the Cognitive State of Patients for the Clinician." *Journal of Psychiatric Research* 12:189–198.

Frostig, M. (1963). *Developmental Test of Visual Perception.* Chicago, IL: Follett.

Goldfarb, A. I., and Antin, S. (1975). Unpublished data. In *The Physiology and Pathology of Human Aging,* ed. R. Goldman and M. Rockstein (New York: Academic Press).

Gonzales-Rothi, L. J., Costett, H. B., and Heilman, K. M. (1984). "Battery of Adult Reading Function." Unpublished, experimental test of the Veteran's Hospital, Gainesville, FL.

Goodglass, H., Gleason, J. B., Bernholtz, N. D., and Hyde, M. R. (1972). "Some Linguistic Structures in the Speech of a Broca's Aphasic." *Cortex* 8:191–212.

Goodglass, H., and Kaplan, E. (1983). *The Assessment of Aphasia and Related Disorders.* Philadelphia, PA: Lea and Febiger.

Granger, C., and Albrecht, G. (1979). "Outcome of Comprehensive Medical Rehabilitation: Measurement by PULSES Profile and Barthel Index." *Archives of Physical Medicine and Rehabilitation* 60:145–154.

Gurland, B. J., Copeland, J., Sharpe, L., and Kelleher, M. (1976). "The Geriatric Mental Status Interview (GMS)." *International Journal of Aging and Human Development* 7:303–311.

Hagen, C. (1984). "Language Disorders in Head Trauma." In *Language Disorders in Adults: Recent Advances,* ed. A. Holland (San Diego, CA: College-Hill).

Halstead, W. C., and Wepman, J. M. (1949). "The Halstead-Wepman Aphasia Screening Test." *Journal of Speech and Hearing Disorders* 14:9–15.

Harvey, R., and Jellinek, H. (1983). "Patient Profiles: Utilization in Functional Performance Assessment." *Archives of Physical Medicine and Rehabilitation* 64:268–271.

Haynes, W., and Greenberg, B. (1976). *Understanding Aphasia.* Danville, IL: Interstate Printers and Publishers.

Helm-Estabrooks, N., Ramsberger, G., Morgan, A. R., and Nicholas, M. (1989). *Boston Assessment of Severe Aphasia.* Austin, TX: Pro-Ed.

Helmick, J., Watamori, T., and Palmer, J. (1976). "Spouses' Understanding of the Communication Disorders of Aphasic Patients." *Journal of Speech and Hearing Disorders* 41:238–243.

Holland, A. (1977). "Comment on Spouses' Understanding of the Communication Disorders of Aphasic Patients." *Journal of Speech and Hearing Disorders* 42:307–308.

Holland, A. (1980). *Communicative Abilities in Daily Living.* Baltimore, MD: University Park Press.

Hooper, E. (1958). *The Hooper Visual Organization Test.* Los Angeles, CA: Western Psychological Services.

Jenkins, J., Jiménez-Pabón, E., Shaw, R., and Sefer, J. W. (1975). *Aphasia in Adults.* 2nd ed. New York: Harper and Row.

Johns, D. (1978). *Clinical Management of Neurogenic Communicative Disorders.* Boston: Little, Brown.

Johnson, G. O., and Boyd, H. F. (1981). *Nonverbal Test of Cognitive Skills.* Columbus, OH: Charles E. Merrill.

Kaplan, E., Goodglass, H., and Weintraub, S. (1976). *Boston Naming Test.* Philadelphia, PA: Lea and Febiger.

Kaplan, E., Goodglass, H., and Weintraub, S. (1983). *Boston Naming Test.* Philadelphia, PA: Lea and Febiger.

Keenan, J., and Brassell, E. (1974). "A Study of Factors Related to Prognosis for Individual Aphasic Patients." *Journal of Speech and Hearing Disorders* 39:257–269.

Keenan, J., and Brassell, E. (1975). *Aphasia Language Performance Scales.* Murfreesboro, TN: Pinnacle Press.

Kertesz, A. (1979). *Aphasia and Associated Disorders: Taxonomy, Localization and Recovery.* New York: Grune and Stratton.

Kertesz, A. (1980). *Western Aphasia Battery.* London, Ontario: University of Western Ontario.

Kertesz, A., and McCabe, P. (1977). "Recovery Patterns and Prognosis in Aphasia." *Brain* 100:1–18.

Kinsella, G., and Duffy, F. (1978). "The Spouse of the Aphasic Patient." In *The Management of Aphasia,* eds. Y. LeBrun and R. Hoops (Amsterdam: Swets and Zeitlinger).

Kirk, S. A., McCarthy, J., and Kirk, W. D. (1968). *Illinois Test of Psycholinguistic Abilities.* Champaign, IL: University of Illinois Press.

LaPointe, L., and Horner, J. (1978). "The Functional Auditory Comprehension Task (FACT): Protocol and Test Format." *FLASHA Journal* (Spring): 27–33.

LaPointe, L., and Horner, J. (1979). *Reading Comprehension Battery for Aphasia.* Austin, TX: Pro-Ed.

Leutenegger, R. (1975). *Patient Care and Rehabilitation of Communication Impaired Adults.* Springfield, IL: Charles C. Thomas.

Levin, H. S., O'Donnell, V. M., and Grossman, R. G. (1979). "The Galveston Orientation and Amnesia Test: A Practical Scale to Assess Cognition after Head Injury." *Journal of Nervous System and Mental Disorders* 167:675–684.

Lezak, M. D. (1983). *Neuropsychological Assessment.* 2nd ed. New York: Oxford University Press.

Linebaugh, C., and Lehner, L. (1977). "Cueing Hierarchies and Word Retrieval: A Therapy Program." In *Clinical Aphasiology: Conference Proceedings,* ed. R. Brookshire (Minneapolis, MN: BRK Publishers).

Lomas, J., Pickard, L., Bester, S., Elbard, H., Finlayson, A., and Zoghaib, C. (1989). "The Communicative Effectiveness Index: Development and Psychometric Evaluation of a Functional Communication Measure for Adult Aphasia." *Journal of Speech and Hearing Disorders* 54: 113–124.

McDearmon, J., and Potter, R. (1975). "The Use of Representational Prompts in Aphasia Therapy." *Journal of Communication Disorders* 8:199–206.

McNeil, M., and Prescott, T. (1978). *Revised Token Test.* Baltimore, MD: University Park Press.

Marquardt, T. P. (1982). *Acquired Neurogenic Disorders.* Englewood Cliffs, NJ: Prentice Hall.

Marshall, R., and Phillips, D. (1983). "Prognosis for Improved Verbal Communication in Aphasic Stroke Patients." *Archives of Physical Medicine and Rehabilitation* 64:597–600.

Mattis, S. (1976). "Mental Status Examination for Organic Mental Syndrome in the Elderly Patient." In *Geriatric Psychiatry,* ed. R. Bellack and B. Karasu (New York: Grune and Stratton).

Metter, E. J., and Hanson, W. R. (1985). "Brain Imaging as Related to Speech and Language." In *Speech and Language Evaluation in Neurology: Adult Disorders,* ed. J. K. Darby (Orlando, FL: Grune and Stratton).

Muller, D., Code, C., and Mugford, J. (1983). "Predicting Psychosocial Adjustment to Aphasia." *British Journal of Disorders of Communication* 18:23–29.

Myers, P. S. (1984). "Right Hemisphere Impairment." In *Language Disorders in Adults: Recent Advances,* ed. A. L. Holland (San Diego, CA: College-Hill).

Nation, J., and Aram, D. (1977). *Diagnosis of Speech and Language Disorders.* St. Louis, MO: Mosby.

Pimental, P. A., and Kingsbury, N. A. (1989). *Mini Inventory of Right Brain Injury.* Austin, TX: Pro-Ed.

Plutchik, R., Conte, H., Lieberman, M., Bakur, M., Grossman, J., and Lehrman, N. (1970). "Reliability and Validity of a Scale for Assessing the Function of Geriatric Patients." *Journal of the American Geriatrics Society* 18:491–500.

Porch, B. (1981). *Porch Index of Communicative Ability.* Austin, TX: Pro-Ed.

Porter, J., and Dabul B. (1977). "The Application of Transactional Analysis to Therapy with Wives of Adult Aphasic Patients." *Journal of the American Speech and Hearing Association* 19:244–248.

Powell, G., Bailey, S., and Clark, E. (1980). "A Very Short Form of the Minnesota Aphasia Test." *British Journal of Social and Clinical Psychology* 19:189–194.

Powell, L., and Courtice, K. (1983). *Alzheimer's Disease.* Reading, MA: Addison-Wesley.

Raven, J. (1963). *Guide to Using the Coloured Progressive Matrices: Sets A, B, Ab.* London: H. K. Lewis.

Reisberg, B., Ferris, S. H., and Crook, T. (1982). "Signs, Symptoms, and Course of Age-Associated Cognitive Decline." In *Aging,* Vol. 19, *Alzheimer's Disease: A Report of Progress,* ed. S. Corkin, K. L. Davis, J. H. Growdon, E. Usdin, and R. L. Wurtman (New York: Raven Press).

Reyes, B. (1995). "Considerations in the Assessment and Treatment of Neurogenic Communication Disorders in Bilingual Adults." In

Bilingual Speech-Language Pathology: An Hispanic Focus, ed. H. Kayser (San Diego, CA: Singular Publishing).

Rosenbek, J. C., LaPointe, L., and Wertz, R. T. (1989). *Aphasia: A Clinical Approach.* Boston: College-Hill.

Ross, J. D., and Ross C. M. (1976). *Ross Test of Higher Cognitive Processes.* Novato, CA: Academic Therapy Publications.

Ross-Swain, D., and Fogle, P. (1996). *Ross Information Processing Assessment-Geriatric.* Austin, TX: Pro-Ed.

Rustad, R. A., DeGroot, T. L., Jungkunz, M. L., Freeberg, K. S., Borowick, L. G., and Wanttie, A. M. (1993). *The Cognitive Assessment of Minnesota.* Tucson, AZ: Therapy Skill Builders.

Sarno, J., and Sarno, M. (1973). "The Functional Life Scale." *Archives of Physical Medicine and Rehabilitation* 54:214–220.

Sarno, M. T. (1969). *Functional Communication Profile.* New York: Institute of Rehabilitation Medicine.

Sarno, M. T., Silverman, M., and Sands, E. (1970). "Speech Therapy and Language Recovery in Severe Aphasia." *Journal of Speech and Hearing Disorders* 13:607–623.

Schuell, H. (1957). "A Short Examination for Aphasia." *Neurology* 7:625–634.

Schuell H. (1966). "A Re-evaluation of the Short Examination for Aphasia." *Journal of Speech and Hearing Disorders* 31:137–147.

Schuell, H. (1973). *The Minnesota Test for Differential Diagnosis of Aphasia.* Minneapolis, MN: University of Minnesota Press.

Schuell, H., Jenkins, J., and Jiménez-Pabón, E. (1964). *Aphasia in Adults.* New York: Harper and Row.

Shewan, C. M. (1980). *Auditory Comprehension Test for Sentences.* Chicago, IL: Biolinguistics Clinical Institutes.

Shewan, C. M., and Bandur, D. L. (1986). *Treatment of Aphasia: A Language-Oriented Approach.* San Diego, CA: College-Hill.

Sklar, M. (1966). *Sklar Aphasia Scale.* Los Angeles, CA: Western Psychological Services.

Spellacy, F., and Spreen, O. (1969). "A Short Form of the Token Test." *Cortex* 5:390–397.

Spreen, O., and Benton, A. (1977). *Neurosensory Center Comprehensive Examination for Aphasia.* Victoria, BC: University of Victoria.

Taylor, M. (1963). *Functional Communication Profile.* New York: New York University Medical Center.

Tifosky, R. (1984). "Assessment of Aphasic Disorders." In *Adult Aphasia,* ed. J. Eisenson (Englewood Cliffs, NJ: Prentice Hall).

Tompkins, C. A. (1995). *Right Hemisphere Communication Disorders: Theory and Management.* San Diego, CA: Singular Publishing.

Ulatowska, H. K., and Bond, S. (1983). "Aphasia: Discourse Considerations." *Topics in Language Disorders* 3:21–34.

Ulatowska, H. K., Freedman-Stern, R. F., Doyle, A. W., Macaluso-Haynes, S., and North, A. J. (1983). "Production of Narrative Discourse in Aphasia." *Brain and Language* 19:317–334.

Ulatowska, H. K., Macaluso-Haynes, S., and Mendel-Richardson, S. (1976). "The Assessment of Communicative Competence in Aphasia." In *Clinical Aphasiology Conference Proceedings,* ed. R. H. Brookshire (Minneapolis, MN: BRK Publishers).

Ulatowska, H. K., North, A. J., and Macaluso-Haynes, S. (1981). "Production of Discourse and Communicative Competence in Aphasia." In *Clinical Aphasiology Conference Proceedings,* ed. R. H. Brookshire (Minneapolis, MN: BRK Publishers).

Wallace, G. L. (1993). "Adult Neurogenic Disorders." In *Communication Disorders in Multicultural Populations,* ed. D. E. Battle (Boston, MA: Andover Medical Publishers).

Wechsler, D. (1955). *Manual for the Wechsler Adult Intelligence Scale.* New York: The Psychological Corporation.

Wechsler, D., and Stone, C. (1948). *Wechsler Memory Scale.* New York: The Psychological Corporation.

Whitney, J. L. (1975). "Developing Aphasics' Use of Compensatory Strategies." Paper presented at the annual convention of the American Speech and Hearing Association, Washington, DC.

Whurr, R. (1983). *Whurr Aphasia Screening Test.* London: M. Phil.

Wisconsin Division of Health (1966). *Communication Status Chart.* Madison, WI: Division of Health.

Chapter 9

Motor Speech Disorders and the Oral Exam

Motor speech disorders is an umbrella term that includes many diverse, neurologically based problems. Those that may come to mind first are the many adult dysarthrias. The cerebral palsies originate in infancy, and the speech impairment that may coexist with the movement disorder is also considered dysarthria. Neuromuscular difficulties may result in swallowing disorders or dysphagia, which may or may not co-occur with speech disorders. Then, there are the apraxias that may affect various parts of the body, in particular the control of oral muscles, leading to oral (nonverbal) apraxia or apraxia of speech (verbal apraxia). All in all we have our work cut out for us in this chapter. In order to adequately cover evaluation and diagnosis of such a broad spectrum of motor disorders, we will discuss each in individual sections of the chapter. This chapter also provides the logical place for discussion of "how to do an oral-motor examination" of a patient. Information important to the diagnosis of motor speech disorders will come, in part, from the oral exam. We will, however, attempt to be generic in our discussion of the oral examination to make it applicable for clients of any age (child to adult) or with any speech-language disorder (e.g., articulation, cleft palate, dysarthria). With our territory now laid before us, let us begin our journey.

Apraxia of Speech in Adults

The Greek word *praxis* means action. The performance of action can go awry with damage to the central nervous system, and the resulting disruption of movement control can affect various body parts and abilities (Wertz, LaPointe, and Rosenbek 1984). Limb apraxia, constructional apraxia, and a myriad of apraxic conditions have been reported; we will focus our discussion on apraxia of speech with brief mention of its close cousin, oral (nonverbal) apraxia.

Cortical damage to the inferior-posterior region of the frontal lobe in the left (dominant) hemisphere can impair oral movements and, in particular, articulate speech production. This condition has been called by many names, but is generally known as *apraxia of speech*. Controversy continues as to whether the disturbance in articulatory programming is the *same* as Broca's aphasia, is a condition that *coexists* with Broca's aphasia, or is a condition that can occur in *isolation* of language impairment (Benson 1979; Johns and LaPointe 1976; Martin 1974). Prevailing opinion, and the perspective of this chapter, is that apraxia is a nonlinguistic speech disorder (Darley, Aronson, and Brown 1975; Wertz, LaPointe, and Rosenbek 1984). It can coexist with other disorders and is frequently observed in concert with aphasia and/or dysarthria. Wertz, Rosenbek, and Deal (1970) found that 65 percent of patients with apraxia of speech also demonstrated aphasia, 14 percent had a combination of apraxia, aphasia, and dysarthria, 13 percent had apraxia only, and 8 percent showed apraxia combined with dysarthria. As we shall see, the differential diagnosis of a patient is important in shaping the appropriate management program. Treatment strategies need to be tailored to the specific type(s) of speech motor programming deficit.

The Characteristics of Adult Apraxia of Speech

According to Kent and Rosenbek (1983), apraxia of speech is the impaired volitional production of articulation and prosody. The articulation and prosodic disturbances, however, do not result from muscle weakness or slowness, but from inhibition or impairment of the central nervous system's programming of oral movements. Wertz, LaPointe, and Rosenbek (1984) traced the evolution of our clinical knowledge regarding the characteristics of apraxia of speech and have discarded much of "what we thought we knew." They state the salient, clinical characteristics of apraxia of speech are as follows:

1. *Effortful, trial and error, groping articulatory movements and attempts at self-correction*
2. *Dysprosody unrelieved by extended periods of normal rhythm, stress, and intonation*
3. *Articulatory inconsistency on repeated productions of the same utterance*
4. *Obvious difficulty initiating utterances.*

Many investigators have analyzed articulation error patterns of persons with apraxia of speech. Clinicians hold that substitution errors occur more frequently than do errors of distortion, omission, or addition. Perceptual studies support this observation, but recent acoustical investigations suggest that articulatory distortions are more commonplace. This revelation challenges our traditional differential diagnostic guideline where we once said apraxics make substitution errors while dysarthrics make errors of distortion. Wertz, LaPointe, and Rosenbek (1984) conclude that, in general, apraxic errors are "in the ballpark" rather than being unrelated to the target sounds. Place and manner of articulation errors predominate (e.g. substitution of a /t/ for a /p/ or substitution of a stop for a fricative), and patients are more likely to substitute voiceless consonants for voiced ones (rather than the opposite). Sequencing difficulties have long been recognized in apraxia of speech. Anticipatory errors, where a phoneme is replaced by one that occurs later in the word (e.g., "lelo" for "yellow"), are more common than perseverative errors (phoneme replaced by earlier one as in "dred" for "dress"). Metathetic errors (switching phoneme positions as in "tefalone" for "telephone") occur infrequently. Articulatory complexity also affects apraxic errors. Consonant errors are more likely than vowel errors, and more errors occur on consonantal clusters than on single consonants. Affricates and fricatives are more often errored than plosives, laterals, or nasals.

Prosodic disturbances in apraxia of speech have been reported by Wertz, LaPointe, and Rosenbek (1984). These disturbances include a tendency toward equal stress, inappropriate pausing between syllables, restriction or alteration of intonational and loudness contours, and an overall slower speaking rate.

Wertz, LaPointe, and Rosenbek (1984) cite other influences on apraxic error patterns that are important to remember in assessing patients, selecting treatment stimuli, and organizing a treatment hierarchy. We list some of them here.

1. *Articulatory accuracy is better for meaningful than nonmeaningful utterances. In testing, then, the use of nonsense syllables may lead to spuriously high error rates. Treatment stimuli should be meaningful.*
2. *Errors increase as words increase in length. Assessment tasks almost always include length comparisons such as having the patient say "zip–zipper–zippering."*
3. *Errors increase as the distance between successive points of articulation increases. The patient, therefore, is more likely to have articulatory difficulties saying, "school" than "stool."*
4. *Articulatory accuracy is better for automatic-reactive than for volitional-purposive speech. In fact, the concept of "volitional" movement appears central to many definitions of apraxia and to the process of differential assessment. The patient with apraxia often exhibits many motor sequences at the involuntary level but is unable to replicate them voluntarily. (Conversely, the dysarthric patient is consistent in movement problems.) In an evaluation, comparison of error rates is often done during automatic tasks like counting and naming the days of the week, and observing spontaneous reactions such as swearing or commenting "I can't say that" versus more purposive speech such as labeling, repeating, conversing, and the like.*
5. *Articulatory accuracy may be better with combined auditory and visual stimulation rather than using only one modality. In working with patients, then, the instructions often begin with "Listen and watch me."*
6. *Imitative accuracy is better than spontaneous accuracy.*
7. *Articulatory accuracy often improves with consecutive attempts at production.*

Oral, nonverbal apraxia can be described as having problems in making volitional oral movements in the absence of significant paralysis or paresis. For example, the patient may have great difficulty when asked by the clinician to "pucker your lips" but may have no difficulty kissing his/her spouse as they part for the day.

Apraxia of speech and this oral, nonverbal form of apraxia may coexist or may occur independently of each other.

Case History and Prognostic Factors

As with any evaluation, we collect case history information on the patient suspected of having apraxia of speech. It should be pointed out that rarely do we know ahead of time that we are going to evaluate a patient with apraxia. More often than not, we are asked to evaluate a patient who sustained brain damage, and a language assessment is of foremost importance. During the testing for aphasia, we may become aware of a motor speech impairment and may test further to diagnose the specific nature and extent of the impairment.

As far as case history information is concerned, marital status, place of residence, social networks, and the like may influence treatment. Prognostic significance has been attributed to some biographical data, such as age, education, premorbid handedness, occupational status at onset and highest occupational level achieved, and premorbid intelligence (Marquardt 1982; Wertz, LaPointe, and Rosenbek 1984).

Medical information helpful in making a differential diagnosis includes localization evidence of damage to the third frontal convolution and the presence of right hemiplegia. Medical data suggestive of a favorable prognosis are damage from a single episode (no previous history of brain damage), a small lesion confined to Broca's area, recent onset, and absence of coexisting medical/health problems.

The Evaluation of Apraxia

As mentioned previously, seldom do we know ahead of time that a patient is apraxic. The speech-language referral merely mentions a brain-damaged adult, so a multitude of coexisting problems *could* be present: aphasia, intellectual impairment, dysarthria, apraxia, and other possibilities. The job of the SLP is to thoroughly evaluate the patient to identify problem areas as well as strengths. In this way, a diganosis will be arrived at based on the patient's characteristics. It is necessary, therefore, that the clinician be knowledgeable about the characteristics of various speech-language disorders. The clinician should plan a battery of measures but maintain flexibility so that as the patient's performance unfolds, planned tests can be altered and additional items can be added to the battery. A typical starting point is elicitation of a spontaneous speech sample and the administration of an aphasia test (see Chapter 8 for possibilities). As suspicions of motor problems become apparent in the patient's speech attempts, the clinician alters testing plans to investigate in detail the possibility of a motor disorder. Both formal and informal measures can be used. Table 9.1 lists areas to include in a thorough evaluation (Marquardt 1982; Wertz, LaPointe, and Rosenbek 1984). Diagnostic questions should unfold in the mind of the clinician: Is there a clinically significant motor speech problem? If so, is it an apraxia or a dysarthria? Which type of apraxia does the patient have? Does the patient have mixed types of apraxia? Which kind of dysarthria is present? Are coexisting motor disorders present?

TABLE 9.1   Typical Assessment Battery
for the Evaluation of Apraxia

Spontaneous speech sample
Aphasia test
Intelligence, cognitive, memory tests, as needed
Articulation test
Oral-peripheral examination
Apraxia battery

Several of the aphasia tests evaluate the articulatory agility, melodic line, phonemic difficulties, and oral-nonverbal skills of patients. The Boston Diagnostic Aphasia Examination (Goodglass and Kaplan 1983) and the Western Aphasia Battery (Kertesz 1980) are examples. Characteristics of apraxia may become evident through such testing of a patient. A spontaneous speech sample should be analyzed, and an articulation test may be given as well. Of extreme importance is the oral-motor examination. The general oral peripheral examination, which we will discuss at the end of this chapter, is supplemented with motor and articulatory tasks to reveal volitional programming deficits. Such tasks or tests should address oral, nonverbal apraxia and apraxia of speech.

Let us now walk through this evaluation process as it relates to apraxia. Although several so-called tests of apraxia exist, few have adequate psychometric properties and normative data. Only one test is commercially available; others are published in professional journals. These tools therefore should be considered informal yet insightful, rather than formal, standardized tests. The tests available for evaluating apraxia of speech are listed in Table 9.2. Let us highlight the components of a few.

TABLE 9.2   Formal and Informal Tests for
Apraxia of Speech in Adults

Test of oral and limb apraxia
   (DeRenzi, Pieczuro, and Vignolo 1966)

Oral apraxia test
   (Darley, Aronson, and Brown 1975)

Test of verbal, oral, and limb apraxia
   (Rosenbek and Wertz 1976)

Apraxia Battery for Adults
   (Dabul 1979)

An oral movement battery
   (Moore, Rosenbek, and LaPointe 1976)

Tests of integrity and consistency of phoneme production
   (Johns and Darley 1970)

Motor Speech Evaluation
   (Wertz, LaPointe, and Rosenbek 1984)

Early, modern attempts to evaluate oral and limb apraxia were developed by DeRenzi, Pieczuro, and Vignolo (1966). Their test included ten oral and ten limb tasks that patients were asked to perform on command or, if necessary, on imitation. Oral items included such gestures as "Stick out your tongue," "Whistle," "Show how you would kiss someone," and the like. A three-point scale of response accuracy was used, and limited norms were available for this test.

Darley, Aronson, and Brown (1975) modified the oral apraxia portion of DeRenzi's test. The expanded version included twenty oral items, an eleven-point rating scale of response accuracy, and the addition of now-famous long words and phrases for eliciting articulatory difficulties (e.g. "gingerbread," "statistical analysis," "zip–zipper–zippering").

Rosenbek and Wertz (1976) expanded the verbal, oral, and limb battery still more. The oral and limb apraxia sections were not greatly modified; an eleven-point rating system was used. The verbal section, however, incorporated new tasks of vowel prolongation and imitation of syllable sequences, as well as the production of words and phrases. Responses were scored and analyzed for phonemic and prosodic errors.

Dabul (1979) designed the Apraxia Battery for Adults with six subtests: diadochokinetic rate, increasing word length, limb apraxia and oral apraxia, latency and utterance time for polysyllabic words, repeated trials, and an inventory of articulation characteristics of apraxia. A variety of methods are used to score these subtests; scores are then used to complete a checklist of apraxia features and to rate the severity of the patient's impairment from mild to profound.

The Motor Speech Evaluation (Wertz, LaPointe, and Rosenbek 1984) is useful in detecting the presence of apraxia of speech or dysarthria and in rating the severity of the condition. The evaluation includes the following tasks: conversation, vowel prolongation, rapid alternating movements, repetition of multisyllabic words, repeated production of the same word, repetition of words that increase in length, repetition of monosyllabic words that begin and end with the same phoneme, repetition of sentences, counting forward and backward, picture description, and oral reading. Several methods of scoring are suggested by the authors; however, severity is rated on a 1–7 scale, with 1 being equivalent to mild and 7 to severe.

The Apraxia Battery for Adults (Dabul 1979) and the Motor Speech Evaluation (Wertz, LaPointe, and Rosenbek 1984) are probably the most widely used instruments for the assessment of apraxia of speech. In using evaluation tools to diagnose a patient, we need to remember the important maxim: A test does not make the decision; a clinician does. There is an art to assessing the motor responses of patients on so-called tests of apraxia. Although attempts have been made to scale or rate the level of accuracy, all such scoring remains subjective. The clinician has a responsibility to evaluate and interpret the patients' efforts competently.

Differentiating Apraxia from Other Disorders

As we stated earlier, apraxia of speech often coexists with other disorders of communication. Differential diagnosis of the many components of a patient's problem is of paramount importance.

Apraxia is often differentiated from aphasia on the basis of the patient's relatively normal auditory comprehension as compared to oral expression difficulties. In actuality, this differentiation is clear-cut for some forms of aphasia but is quite muddled for others. Recall that apraxia of speech often co-occurs with Broca's aphasia. Rosenbek, LaPointe, and Wertz (1989) explain the issue this way:

> *Goodglass and Kaplan's (1983) rating scale of speech characteristics shows Broca's aphasic patients have disrupted melodic line and articulatory agility. We consider these signify disturbed prosody and the effortful, groping articulatory movements, articulatory inconsistency, and difficulty initiating utterances that constitute apraxia of speech. The short phrase length, disrupted grammatical form, tendency to produce primarily content words, word-finding problems, and mild auditory comprehension deficits represent Broca's aphasia. Thus, two disorders, apraxia of speech and Broca's aphasia, coexist. Some have difficulty in accepting the coexistence of disorders and elect to combine all symptoms into one disorder, Broca's aphasia. (88)*

On occasion, patients with apraxia of speech have sufficient phrase length and grammatical form to appear somewhat "fluent," despite their prosodic and articulatory difficulties. Errors may mimic literal paraphasias. Table 9.3 summarizes symptoms that differentiate apraxia from fluent, conduction aphasia, as discussed by Rosenbek, LaPointe, and Wertz (1989).

Apraxia is differentiated from the language of confusion and generalized intellectual deterioration on the basis of more intact orientation, memory, and learning abilities. The reader should refer to Table 8.5 from Chapter 8 for examples of cognitive tests that might be used to make such a differential diagnosis.

Apraxia, classically, is differentiated from dysarthria by the preponderance of phonemic substitutions compared to distortion errors (Johns and Darley 1970) and intact neuromuscular functioning with the exception of facial weakness and hemiplegia. Table 9.4 provides information useful in making a differential diagnosis of dysarthria and apraxia of speech.

Patients with apraxia of speech can generally anticipate their errors and can also recognize them once emitted. Perhaps this explains, in part, the many retrials and false starts heard in the speech of apraxics. The effortful articulatory groping and repetitive attempts may, at times, be reminiscent of stuttering secondary

TABLE 9.3   Differential Diagnosis of Conduction Aphasia and Apraxia

Conduction Aphasia	Apraxia
High proportion of sequencing errors	Low proportion of sequencing errors
Unpredictable substitutions	Predictable substitutions
Intact prosody	Abnormal prosody
Easy speech initiation	Difficult speech initiation, often struggled
Association with posterior brain lesion	Association with anterior brain lesion

TABLE 9.4   Differential Diagnosis of Dysarthria and Apraxia

	Dysarthria	Apraxia
Definition	There are distinct patterns of speech owing to weakness, slowness and incoordination of speech muscles. Oral movements are disrupted and reflect different types of neuropathology.	There are articulation errors, in the absence of muscle slowness, weakness, incoordination, owing to disruption of cortical programming for the *voluntary* production of speech sounds
Oral peripheral examination	There is obvious defectiveness: slow, weak, and incoordinated. *Vegetative* functions (sucking, chewing), as well as speech movements, are disturbed.	There is no obvious dysfunction except when person is asked to execute *voluntary* movements. Vegetative functions are performed adequately.
Articulation	There is simplification: a. Distortions b. Substitutions Errors are consistent. More complex units (clusters of consonants) are more difficult. There are more errors in final position. Errors are consistent with neurological record. Severity is related to extent of neuromuscular involvement.	Complications are: a. Transpositions, reversals b. Perseverative and anticipatory errors c. Fewer distortions, more substitutions, intrusive additions Errors increase proportionate to word weight (grammatical class, difficulty of initial consonant, position in sentence and word length). There are fewer errors in spontaneous performance. Inconsistency is key sign.
Repeated utterance	Same performance obtains.	Person makes repeated attempts and may achieve correct performance. Person appears to grope or struggle for correct production.
Rate	There is deterioration of performance with increased rate. There is slow rate of speech.	Performance improves at faster rate. There are disturbances of prosody: stutteringlike struggle reactions; slow, labored speech during voluntary attempts.
Response to stimulation	Person may alter performance slightly to match auditory-visual model. Best response is to demonstration of specific articulatory gestures.	Best performance obtains if person sees and hears model. Person does better if provided one stimulation and given several chances to match the model.

behaviors. This raises the question of a relationship between neurogenic stuttering (see Chapter 7) and apraxia of speech. Although we do not know the nature of this relationship, if any, it is worth considering in making a differential diagnosis.

Case Example. *Mr. Nils Elander was referred to the hospital-based speech-language pathologist for testing. Evidence from the neuroradiology department showed a left hemisphere thromboembolic infarct. Speech and language improvement was rapid during the two weeks postinfarct. A predischarge reevaluation was performed by the clinician. Mr. Elander presented with mild Broca's aphasia and a moderate coexisting apraxia of speech. Numerous techniques were tried on a trial and error basis to see what stimulation and assistance aided Mr. Elander in initiating difficult words that occurred randomly, as well as at the beginning of utterances. The clinician was able to refer Mr. Elander for out-patient treatment at another facility. The report forwarded to that facility included specific recommendations as to the future direction of treatment. These recomendations included multimodality prestimulation, first phoneme cueing, and use of baton gestures or finger-tapping to impose rhythmical fluency.*

Developmental Apraxia of Speech

Developmental apraxia of speech is a poorly understood and controversial speech disorder in children. These children typically have little or no intelligible speech, yet they seem to posess adequate language comprehension skills and intelligence. Additionally, there is no clear evidence of muscular paresis or paralysis. The term *apraxia*, itself, emphasizes that these children have articulatory or motor programming deficits rather than any central language impairment. Presumably, the brain damage leading to these speech difficulties occurred before the onset of speech development, hence the diagnostic label of *developmental apraxia.*

Differential Diagnosis

Yoss and Darley (1974), in a classic article on the topic, reported that five predictors help differentiate developmental apraxia of speech from more typical "defective articulation" disorders. These predictors are as follows:

1. Neurologic findings, such as difficulty in fine motor coordination, gait, and alternating motion rates of the tongue and extremities (often manifested as a generalized dyspraxia)
2. Two- and three-feature articulation errors (for example, /p/ for /ð/ involves an error in place, voicing, and continuancy), prolongations and repetitions of sounds and syllables, distortions, and additions in repeated speech tasks
3. Distortions, omissions, additions, and one-place errors in spontaneous speech
4. Slower than normal rate on measurements of oral diadochokinesis
5. Poor maintenance of syllable sequences and shapes; polysyllabic words altered by addition, omission, or revision of syllables.

Yoss and Darley also reported that children with developmental apraxia of speech make more errors involving the voiced/voiceless feature than do children with defective articulation and that slower rates and equalization of stress patterns disrupt prosody. They often found coexisting oral apraxia in the children, as evidenced by difficulty performing volitional oral movements, such as puckering or biting the lower lip.

Crary (1988) elaborates on the symptomatology, stating that children with developmental apraxia exhibit slow and irregular alternating motion rates (diadochokinesis). They possess a reduced sound inventory, including vowels, and have obvious prosodic deficits, including slow rate, excess stress, prolonged sounds and pauses, postural/articulatory groping, and unusual intonational contours.

Other authors have cited nasal resonance and nasal emission as characteristics of developmental apraxia of speech (Hall, Hardy, and LaVelle 1990; Morley 1957). Presumably, the velopharyngeal mechanism performs inadequately during complex, rapid, sequential speech. Nasality, then, is more pronounced with conversational speech as opposed to single-word utterances.

Prognosis

Yoss and Darley (1974), after reviewing the literature and case study presentations, report that treatment involves "an inordinate amount" of time with minimal improvements being achieved. The children reportedly seldom carry over to contextual speech the level of self-monitoring attained at the syllable and single-word levels in the treatment program. Sequencing difficulties, at the heart of the disorder, appear to hinder progress in all realms.

Blakeley (1983) believes that parents should be advised of the nature and severity of their child's apraxia of speech and should be given an estimate of the number of years that speech habilitation may take. Blakeley states that three to ten years of treatment are likely. As adults, these individuals may continue to have difficulty with motorically complex words.

Crary (1988) also discussed the prognosis for the future of a child with developmental apraxia of speech. He says that about 40 to 50 percent of these children are at risk for subsequent academic difficulties. Reading and writing skills seem to be particularly affected.

Case History Indicators

Square and Weidner (1981) reviewed case history information on children diagnosed as having developmental apraxia of speech and found some commonalities. Parents reported that auditory responses of the infants seemed normal but that early vocal patterns were suspect. The parents often said little, if any, babbling occurred. If babbling was done by the infant, parents reported its phonetic pattern to have been undifferentiated. The infant was often described as a "quiet baby." Feeding differences were also reported by the mothers. Babies were said to prefer liquids and soft foods. Some were described as "lazy chewers." As regards general motor development, reports suggest clumsiness, developmental immaturity, and possible "soft" neurological signs. As a toddler, there remained little or no attempt to imitate sounds or words.

Assessing Developmental Apraxia

Miller (1986), recognizing the ill-defined nature of developmental apraxia, states that assessment is a process of excluding other disorders and including, or identifying, apraxic signs and symptoms. Miller calls for a multidisciplinary evaluation of the child. The medical evaluation will seek to exclude other causes of the motor impairment, such as neoplastic disease, degenerative conditions, cerebral palsy, acquired CNS damage, and the like. The psychological evaluation will exclude general mental retardation, autism, and behavioral-emotional problems (however, it is recognized that behavioral problems are often a consequence of the child's apraxia). The primary sensorimotor evaluation will exclude problems of muscular tone, strength, speed, and sensation. Miller goes on to discuss numerous subtests that may be part of an extensive assessment battery. The interested reader is referred to this detailed discussion.

Commercially available, the Screening Test for Developmental Apraxia of Speech (Blakeley 1980) is useful with children ages four through twelve. It assesses expressive language discrepancy, vowels and diphthongs, oral-motor movement, verbal sequencing, motorically complex words, articulation, transpositions, and prosody.

Crary (1988) suggests areas important for the SLP to tap in the assessment of developmental apraxia of speech. We have summarized these areas into a list, displayed in Table 9.5. We concur completely with his evaluation suggestions.

TABLE 9.5   Areas to Assess in Development Apraxia

Motor Assessment

Facial/limb praxis
Oral apraxia on simple and complex tasks
Lingua-mandibular and labial-mandibular synkinesis
Velar function
Oral reflexes
Facial mimicry tasks

Motor-Speech Assessment

Diadochokinesis
Nasal resonance (and further tests, if noted)
Standard articulation tests
Phonological analysis (distinctive features and phonological error processes)

Prosody Assessment

Stress patterns
Intonation patterns
General fluency and articulatory flow

Language Assessment(s)

Auditory memory assessment

Let us now describe the assessment procedure advocated by Square and Weidner (1981). Pertinent topics to discuss with parents in the case history interview include the early vocal patterns used during infancy (babbling), feeding difficulties, and general motor development. The evaluation of the child incorporates both speech and nonspeech tasks. Regarding speech tasks, a spontaneous speech sample should be analyzed. A traditional articulation test may be given, as well as the spontaneous "tell a story" version available with many articulation tests. Next, the clinician engages the child in various repeated speech tasks. Have the client repeat CVC words using frequently occurring and complex consonants, such as /f, k, l, r, z, s, v, g, ʃ, θ, tʃ, ʒ/. Sample CVC words include: *lake, sack, shoes, thick,* and *chop.* Next, have the client repeat CVC nonsense syllables using the same consonants. Using the carrier phrase, "I had a _____," have the client repeat polysyllabic words, such as *butterfly, popsicle, hamburger, mosquito, basketball, firetruck,* and so forth. Finally, do diadochokinetic testing, in the usual manner. The nonspeech tasks recommended by Square and Weidner are volitional oral movements and sequential volitional oral movements (both two- and three-item sequences). Table 9.6 lists some suggested nonspeech oral movements for the client to perform.

We would like to conclude this section with a reminder. In testing for developmental apraxia of speech, the clinician must, among other things, carefully observe the level of articulatory effort and the pattern of errors that the client makes.

TABLE 9.6 Nonspeech Tasks for Assessing Developmental Apraxia

Volitional Oral Movements

Stick out your tongue.
Try to touch your nose with your tongue.
Try to touch your chin with you tongue.
Bite your lower lip.
Pucker your lips.
Puff out your cheeks.
Show me your teeth.
Click your teeth together.
Wag your tongue from side to side.
Clear your throat.
Cough.
Whistle.
Show me that you're cold by making your teeth chatter.
Smile.
Show me how you would kiss a baby.
Lick your lips.

Sequenced Volitional Oral Movements: Two Items

Puff your cheeks, then smile.
Pucker your lips, then wag your tongue.

Sequenced Volitional Oral Movements: Three Items

Puff out your cheeks, show me your teeth, then pucker your lips.

No test score will indicate a diagnosis of apraxia. The decision rests with the diagnostic skill, albeit somewhat subjective, of the SLP.

The Adult Dysarthrias

All the diverse structures and systems that combine to produce speech are planned and regulated by the nervous system. Any damage or disease involving this regulatory system may disrupt the processes of respiration, phonation, articulation, and resonation and thus ultimately affect the normally swift movements of the speech mechanism. Two types of motor speech disorders are apraxia of speech, which we have discussed, and dysarthria. Let us now turn our attention to a discussion of the clinical forms of dysarthria.

As defined by Marquardt (1982), *dysarthrias* are neuromuscular speech disorders arising from motor pathway damage at singular or multiple sites from the cortex to the muscle. The entire speech production mechanism, including respiratory, phonatory, articulatory, and resonatory processes may be affected (as in Parkinson's disease). Likewise, disruption may be confined to specific musculature (as in Bell's palsy of the face).

Differential Diagnosis

Novice clinicians often have difficulty differentiating the two motor speech disorders: apraxia and dysarthria. The underlying neuromotor impairment is clearly different and site of lesion knowledge will go far in sorting out the two possibilities. Yet, going only on clinical (behavioral) signs that the patient displays, the diagnosis is not nearly as clear-cut as many textbooks imply. Review Table 9.4, which lists distinguishing characteristics of patients with apraxia of speech and dysarthria. Complicating the differential diagnosis is the fact that the two disorders can co-occur.

Differential diagnosing also involves categorizing the patient's symptoms by type of dysarthria. Again, this often proves to be a difficult task for many clinicians, not just the novice student. The type of dysarthria demonstrated will depend upon the site of lesion within the motor pathways. The landmark investigation that delineated the types of dysarthria, prominent speech dimensions, and neurological disruption was conducted at the Mayo Clinic and published in the book *Motor Speech Disorders* (Darley, Aronson, and Brown 1975). An understanding of the types of dysarthria is paramount to the assessment process and the differential diagnosis. Using the information from this book, we present a synopsis of the characteristics of each type of dysarthria. We are assuming, however, that the reader has an understanding of the nervous system and neuroanatomical terminology.

Flaccid Dysarthria
Flaccid dysarthrias result from disorders (or lesions) of the lower motor neuron system. The muscle-movement problem may be progressive, as in myasthenia gravis, or may affect the bulbar motor units, as in the bulbar palsies. In bulbar palsy, a

common form of flaccid dysarthria, the muscles are weak, hypotonic (flaccid), and hyporeflexive and may be atrophied. Spontaneous twitches or dimpling of the skin over the muscle may be noted (fasciculations and fibrillations). Often the bulbar palsy is due to damage of one cranial nerve, and the muscular problems are confined to the body region or group of muscles served by that nerve. For example, in facial palsy (also known as Bell's palsy), the damage to one of the facial nerves (cranial nerve VII) results in a drooping facial expression, inability to raise the corner of the mouth during a smile, infrequent blinking, lowering of the eyebrow, and inability to wrinkle the forehead on the affected side. In hypoglossal palsy, there is damage to cranial nerve XII, and the tongue becomes flabby, atrophied/shrunken, and wrinkled. The client will be unable to perform many of the tongue maneuvers asked during the oral peripheral examination. Damage may be due to multiple cranial nerve involvement as well. This type of flaccid dysarthria is known as generalized bulbar palsy. It would not be uncommon in this condition for the lips, tongue, jaw, velum, pharynx, and larynx to be affected in varying degrees.

Speech abnormalities that are often observed in the bulbar palsies include hypernasality, imprecise articulation of consonants, breathiness, monopitch, and nasal emission. Other characteristics are certainly seen in these patients. We have only attempted to highlight some of the most prominent.

Spastic Dysarthria

Spastic dysarthrias result from disorders of the upper motor neuron system—in particular, the pyramidal system. As a result, there can be whole extremity damage (as in cortical lesions) or generalized damage (as from lesions of the internal capsule). The damage may be unilateral, as often seen following a stroke where the patient has aphasia and hemiparesis, or the damage may be bilateral. If bilateral, we often use the classification *pseudobulbar palsy*, as the bulbar system is affected indirectly. Muscular symptoms include spasticity, weakness, limited range of motion, slowness of movement, and hyperreflexia.

Deviant speech dimensions include imprecise consonant articulation, monopitch, reduced stress, harsh voice quality, monoloudness, low-pitched voice, and slow speech rates. Again, we have only attempted to list some of the more prominent and severe symptoms.

Ataxic Dysarthria

Disease or damage to the cerebellum can result in ataxic dysarthria. In ataxia, there is inaccuracy of movement (affecting force, range, timing, and direction of movements), slowness of movement, and hypotonia (flabby muscles). Speech characteristics include imprecise consonant articulation, use of excess and equal stress patterns, and irregular articulatory breakdowns, among others.

Hypokinetic Dysarthria

Disorders of the extrapyramidal system, such as in the basal ganglia complex, often result in hypokinesia, a reduction of movement. A commonly encountered disease causing hypokinesia is Parkinson's. There seem to be six characteristic signs of hypokinetic dysarthria: (1) slowness of movement; (2) limited range of motion; (3) paucity of movement, where the patient may have difficulty initiating a movement and may experience false starts, arrests of movement, or even immobility; (4) rigidity or hypertonicity (may be intermittent); (5) loss of automatic aspects of movement; and (6) presence of rest tremors. Deviant speech dimensions often seen in patients with Parkinsonism highlight the movement difficulties of the hypokinetic dysarthrias. The most deviant are monopitch, reduced stress patterns, monoloudness, imprecise consonant articulation, inappropriate silences, and short rushes of speech. Other, less deviant characteristics exist as well.

Hyperkinetic Dysarthria

Hyperkinetic dysarthrias result from disorders of the extrapyramidal system. The hallmark of these disorders is the presence of abnormal involuntary movements—some are quick movements and others are classified as slow. In the short space we have in this textbook, we cannot completely describe the numerous forms of both quick and slow hyperkinesias. The interested reader is urged to study further. We will, however, summarize some of the most distinguishing and deviant speech characteristics, averaged over the various subtypes. These include imprecise consonants, variable (or perhaps slow) rate, monopitch, harsh or strained voice quality, inappropriate silences, distorted vowels, and excess loudness variation.

Mixed Dysarthrias

Mixed dysarthrias, as the name implies, result from involvement of several motor systems. Often mixed dysarthrias are associated with syndromes or particular diseases, such as amyotrophic lateral sclerosis, multiple sclerosis, and Wilson's disease. Owing to the mixed nature of these dysarthrias, it is almost impossible to summarize characteristic speech disturbances. The reader is again urged to study this vast topic further. Books about adult dysarthrias include those by Darley, Aronson, and Brown (1975), Marquardt (1982), McNeil, Rosenbek, and Aronson (1984), Perkins (1983), and Yorkston, Beukelman, and Bell (1988).

The Appraisal of Dysarthria

As evident from the various speech characteristics associated with the types of dysarthria, the patient may have difficulty with any or all of the speech production processes. Consequently, the clinician must assess features of respiration, phonation, articulation, and resonation.

Such an appraisal follows along the lines of a voice evaluation. This topic will be dealt with more thoroughly in Chapters 10 and 12. Suffice it to say that we need to take note of any inhalatory noises, poor breath support, poor management of the airstream, abnormal vocal loudness and stress patterns, abnormal vocal pitch and inflectional patterns, and abnormal vocal-resonatory qualities.

Regarding the articulatory impairment that is often present in the dysarthrias, the clinician should analyze a sample of spontaneous speech and/or have the patient read aloud. Standard articulation tests, either single-word or sentence versions, are also useful in documenting phoneme errors. Distortion is the most common articulatory error in dysarthric speech. Unlike the difficulties seen in apraxia of speech, the imprecision of consonantal articulation is usually consistent in dysarthria.

In addition to the voice test (which includes appraisal of respiration, phonation, and resonation) and the articulatory assessment, a thorough evaluation of a patient with dysarthria should include an oral peripheral examination and a special "dysarthria test," which involves appraisal of both speech and nonspeech motor functions. So-called tests of dysarthria are helpful in assessing the severity of the disorder, as well as the type of dysarthria.

The thirty-eight speech dimensions used in the original Mayo Clinic study may be rated by the clinician (Darley, Aronson, and Brown 1975). A patient's speech performance is rated on each dimension using a seven-point equal-appearing interval scale of severity (1 = normal, 7 = very severe). The thirty-eight dimensions pertain to pitch, loudness, vocal quality, respiration, prosody, articulation, and an overall or general impression of intelligibility and bizarreness.

Although there is no score or profiling system, per se, the clinician can match a patient's performance to the "standard" characteristics and thereby determine the type of dysarthria. We would add that the rating of all thirty-eight dimensions is likely to be time consuming.

The Frenchay Dysarthria Assessment (Enderby 1980; 1983) profiles oral-motor performance for the various diagnostic categories, such as spastic—upper motor neuron, flaccid—lower motor neuron, extrapyramidal, cerebellar, and mixed neurological lesions. Clinicians may find this helpful in differential diagnosis decision making. Normed on patients aged twelve to adult, performances are rated on eleven sections: reflex, respiration, lips, jaw, palate, laryngeal, tongue, intelligibility, rate, sensation, and associated factors.

The Motor Speech Evaluation (Wertz, LaPointe, and Rosenbek 1984) is useful in detecting the presence of apraxia of speech or dysarthria. A severity rating is also generated on a scale of 1 (mild) to 7 (severe). The components of this test were discussed earlier in the chapter as part of the adult apraxia section, and we will not repeat that information here.

The Assessment of Intelligibility of Dysarthric Speech (Yorkston and Beukelman 1981) has the patient read words and sentences. Several measures can be derived, including intelligibility for single words, intelligibility for sentences, speech rate, rate of intelligible speech, rate of unintelligible speech, and a communication efficiency ratio. Classification by type of dysarthria is also possible with this test. Also available is the Computerized Assessment of Intelligibility of Dysarthric Speech (Yorkston, Beukelman, and Traynor 1984). The software provides for efficient quantifying of single-word intelligibility, sentence intelligibility, and speaking rates without tedious stimuli selection or computation.

One diagnostic task to which many authorities attribute importance is that of diadochokinetic testing, also known as assessing alternating motion rates (AMRs). Darley, Aronson, and Brown (1975), in particular, state that the rhythm and speed with which alternating motion rates can be performed are helpful in sorting out the various types of dysarthrias. They acknowledge that differential diagnosis may be difficult from only a conversational sample of speech. AMRs, on the other hand, seem to "stress" the motor system and, consequently, reveal the difficulties of movement more clearly.

Diadochokinesis, or AMRs, typically involves the repetition of the sounds "puh," "tuh," and "kuh" as fast and evenly as possible. The instructions to the patient should stress this notion of "fast and even." Information that is important to the clinician includes the rate, regularity, and duration of the alternate movements of the articulators.

According to Darley, Aronson, and Brown (1975), a slow, regular diadochokinetic rate is highlighted in spasticity. For ataxia, alternate motion rates underscore the irregular breakdowns in articulatory precision. It is characteristic to hear fluctuating changes in the intervals between syllables, as well as variations in their duration and loudness. Rate of syllable production varies from normal to slow. In hypokinetic Parkinsonism, alternate motion rates may begin at a slow rate and then accelerate to a rapid, yet usually regular, rhythm. Imprecise articulation due to limited excursions of movement (i.e., hypokinesia) may produce the sound of a continuous blur. Hyperkinetic dysarthrias take on many different forms; AMRs are usually irregular, slow, and perhaps interrupted by arrests of speech.

We offer one final note about appraisal. The patient with dysarthria is not expected to have language, cognitive, intellectual, memory, or learning deficits unless such deficits are associated with the disease process that produced the dysarthria. The clinician, however, should be alert to deficits in these areas and should include appropriate language-cognitive tests in the assessment battery, if necessary.

Prognosis

Marquardt (1982) states that no efficacy or prognosis studies have been completed for dysarthria. Prevailing thought, however, is that the prognosis is naturally worse when dysarthria is part of a progressive or degenerative neurological condition. Prognosis should be good when the extent of damage to the nervous system is limited. In addition, prognosis would seem to be affected by the medical treatment applied. Although they do not cure the dysarthria, many pharmacological or surgical treatments can have enormous impact on the patient's motor functioning. Lastly, we believe that the emotional and environmental aspects of the patient shape treatment outcome.

> Case Example. *A 49-year-old male was referred following a bilateral brain stem infarct with resultant quadriplegia and dysarthria. Appraisal procedures included case history, oral peripheral examination, acquisition of a speech sample, recording of a standard reading passage, and auditory testing. The oral peripheral examination revealed bilateral facial and velopharyngeal weakness and weakness of the left side of the tongue. Diadochokinetic rates, intelligibility of conversational*

speech, and intensity and frequency ranges were moderately reduced. Voice qual-
ity was breathy. A moderate bilateral sensorineural hearing loss was present. No
cognitive or language deficits were evident from a mental status examination.
Since there was no indication of hemispheric brain damage and the primary mus-
cular deficit was weakness, the diagnosis was moderate flaccid dysarthria sec-
ondary to brain stem infarct. (Marquardt 1982, 64)

Cerebral Palsies and Dysarthria in Children

Brain damage sustained before, during, or shortly after birth can produce movement
disorders, known as *cerebral palsies*. Movement can be mildly affected or severely
crippled. When the muscles underlying speech are affected, we may say that the person has dysarthria (a motor speech disorder) subsequent to the cerebral palsy.

Although various classification systems for cerebral palsy have been proposed, DiCarlo and Amster (1984) prefer the six principal symptom areas: (1) Spasticity is characterized by hyperactivity of the stretch reflex. It is secondary to a
lesion in the cerebral cortex that causes a loss of control and differentiation of fine
voluntary movements with increased muscle tone. (2) Athetosis is involuntary
writhing or squirming movements that are irregular, coarse, relatively continuous,
and somewhat rhythmic. It is secondary to damage in the extrapyramidal system,
often the basal ganglia complex. (3) Cerebellar ataxia is incoordination and poor
balance owing to cerebellar dysfunction. (4) Rigidity is a "lead pipe" characteristic of affected muscles and often resembles a severe form of spasticity. (5) Tremors,
either athetoid or rigid, involve generalized trembling of the extremities. (6) Flac-
cidity, as a form of cerebral palsy, is due to damage to the sensorimotor cortex. Affected muscles are unable to contract except reflexively. Perhaps 90 percent of the
cases of cerebral palsy are of the first three types, with spasticity overwhelmingly
being the most common (DiCarlo and Amster 1984).

Many excellent sources are available to the interested reader that thoroughly
discuss the multiple aspects of cerebral palsy (Cruickshank and Raus 1966;
McDonald and Chance 1964; Mysak 1980).

The Assessment of a Child with Cerebral Palsy

All authorities on cerebral palsy strongly advocate the multidisciplinary approach
to assessment, diagnosis, and intervention. Certainly the SLP will not assess motor
function and abnormal reflexology without the aid of a physical therapist or other
health care professional. Such information, however, is necessary to shape the feeding and prespeech stimulation programs that the infant may need, the handling and
positioning techniques that need to be applied, and the facilitating and inhibiting
techniques that might be incorporated in the speech rehabilitation program.

The child with cerebral palsy typically presents with a host of impairments—
orthopedic, sensory, intellectual, socioemotional, and so forth. Of interest for this
chapter is the assessment of communication skills and deficits.

DiCarlo and Amster (1984) state that a review of the literature clearly documents that children with cerebral palsy (particularly athetosis) have higher auditory detection thresholds, poorer speech reception thresholds, and poorer speech discrimination than do normal children. A complete audiological evaluation, then, should be part of every evaluation session.

Capute (1974) reports that about 50 to 60 percent of the cerebral palsied population show some degree of mental retardation, while the rest possess normal intellectual capabilities. Impaired language development, learning difficulties, and academic problems often occur in children with cerebral palsy. Etiological reasons may be numerous. Certainly, the SLP must assess cognitive development and linguistic attainment in a cerebral palsied client. Procedures discussed in Chapters 4 and 5 should be utilized.

Speech is a dynamic process requiring highly skilled coordination of the articulatory movements for the production and sequencing of sounds into utterances. It is of no surprise, then, that speech impairments are common among children with cerebral palsy. Hopkins, Bice, and Colton (1954) state that about 70 percent of cerebral palsied children exhibit speech disorders; athetoid and ataxic forms seem to be particularly deleterious to speech. However, there appears to be insufficient evidence for the notion that these speech impairments are so distinctive as to justify the concept of *cerebral palsied speech*. This myth was laid to rest in Chapter 6 when we discussed articulatory and phonological speech disorders. The assessment tools discussed in that chapter are certainly applicable to the child with cerebral palsy. Respiration, phonation, and rhythm are likely to be affected as well and must be assessed by the clinician. The ultimate measure of speech effectiveness is its intelligibility; a severity rating scale may be one aspect of the assessment battery. Lastly, we would remind the clinician that an oral peripheral (oral-motor) examination be done. How to do this is the subject of our next section.

The Oral Peripheral Examination

An examination of a client's oral cavity and surrounding area is a routine part of every speech-language evaluation. Regardless of the client's particular communication impairment, the findings of the oral peripheral examination may help shape a theory of etiology, diagnosis, and prognosis for change and provide a direction that the treatment should take. In order to avoid repetition in the chapters of this book, we thought it best to consolidate our discussion of the oral peripheral examination into one place. Since the oral peripheral examination not only looks at structures but also assesses the function of those structures from a motoric point of view, we thought it most appropriate to include it in our discussion in this chapter on motor speech disorders. Indeed, the oral peripheral examination is often called the oral-motor exam, a reflection of the importance of motoric integrity for normal speech production.

As we said, it is common practice to inspect a client's oral region to determine its structural and functional adequacy for speech. To provide an example of typical data gathered during an oral peripheral examination, we have included notes hastily scribbled during an evaluation of a nine-year-old boy with a hoarse voice and several articulation errors:

> *Lips look okay. No asymmetry of face. Slight open bite; poor dental hygiene (lots of cavities and tartar build-up). Tongue has good mobility, no paralysis or sluggishness; can protrude, wiggle from side to side swiftly, and touch the alveolar ridge; can even curl and groove. Hard palate seems OK, no scars. Soft palate has good tissue supply; elevated fine, no asymmetry. Palatine tonsils are really enlarged, filling the whole isthmus between the fauces. Pharynx looks inflamed (possible postnasal drip?). Good gag reflex. Wonder why he has mandible thrust to left side on /ʃ/ and /tʃ/?*

Note the systematic nature of the inspection. Although the period of observation was relatively brief—an oral examination is generally completed in less than two minutes—the clinician has a sound basis for making a referral to a laryngologist. Now we shall present a rather detailed procedure for conducting an oral examination.

Tools You Will Need

You will need a light source; a small flashlight is good (we avoid the head mirror because it makes us look like a physician). Next, we obtain a supply of wooden tongue depressors; the individually wrapped ones are best for sanitary purposes (and cherry and grape flavored tongue depressors are available in a junior size from the Super Duper School Company, Department C, P.O. Box 24997, Greenville, SC 29616). Since we are living in the age of AIDS and other contagious diseases, the prudent clinician will wear sterile gloves, or at least use a finger cot, when palpating the roof of the client's mouth. Finally, your kit might include several pads of cotton gauze (for holding onto tongues), a few candy suckers, and a mirror. For more elaborate or specialized examinations, additional materials may be needed. These might include cotton-tipped applicators, various flavor vials for taste sensation, oral stereognostic forms, bite blocks, a syringe of water, some cookies or crackers, and the like.

Areas to Be Assessed

It is important to be *systematic* and *swift* when conducting an oral examination. This demands considerable practice. Use every opportunity to scrutinize normal-speaking persons of all ages, not only to perfect your technique and observational skills but also to establish a frame of reference on the range of normal structural and functional variation. The following outline is presented as a guide for conducting a typical oral peripheral examination:

1. *Lips and Lip Movement.* Inspect the lips first for relative size, symmetry, and scars. Can the client smile, pucker his lips, and retract them? Can she close her lips tightly for the sounds /p/, /b/, /m/? Can she utter the nonsense syllable "puh" at least once per second (Fletcher 1972)?

2. *Jaws.* Scrutinize the client's jaw in a state of rest; observe for symmetry. Can he/she open and close his/her mandible at least once per second? Does his/her mandible deviate to the right or the left on opening? Assess mandibular strength by having him/her attempt to open or move his/her jaw laterally against resistance.

3. *Teeth.* Inspect the client's bite during a state of rest. A normal dental bite is characterized by the upper incisors' overlapping the lower incisors by not more than one half of their vertical dimension. Is there an open, under-, or overbite? Does the client have cavities, jumbled teeth, gaps between teeth, or more than the normal complement of teeth? Does he/she wear a dental prosthesis?

4. *Tongue.* Note the size of the tongue relative to the oral cavity. Observe for symmetry of structure and during movement. Is there any scarring, atrophy, or fasciculations? Can the client protrude and retract his/her tongue, wiggle it from side to side, and touch the alveolar ridge without random movement or extraordinary effort? Inspect the tip of tongue and the frenulum for any evidence of tongue tie. (Some clients, especially those presenting with neuromuscular problems, may find it difficult to elevate the tip of their tongue to the alveolar ridge on command. We use a sucker, placing the moistened candy behind the upper incisors and encouraging the client to go after it. A spot of peanut butter or a tiny paper wedged high between the central incisors can also be used.) Can he/she trill his/her tongue when the mandible is stabilized? Test for diadochokinesis by having him/her utter "tuh"; can he/she say one per second? (Norms for diadochokinesis may be found in Bloomquist 1950; Canning and Rose 1974; and Fletcher 1972. Fletcher's norms are commonly used.) Be sure to look for regularity as well as rate in any tongue movement task. Is there any evidence of tongue thrust? (An open bite might alert you to this possibilty.) When he/she swallows, does he/she have an exaggerated lip seal? Does his/her tongue protrude beyond the incisors? Is there no apparent bunching in the masseter muscle? (If the answers to these last three queries are positive, then the client may be a tongue thruster.)

5. *Hard Palate.* Note the shape (is it flat? high and arched?) and width of the hard palate. Are there any scars present? Is there any blue coloration to the palate? Can you palpate solid bone under the tissues at the palatal midline? Can the client produce /r/ and /l/?

6. *Soft Palate and Velopharyngeal Closure.* Inspect the velum for total size, scars, and symmetry of movement. Is it bifid? Look carefully for any variations in color, such as bluish borders or striations. Does the soft palate move back and up toward the posterior pharyngeal wall? What is the size of the velum relative to the depth of the pharynx (= effective velar length)? Estimate the location of the velar dimple (formed by the insertion of velar muscles) and calculate its distance along the velar length (80 percent is normal, less may indicate velopharyngeal inadequacy). Can you visualize lateral movement of the velum? Can the client whistle or puff up his/her cheeks? (Chapter 11 presents details of assessing velopharyngeal competency as it relates to hypernasality and nasal emission.)

7. *Fauces.* Inspect the pillars for scars, the status of the palatine tonsils, and the width of the isthmus. Check the general condition of the oropharynx.

8. *Others.* Observe the client's breathing during speech and at rest. Is there an obstruction of the nasal passages? Is the client a mouth breather? Observe the facial muscles: Is a nasolabial fold flattened? Does an eyelid droop (ptosis)? Is one side of the face smooth and devoid of normal creases? Is there anything unusual about the appearance of the individual's head or spacing of the facial features?

The preceding outline is typical of the methodical process that clinicians do, albeit swiftly, with all clients. Several formalized procedures and recording forms have been developed to assess oral peripheral function for speech. The interested reader is referred to the popular works of Dworkin and Culatta (1980), Mason and Simon (1977), Ruscello et al. (1982), Siegel and Hanlon (1983), and St. Louis and Ruscello (1981).

There are other, perhaps less-well-known, procedures that we would like to mention as well. Bosma's (1976) excellent tutorial article describes in detail the oral-motor actions necessary to speak, feed, and maintain the proper head and body positions. Bosma discusses the importance of a case history in the evaluation of oral-motor function and provides guidelines for a complete examination of the oral-motor system, including facial and suspensory muscles, tongue, pharynx, palate, submental muscles, and the craniocervical postural system.

Sonies et al. (1987) developed an oral-motor function scale that assesses three areas: oral anatomy, physiology, and speech. There are ten categories covering these three areas, and each is rated on a four-point severity scale (1 = normal, 2 = mild, 3 = moderate, 4 = severe). Some weighting of measures is done to obtain a profile of performance. Anatomy ratings include assessment of the appearance of facial bones, tissues, and oral facial symmetry. Physiology ratings include assessment of range of motion, strength, precision, and speed of lingual, labial, palatal, velar, and facial muscles along with assessment of oral sensation. Swallowing function, a subcomponent of the scale, is assessed from a questionnaire, an ultrasound visualization of the swallowing act, mealtime observations, and a medical history. Speech ratings include articulation, voice, fluency, and diadochokinetic rate.

It now may be obvious to the reader that some assessment scales are more detailed than others and that some seem to weigh heavily certain aspects of the total oral peripheral examination. This certainly is the case. If the clinician is interested in assessing swallowing function, then in addition to the scales mentioned, the works of Bell and Goepfert (1977), Larsen (1972), and Logemann (1983) should be consulted. Patients with motor speech disorders may need more in-depth testing, as this chapter has pointed out. For example, oral-motor abilities of a patient with apraxia of speech may be appraised by the tests of Dabul (1979) or of Wertz, LaPointe, and Rosenbek (1984), whereas the Frenchay Dysarthria Assessment (Enderby 1980, 1983) may prove useful with a dysarthric patient. Several informal assessment instruments purport to test the integrity of the cranial nerves. Examples of such cranial nerve batteries are the Bulbar-Cranial Nerve Examination (Rancho Los Amigos Hospital 1966) and the example protocol provided by Marquardt (1982). Likewise, clinicians working in cleft palate centers typically have examination forms specific for oro-facial anomalies (Bzoch 1979; Rampp, Pannbacker, and Kinnebrew 1984).

To conclude our discussion of the oral peripheral examination, we would like to say that at some point in the not-too-distant future, the diagnostician may have instruments that measure tongue, lip, and other movements very precisely (Barlow and Abbs 1983; Porter and Lubka 1980). Remember, though, one swallow does not make a summer, and one deviancy in the oral area does not necessarily cause disordered speech.

Dysphagia

The role and scope of practice in speech-language pathology includes the evaluation and management of swallowing disorders in persons regardless of whether there is a concomitant communication disorder (ASHA 1987). As the majority of adult and pediatric feeding and swallowing difficulties are associated with neurologic conditions, an overview of dysphagia assessments is included in this chapter.

According to the American Speech, Language, and Hearing Association's 1992 omnibus survey, SLPs report that patients exhibiting dysphagia comprise 11 percent of their caseloads (Slater 1992). The definition provided by ASHA (1987) is encompassing:

> *Dysphagia is a swallowing disorder characterized by difficulty in oral preparation for the swallow or in moving material from the mouth to the stomach. Subsumed in this definition are problems in positioning food in the mouth and in the oral manipulation preceding the swallow including suckling, sucking and mastication. (57)*

The four most common etiologies associated with dysphagia in adults are (in order of occurrence): stroke, traumatic brain injury, spinal cord injury, and brain tumor (Cherney 1994).

Normal Deglutition in the Adult

The purpose of swallowing is to transport food and other materials from the oral cavity to the stomach without allowing entry of substances into the airway. Safe swallowing entails precise coordination of neuromuscular events including those in the brain, brainstem, cranial nerves, and muscles of the oral cavity, pharynx, and esophagus (Tuchman 1994).

Swallowing is considered a three-phase process by most authorities (Miller 1982; Tuchman 1994) although the first phase may be subdivided for clinical utility into the preparatory stage and transport stage (Leopold and Kagel 1983; Logemann 1983). Normal feeding begins with the *oral phase,* specifically the oral preparation stage, which is under volitional control and so may be manipulated in a therapeutic regime. Oral preparation reduces food to a consistency appropriate for swallowing. Lips are closed, the tongue manipulates the food in the mouth as muscles of mastication move the jaw, the teeth tear and crush the morsels, and saliva is mixed with the mass of food forming a cohesive *bolus.* Duration of oral preparation is highly variable, depending on the consistency of the food and the time spent tasting it. Oral preparation provides much of the pleasure from eating, and so it is an important psychological consideration when working with a patient with dysphagia (Logemann 1983). Liquid diets bypass this pleasurable subphase.

When readied, the bolus is manipulated to the back of the oral cavity, near the faucial pillars. This transport stage is the second part of the oral phase, and it too is considered under volitional control by way of hypoglossal, cranial nerve XII. Tongue muscles nestle the bolus then elevate and retract to propel the bolus to the back of the oral cavity. The swallowing reflex is believed to be triggered by tongue action as the bolus passes the anterior faucial pillars, although little is understood of this elicitation. Triggering of the swallowing reflex is crucial to a safe swallow but the importance of healthy tongue manipulation cannot be underestimated. Logemann (1983) explains that with impaired tongue action

> *the food will spread through the oral cavity as the patient attempts to move it back-ward. Some food drips down into the pharynx as the patient struggles to control the food and initiate the swallow. The food dripping into the pharynx prematurely may be aspirated before the swallow, or may come to rest in the valleculae and pyriform sinuses. Where the food lands will depend on the patient's posture, the amount of food and the consistency of the food.* (6)

From this, the astute reader will discern areas of behavioral assessment and variables to systematically manipulate in the evaluation and treatment of a person with dysphagia. Worthy of mention is that the oral phase of swallowing lasts approximately one second, regardless of the person's age, gender, or the consistency of the food being swallowed.

As the swallowing reflex is triggered, there is a pharyngeal response. Events in this *pharyngeal phase* are automatic and mediated primarily by the glosso-pharyngeal (IXth) cranial nerve and the brainstem. Logemann (1983) identifies four sequential, split-second neuromuscular activities in the pharyngeal phase: (1) velopharyngeal closure to separate breathing from swallowing; (2) peristalic action of the pharyngeal constrictor muscles to clear food from the pharynx; (3) elevation and closure of the larynx to protect food from entering the airway; and (4) relaxtion of the muscles encircling the top of the esophagus. Each event lasts a fraction of a second with the total pharyngeal phase occurring in one second. This duration does not vary with age, gender, or food consistency. Potential to reestablish a patient's normal pharyngeal phase is a key assessment/prognostic feature of a dysphagia evaluation: In the pharyngeal phase, food is propelled into the esophagus and the airway is protected.

Once the bolus has entered the esophagus, it cannot be controlled volitionally and does not respond to exercise programs (Logemann 1983). This *esophageal phase* of swallowing begins when the bolus enters the esophagus and ends when the bolus passes through the lower esophageal valve and into the stomach. Duration of this phase varies from eight to twenty seconds and often lengthens with age.

Cherney (1994) provides additional details of swallowing patterns in healthy and frail aged adults.

Assessment of Adult Swallowing Disorders

Several protocols for assessing adult dysphagia are available (Cherney 1994; Fleming and Waver 1987; Larsen 1972; Logemann 1983; Longstreth 1986; Miller 1984). Three protocols will be highlighted in this chapter.

The BELZ Dysphagia Scale (Longstreth 1986) rates twelve categories on a 0–3 scale. The rating categories include a clinical swallowing evaluation, otolaryngology examination, cognition/communication status, physical status, pulmonary function, chest x-ray, videofluoroscopic evaluation of swallowing physiology, tracheostomy tube status, diet consistency, tube feeding, respiratory tract treatments, and gastrointestinal function.

The Fleming Index of Dysphagia (FID) (Fleming and Waver 1987) is a computerized index. Responses to questions and prompts are inputted; each item is assigned an impact score, and these scores are combined with severity ratings and problem codes to determine the severity of dysphagia, the urgency for treatment, and suggestions for patient management.

The Clinical Evaluation of Dysphagia (CED) from the Rehabilitation Institute of Chicago (Cherney, Pannell, and Cantieri 1994) outlines the areas to assess for the SLP. Typically, a prefeeding evaluation is first done when a patient is high risk for aspiration (e.g., patients who are not yet eating orally or those with tracheostomies).

The evaluation of prefeeding skills on the CED includes collecting a complete history of the problem and observing oral, pharyngeal, and laryngeal structures and functions. From this, the SLP decides the patient's potential for oral intake and the need for further evaluation and referral. The CED's prefeeding evaluation form guides the clinician in the collection and documentation of the following relevant information:

1. Medical/nutritional status (Inquire about diseases, surgeries, medications, and swallowing complaints.)
2. Respiratory status (Ascertain rate [normal = 12–16 breaths per minute] and note any chronic coughing or shortness of breath.)
3. History of aspiration
4. Type and size of tracheostomy, if any
5. Level of responsiveness (Assess ability to follow directions.)
6. Behavioral characteristics
7. Current feeding methods (Describe type of feeding [oral, nasogastric tube, gastrostomy tube, percutaneous endoscopic gastrostomy], when tube was placed, and the frequency and amount of food intake.)
8. Positioning (Note habitual body, head, and neck positions and any motor control problems; determine the best feeding position without giving food [maximal airway protection is upright at ninety degrees with head tilted forward] and what is needed to achieve that position comfortably [use of wedges, pillows, other supports].)
9. Observation of oral motor, pharyngeal, and laryngeal functioning (Perform a thorough oral motor examination, include observations on quality and strength of the voice.)

10. Cough (Note the presence or absence of both involuntary and elicited coughs.)

11. Gag reflex (Elicit reflex and note its strength bilaterally.)

12. Voluntary swallow (Assess ability to perform a dry swallow on command; feel and watch for laryngeal elevation.)

13. Other observations (Observe presence of drooling, mouth odors, and abnormal reflexes that may affect feeding.)

14. Response to stimulation (Note adequacy of lip closure, lip protrusion, response to touching by a spoon, and the like.)

15. Recommendations and goals

Although it may be determined after this assessment that a patient should remain "NPO" (nothing per oral; nutrition must be accomplished through other means), treatment may be recommended to improve prefeeding skills with the anticipation of improvement and future reassessment.

Next, a clinical evaluation of dysphagia can be performed on patients who can tolerate at least one food consistency. The nature of this evaluation differs substantially for patients of differing levels; Cherney, Pannell, and Cantiere (1994) provide guidelines for patients with severe dysphagia, those with a tracheostomy, and those receiving an oral diet.

The CEP guides the SLP in observing (or inferring) behaviors during swallowing, from the oral phase through the pharyngeal phase. Six different food consistencies can be evaluated; Table 9.7 lists sample foods. The clinician documents

TABLE 9.7   Foods and Food Consistencies Used in Evaluating Dysphagia

Thin liquids

water, apple juice

Thick liquids

tomato juice, cream soups, yogurt

Pureed foods

applesauce, pureed canned fruit, pudding

Ground foods

rice, scrambled eggs, tuna, ground chicken, hamburger

Chopped solids

tender bits of meats, vegetables

Regular solids

(usual table foods)

his/her observations and rates the performance (ranging from adequate to nonfunctional) for each structure (lips, tongue, mandible, and so forth) and for each phase of swallowing.

The clinican often works with a multidisciplinary team to further evaluate swallowing competence. Imaging studies, particularly videofluoroscopic evaluations, are necessary to judge motoric adequacy and potential for aspiration. The role of the SLP in imaging analyses is described by Logemann (1983) and others.

Two questions must be addressed after the thorough diagnostic workup of a patient with dysphagia. First, what type of nutritional management is appropriate for the patient—oral versus nonoral feeding—both now and in the long term? Second, should treatment include direct or indirect work on swallowing? Principles of direct-versus-indirect efforts are discussed by Logemann (1983). The reader is encouraged to further study this burgeoning area of adult dysphagia rehabilitation.

Pediatric Feeding and Swallowing Disorders

Voluminous literature exists on disorders of sucking, feeding, and swallowing in infants and children, much of it focusing in speech pathology on the optimal handling of infants with cerebral palsy (Morris 1977; Morris and Klein 1987; Mueller 1972). In addition to neuromotor feeding difficulties evident from birth, as may be the case in cerebral palsy, other forms of dysphagia become evident with the passage of time. Neurologic conditions of childhood associated with feeding disorders are cited in Table 9.8 (Ichord 1994).

According to Lefton-Greif (1994), the ultimate goal of a feeding and swallowing assessment is to develop a management protocol that enables safe and efficient feeding that is enjoyable for both the child and the caregivers. Adequate nutrition and hydration goals must be achieved without compromise of airway safety. These goals are best met through a team approach including, at a minimum, the physician, key nursing staff, and a nutritionist.

Groher (1984) proposes five goals of a clinical evaluation: (1) establish a possible cause of dysphagia, (2) assess the child's ability to protect the airway, (3) determine the practicality of oral feeding and/or recommend alternative methods of nutrition, (4) determine the need for additional diagnostic tests, and (5) establish baseline clinical data. To accomplish these goals, pediatric feeding and swallowing evaluations should include four primary components: a careful history, examination of the oral motor mechanism, observation of a trial feeding, and specialized imaging studies as clinically indicated (Groher 1984; Lefton-Greif 1994). An overview of each component is presented.

Case History

Medical records help identify medical, neurological, developmental, and etiological factors that predispose the child to dysphagia. Likewise, knowledge of medications, syndromes, and systemic problems (e.g., cardiopulmonary and respiratory

**TABLE 9.8   Neurologic Conditions of Childhood
Associated with Dysphagia**

Dysfunction of cortex or basal ganglia

static encephalopathy (e.g., in utero intoxications,
     chromosomal defects, CNS infection, cerebrovascular
     accidents, trauma)
progressive encephalopathy (e.g., Wilson's disease, HIV,
     multiple sclerosis, drug-induced movement disorders)

Brainstem

congenital CNS anomalies
tumors of brainstem or posterior fossa
trauma
brainstem encephalitis

Cranial nerves

trauma (asilar skull fracture)
motor neuron disease (poliomyelitis, progressive bulbar
     paralysis of childhood, spinal muscular atrophy)
tumors (schwannoma, neurofibromatosis)
toxins (diphtheria, heavy metals)

Neuromuscular junction

myasthenia gravis
drugs/intoxications (e.g., tetanus, streptomycin,
     bacitracin, beta blocker, phenothizines)

Muscle

congenital (e.g., muscular dystrophy)
errors of metabolism
endocrine (e.g., hyperthyroidism, hypothyroidism)

Esophageal motility

associated with CNS dysfunction
induced by reflux esophagitis
drug induced (e.g., beta adrenergics, muscle relaxants
     associated with myopathies

distress) that increase demands on pharyngeal function and boost nutritional requirements is necessary (Lefton-Greif 1994).

  The mother or primary caregiver/feeder can provide details of the feeding history. The SLP needs to know the child's current oral feeding patterns: types of food
and liquids tolerated, manner of presentation, feeding position, duration of meals
(10–30 minutes is best), frequency of meals, total intake, and the like. If the client
is tube fed, the SLP needs details on the type of feeding tube, when it was initiated,

formula amount per feeding, feeding schedule, position during feeding, and use of and response to oral stimulation.

Oral Motor Examination

The SLP should observe the child at rest, noting body tone and posture. If in an acute care setting, baseline respiratory rates, heart rates, and pulse oxygen levels can easily be obtained (changes in these physiologic patterns during feeding may indicate general intolerance or airway compromise). Look for clinical signs of oral or pharyngeal dysfunction, such as drooling, coughing, and upper aerodigestive tract noises. As discussed earlier in this chapter, a thorough oral motor examination is performed (excellent guidelines are provided by Bell and Goepfert 1977; Bosma 1976; Larsen 1972; Logemann 1983). The lips, tongue and velum are evaluated for precision, strength, range, and symmetry of movement. Cranial nerves screened for oral phase function include V, VII, X, and XII (Logemann 1983). The pharyngeal phase of deglutition is dependent on muscles innervated by cranial nerves IX, X, and XI. Oral sensations and laryngeal functions are also assessed.

Observation of a Trial Feeding

The SLP should observe a regularly scheduled mealtime. As Lefton-Greif (1994) states,

> The parent should feed the child using foods, utensils, special adaptations (e.g., thickening formula or cutting a large hole in the nipple), and positioning equipment used at home. The child is monitored for clinical signs associated with aspiration, including: cough, choke, and/or gag episodes; changes in vocal quality or upper aerodigestive tract noises; episodes of oxygen desaturation; and episodes of apnea or bradycardia. (106)

Observation of a trial feeding allows the clinician to define patterns of oral intake, positioning, and optimal stimuli for feeding (i.e., bolus characteristics of size, texture and temperature).

Indications for Specialized Studies

When to proceed with special tests and imaging procedures is a decision reached by the multidisciplinary team. The child must be medically stable (and able to risk an episode of aspiration); usually there is some prognosis for change in the current feeding regime. A videofluoroscopic evaluation of swallowing function is a common method of imaging the oral and pharyngeal phases of the swallow. Many factors affect oral and pharyngeal performance, including the rate and manner of food presentation (which is mixed with barium for image enhancement). The evaluation itself often manipulates bolus characteristics (texture, amount, temperature), manner of presentation (bottle, spoon, cup), and special adaptations (positioning, specific modifications of feeding devices). Test protocols and assessment forms are available in the literature, including those provided by Benson and Lefton-Greif (1994).

Although videofluoroscopy is the routine method of evaluating swallowing, other technologies are available. Benson and Tuchman (1994) discuss other diagnostic tests, including ultrasonography, manometry, electromyography, and nuclear scintigraphy.

Bibliography

ASHA (1987). "Ad Hoc Committee on Dysphagia Report." *ASHA* 29:57–58.

Barlow, S., and Abbs, J. (1983). "Force Transducers for the Evaluation of Labial, Lingual, and Mandibular Motor Impairments." *Journal of Speech and Hearing Research* 26:616–621.

Bell, K., & Goepfert, H. (1977). "Rehabilitation of Head and Neck Cancer Patients to Deglutinate." *Texas Journal of Audiology and Speech Pathology* 2:3–5.

Benson, D. F. (1979). *Aphasia, Alexia, and Agraphia.* New York: Churchill Livingstone.

Benson, J. E., and Lefton-Greif, M. A. (1994). "Videofluoroscopy of Swallowing in Pediatric Patients: A Component of the Total Feeding Evaluation." In *Disorders of Feeding and Swallowing in Infants and Children: Pathophysiology, Diagnosis, and treatment,* ed. D. N. Tuchman and R. S. Walter (San Diego, CA: Singular Publishing).

Benson, J. E., and Tuchman, D. N. (1994). "Other Diagnostic Tests Used for Evaluation of Swallowing Disorders." In *Disorders of Feeding and Swallowing in Infants and Children: Pathophysiology, Diagnosis, and treatment,* ed. D. N. Tuchman and R. S. Walter (San Diego, CA: Singular Publishing).

Blakely, R. W. (1983). "Treatment of Developmental Apraxia of Speech." In *Current Therapy Communication Disorders: Dysarthria and Apraxia,* ed. W. H. Perkins (New York: Thieme-Stratton).

Bloomquist, B. (1950). "Diadochokinetic Movements of Nine-, Ten-, and Eleven-Year-Old Children." *Journal of Speech and Hearing Disorders* 15:159–164.

Bosma, J. F. (1976). "Sensorimotor Examination of the Mouth and Pharynx." In *Frontiers of Oral Physiology,* ed. Y. Kawamura (Basel, Switzerland: Kerger).

Bzoch, K. (1979). *Communicative Disorders Related to Cleft Lip and Palate.* Boston, MA: Little, Brown.

Canning, B., and Rose, M. (1974). "Clinical Measurements of the Speed of Tongue and Lip Movements in British Children with Normal Speech." *British Journal of Disorders of Communication* 9:45–50.

Capute, A. J. (1974). "Developmental Disabilities: An Overview." *Dental Clinics of North America* 18:557–577.

Cherney, L. R. (1994). "Dysphagia in Adults with Neurologic Disorders: An Overview." In *Clinical Management of Dysphagia in Adults and Children* (2nd ed.), ed. L. R. Cherney (Gaithersburg, MD: Aspen Publishers).

Cherney, L. R., Pannelli, J. J., and Cantiere, C. A. (1994). "Clinical Evaluation of Dysphagia in Adults." In *Clinical Management of Dysphagia in Adults and Children* (2nd ed.), ed. L. R. Cherney (Gaithersburg, MD: Aspen Publishers).

Crary, M. A. (1988). "A Multifaceted Perspective on Developmental Apraxia of Speech." Paper presented to the convention of the Speech and Hearing Association of Alabama, Orange Beach, AL.

Cruickshank, W. M., and Raus, G. M. (1966). *Cerebral: Its Individual and Community Problems.* 2nd ed. Syracuse: Syracuse University Press.

Dabul, B. (1979). *Apraxia Battery for Adults.* Tigard, OR: C. C. Publications.

Darley, F. L., Aronson, A. E., and Brown, J. R. (1975). *Motor Speech Disorders.* Philadelphia, PA: W. B. Saunders.

DeRenzi, E., Pieczuro, A., and Vignolo, L. A. (1966). "Oral Apraxia and Aphasia." *Cortex* 2:50–73.

DiCarlo, L. M., and Amster, W. W. (1974). "Communication Therapy for Problems Associated with Cerebral Palsy." In *Communication disorders: Remedial principles and practices* (2nd ed.), ed. S. Dickson (Glenview, IL: Scott, Foresman).

Dworkin, J. P., and Culatta, R. A. (1980). *Dworkin-Culatta Oral Mechanism Examination.* Nicholasville, KY: Edgewood Press.

Enderby, P. (1980). "Frenchay Dysarthria Assessment." *British Journal of Disorders of Communication* 15:165–173.

Enderby, P. (1983). "The Standardized Assessment of Dysarthria Is Possible." In *Clinical Dysarthria,* ed. W. R. Berry (San Diego, CA: College-Hill).

Fleming, S., and Waver, A. (1987). "Index of Dysphagia: A Tool for Identifying Deglutition Problems." *Dysphagia* 1:206–208.

Fletcher, S. (1972). "Time-by-Count Measurement of Diadochokinetic Syllable Rate." *Journal of Speech and Hearing Research* 15:763–770.

Goodglass H., and Kaplan, E. (1983). *The Assessment of Aphasia and Related Disorders.* Philadelphia, PA: Lea and Febiger.

Groher, M. (1984). *Dysphagia: Diagnosis and Management.* Boston: Butterworths.

Hall, P. K., Hardy, J. C., and LaVelle, W. E. (1990). "A Child with Signs of Developmental Apraxia of Speech with Whom a Palatal Lift Prosthesis Was Used to Manage Palatal Dysfunction." *Journal of Speech and Hearing Disorders* 55:454–460.

Hopkins, T. W., Bice, H. V., and Colton, K. C. (1954). *Evaluation and Education of the Cerebral Palsied Child.* Washington, DC: International Council for Exceptional Children.

Ichord, R. N. (1994). "Neurology of Deglutition." In *Disorders of Feeding and Swallowing in Infants and Children: Pathophysiology, Diagnosis, and treatment,* eds. D. N. Tuchman and R. S. Walter (San Diego, CA: Singular Publishing).

Johns, D. F., and Darley, F. L. (1970). "Phonemic Variability in Apraxia of Speech." *Journal of Speech and Hearing Research* 13, no 3:556–583.

Johns, D. F., and LaPointe, L. L. (1976). "Neurogenic Disorders of Output Processing: Apraxia of Speech." In *Studies in Neurolinguistics I,* ed. H. Whitaker and H. A. Whitaker (New York: Academic Press).

Kent, R. D., and Rosenbek, J. C. (1983). "Acoustic Patterns of Apraxia of Speech." *Journal of Speech and Hearing Disorders* 26:231–248.

Kertesz, A. (1980). *Western Aphasia Battery.* London, Ontario: University of Western Ontario.

Larsen, G. (1970). "Rehabilitation of Dysphagia Paralytica." *Journal of Speech and Hearing Disorders* 37:187–194.

Lefton-Greif, M. A. (1994). "Diagnosis and Management of Pediatric Feeding and Swallowing Disorders: Role of the Speech-Language Pathologist." In *Disorders of Feeding and Swallowing in Infants and Children: Pathophysiology, Diagnosis, and Treatment,* ed. D. N. Tuchman and R. S. Walter (San Diego, CA: Singular Publishing).

Leopold, N. A., and Kagel, M. C. (1983). "Swallowing, Ingestion and Dysphagia: A Reappraisal." *Archives of Physical Medicine and Rehabilitation* 64:371–373.

Logemann, J. (1983). *Evaluation and Treatment of Swallowing Disorders.* San Diego, CA: College Hill.

Longstreth, D. (1986). "The BELZ Dysphagia Scale." Paper presented at the annual convention of the American Speech-Language-Hearing Association, Detroit, MI.

McDonald, E. T., and Chance, B. (1964). *Cerebral Palsy.* Englewood Cliffs, NJ: Prentice Hall.

McNeil, M. R., Rosenbek, J. C., and Aronson, A. A. (1984). *The Dysarthrias: Physiology, Acoustics, Perception, Management.* San Diego, CA: College-Hill.

Marquardt, T. P. (1982). *Acquired Neurogenic Disorders.* Englewood Cliffs, NJ: Prentice Hall.

Martin, A. D. (1974). "Some Objections to the Term Apraxia of Speech." *Journal of Speech and Hearing Disorders* 39:53–64.

Mason, R. M., and Simon C. (1977). "An Orofacial Examination Checklist." *Language, Speech, and Hearing Services in Schools* 8:155–163.

Miller, A. J. (1982). "Deglutition." *Physiologic Review* 62:129–184.

Miller, N. (1986). *Dyspraxia and Its Management.* Rockville, MD: Aspen.

Miller, R. (1984). "Evaluation of Swallowing Disorders." In *Dysphagia Diagnosis and Management,* ed. M. E. Groher (Stoneham, MA: Butterworth).

Moore, W. M., Rosenbek, J. C., and LaPointe, L. L. (1976). "Assessment of Oral Apraxia in Brain-Injured Adults." In *Clinical Aphasiology: Conference Proceedings,* ed. R. H. Brookshire (Minneapolis, MN: BRK Publishers).

Morely, M. E. (1957). *The Development and Disorders of Speech in Children.* London: Livingston.

Morris, S. E. (1977). *Program Guidelines for Children with Feeding Problems.* Madison, WI: Childcraft Education Corporation.

Morris, S. E., and Klein, M. D. (1987). *Pre-Feeding Skills: A Comprehensive Resource for Feeding Development.* Tucson: AZ: Therapy Skill Builders.

Mueller, H. (1972). "Facilitating Feeding and Prespeech." In *Physical therapy services in the developmental disabilities*, ed. P. H. Pearson and C. E. Williams (Springfield, IL: Charles C. Thomas).

Mysak, E. D. (1980). *Neurospeech Therapy for the Cerebral Palsied: A Neuroevolutional Approach.* New York: Teachers College Press.

Perkins, W. H. (1983). *Current Therapy of Communication Disorders: Dysarthria and Apraxia.* New York: Thieme-Stratton.

Porter, R., and Lubka, J. (1980). "The Linguameter: A Device for Investigating Tongue-Muscle Control." *Journal of Speech and Hearing Research* 23:490–494.

Rampp, D. L., Pannbacker, M., and Kinnebrew, M. C. (1984). *VPI Velopharyngeal Incompetency: A Practical Guide for Evaluation and Management.* Austin, TX: Pro-Ed.

Rancho Los Amigos Hospital (1966). "Bulbar-Cranial Nerve Examination." Unpublished, prepared by the Physical Therapy Department, Rancho Los Amigos Hospital, Los Angeles, CA.

Rosenbek, J. C., LaPointe, L., and Wertz, R. T. (1989). *Aphasia: A Clinical Approach.* Boston, MA: College-Hill.

Rosenbek, J. C., and Wertz, R. T. (1976). Veterans Administration Workshop on Speech Motor Disorders, Madison, WI.

Ruscello, D. M., St. Louis, K. O., Barry, P., and Barr, K. (1982). "A Screening Method for Examination of the Peripheral Speech Mechanism." *Folia Phoniatrica* 34:324–330.

Siegel, G., and Hanlon, J. (1983). "Magnitude Estimation of Oral Cavity Distances." *Journal of Speech and Hearing Research* 26:574–578.

Slater, S. C. (1992). "1992 Omnibus Survey: Portrait of the Professions." *ASHA* 34:61–65.

Sonies, B. C., Weiffenbach, J., Atkinson, J. C., Brahim, J., Macynski, A., and Fox, P. C. (1987). "Clinical Examination of Motor and Sensory Functions of the Adult Oral Cavity." *Dysphagia* 1:4.

Square, P., and Weidner, W. E. (1981). *Differential Diagnosis of Developmental Apraxia.* Paper presented to the convention of the Speech and Hearing Association of Alabama, Birmingham, AL.

St. Louis, K., and Ruscello, D. (1981). *The oral speech mechanism examination.* Baltimore, MD: University Park Press.

Tuchman, D. N. (1994). "Physiology of the Swallowing Apparatus." In *Disorders of Feeding and Swallowing in Infants and Children: Pathophysiology, Diagnosis, and treatment*, ed. D. N. Tuchman and R. S. Walter (San Diego, CA: Singular Publishing).

Wertz, R. T., LaPointe, L. L., and Rosenbek, J. C. (1984). *Apraxia of Speech in Adults: The Disorder and Its Management.* New York: Grune & Stratton.

Wertz, R. T., Rosenbek, J. C., and Deal, J. (1970). "A Review of 228 Cases of Apraxia of Speech: Classification, Etiology, and Localization." Paper presented at the convention of the American Speech and Hearing Association, New York.

Yorkston, K. M., and Beukelman, D. R. (1981). *Assessment of Intelligibility of Dysarthric Speech*, Tigard, OR: C. C. Publications.

Yorkston, K. M., Beukelman, D. R., and Bell, K. R. (1988). *Clinical Management of Dysarthric Speakers.* Boston, MA: College-Hill

Yoss, K., and Darley, F. L. (1974). "Developmental Apraxia of Speech in Children with Defective Articulation." *Journal of Speech and Hearing Research* 17:399–416.

Chapter 10

Laryngeal Voice Disorders

There were major changes in the assessment and treatment of voice disorders in the early part of this century. The speech pathologist became involved in the processes of diagnosis and remediation that were previously the province of physicians and singing teachers (Stemple 1984). Recently, there has been increased research in the area of normal and disordered vocal physiology, including investigations of possible differences among culturally diverse groups (DeJarnette and Holland 1993). Assessment and treatment are being changed further by the technological advances in microcomputers and electronics. Thus, today we possess insights into the vocal mechanism that we did not have even a decade ago. New instruments are available for diagnosis and treatment that help to objectify behaviors that were previously unobservable and fleeting. It is an exciting time for those clinicians who deal with voice disorders.

The proliferation of new instrumentation and research, however, should not obscure the fact that we have developed some very effective clinical procedures over the years that do not require equipment. Many authorities continue to believe that it is the listening skill and judgment of the well-trained clinician that are the most important tools in a voice evaluation. Voice diagnosis combines the subjective and the objective as does all clinical work, and the clinician must be able to shift from the mental set of the scientist to that of the wine taster and back again. In this chapter, we will touch upon both subjective and objective aspects of vocal assessment.

Many adults and some children are referred to the speech pathologist by their physician for voice disorders resulting from medical difficulties or surgical intervention. The incidence of laryngeal pathologies in children seems to vary as a function of gender and ethnicity, and so the clinician will benefit from good skills for multicultural interaction. Dobres et al. (1990) examined medical charts in an admittedly modest-sized sample and discerned that Asian Americans have the greatest male-to-female incidence ratio (4.3:1), whites the second greatest (1.8:1), and African Americans the lowest (1.4:1). Of thirty laryngeal pathologies, it is worth noting that vocal nodules were more prevalent in White male children as compared to White females. Asian American gender differences were in the same direction, but the opposite pattern was seen among African American children, females showing a higher incidence.

The clinician also frequently comes in contact with children as the result of screening large numbers of youngsters in school settings or by teacher/parent referral. Prevalence figures for voice disorders among school-age children vary considerably. Silverman and Zimmer (1975) report that 23.4 percent of the primary-grade children they evaluated possessed chronically hoarse voices, while Wilson and Rice (1977) postulate that 1 percent of the school-age population needs voice therapy. Other studies range between 4 and 6 percent. From our experience, it would appear that substantially less than 1 percent of school-age children are presently receiving voice therapy (Deal, McClain, and Sudderth 1976). For a variety of reasons, including fear of working with voice cases and self-perceived lack of training, the practicing speech clinician is not identifying the number of voice cases that the experts predict actually exist (Shearer 1972).

The Nature of Vocal Disturbances

The imprecision of labels, which is the bane of voice study, begins with the term *voice* itself. Some definitions restrict the term to the generation of sound at the level of the larynx, while others include the influence of the vocal tract upon the generated tone, and still others broaden the definition to ultimately include aspects of tonal generation, resonation, articulation, and prosody. In this chapter, we will limit our discussion of voice to disorders affecting the laryngeal mechanism. Cancer of the larynx, its subsequent medical treatment, and the speech rehabilitation of a person so affected is a voice disorder that warrants a chapter unto itself (see Chapter 11). Disorders of resonance will be discussed in Chapter 12.

A framework to conceptualize voice and voice disturbance is shown in Figure 10.1. The auditory characteristics of pitch, loudness, and quality constitute one dimension of our paradigm. These are the primary perceptual attributes of the voice and relate generally to the fundamental frequency, amplitude, and complexity of the signal.

Pitch that is too high, too low, too invariant, or inappropriately variant for the speaker or the circumstances constitutes a voice disorder. The loudness of the speaking voice is usually judged according to the speaking circumstance, with the aberrant ranging from the total lack of voice (aphonia) to the inappropriately loud. For our purposes, the term *quality* refers to the perceived pleasantness, or appeal, of the voice. Although this perception is linked to both the phonatory and resonatory characteristics of the speaker, we will consider only the disturbance of phonation in this chapter. Many terms have been used to describe vocal quality, yet roughness/hoarseness and breathiness seem to be the two most widely accepted.

The physical systems that most directly influence the vocal production are the respiratory, phonatory, and resonatory-articulatory systems, but they are not the

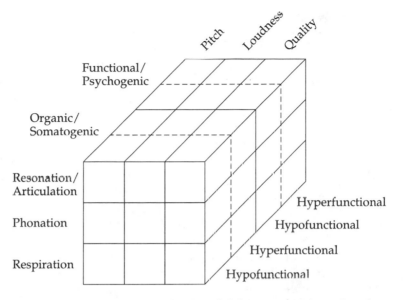

FIGURE 10.1   An Organizational Schema of Voice Disorders

only systems that influence the voice. Luchsinger and Arnold (1965) discuss the impact of the endocrine and neural systems on voice production.

The respiratory system provides the motive force for voice production, and ultimately the resultant airstream becomes the vibrator that embodies all of the characteristics that the ear eventually senses. The importance of the airstream to vocal production is not really the issue at this point, but there is some question as to the influence of the respiratory mechanism upon the various vocal characteristics. It appears that the respiratory mechanism must be capable of the following:

1. Providing an adequate amount of air so that the speaker can sustain speech with ease to allow for natural phrasing and prosodic factors
2. Providing adequate control of the flow of air so that the mechanism can, when necessary, either initiate or arrest the speech signal
3. Providing an airstream that is not so indebted to active muscle contraction that it encourages unnecessary muscle tension in the respiratory and phonatory mechanisms

Knowledge of the elements of laryngeal function is crucial in guiding the diagnostic process. In order to be an efficient sound source, the larynx must perform a valving action upon the flow of air that establishes alternate, regular pressure changes within the body of air. In order to do this, the vocal folds must be capable of (1) performing a wide range of valving actions, from completely open and unrestricted to closed and totally restricted; (2) valving completely along the length of the vocal folds; and (3) closing and opening during phonation with just the right amount of energy to avoid extreme tension during the closing phase; (4) moving in a natural way that is free from superimposed and undue tension; and (5) making small, subtle, instantaneous adjustments, done continuously to alter the various vocal characteristics (these adjustments must allow for a variety of cyclic variations in the potential time of glottal opening and closing, from the long closing time of the glottal fry to the short closing time of the falsetto voice). The vocal folds must also be (1) of approximately equal size and shape so that they can move in synchrony with one another and (2) of appropriate size (length and mass) for the age and sex of the person.

The glottal tone is complex and rich in higher harmonics, but it is only through the resonant and damping effects of the vocal tract that the speech sounds achieve their identity. In order for the resonating chambers of the vocal tract to be efficient, they must be flexible in size, shape, texture, and relationship with one another. The effect of the resonators upon the laryngeal valve has been discussed by several writers (Curtis 1968; Wendahl and Page 1967), but the exact nature of this relationship has yet to be determined.

The term *functional* should imply more than the simple absence of measurable organic deviation; it should imply that the diagnostician has found some active agent of etiology and that the agent is nonorganic. We agree with Powers (1971) that the term *functional* has unfortunately come to mean diagnosis by default. Voice disorders offer an interesting testing ground for the traditional organic-functional dichotomy. This separation does not stand up on almost any basis. Murphy (1964) points out the continuous nature of vocal disorder etiologies.

Figure 10.1 identifies functional/psychogenic and organic/somatogenic as clinically meaningful categories. The term *functional* refers to those disorders where the learned, psychic, or maladaptive behavior has resulted in faulty vocal production, but not in physical alteration. If physical change has resulted from the functional cause, however, the proper designation is *psychogenic*. Similarly, if the original factor was physical or organic, then the term *organic* is justified; but if the physical difference results in behavioral change—that is, emotional response or faulty compensatory adjustments—the term *somatogenic* is appropriate (Murphy 1964).

The terms *hyperfunctioning* and *hypofunctioning* refer, respectively, to an excess or insufficiency of laryngeal tension and, as such, could apply to a wide variety of organic or functional disorders.

The term *voice disorders*, then, refers to abnormal pitch, loudness, or vocal quality according to sex, age, status, temporary physiological state, purpose of the speaker, and elements of the speaking circumstances. Vocal disorders may be primarily organic or functional and may be affected by any of the primary systems.

The Presenting Complaint and Case History Intake

Before beginning our discussion of the diagnostic format, let us restate that this chapter will not cover the anatomy and physiology of the mechanisms of vocal production. Such information is offered in many sources and should be studied carefully before undertaking voice diagnosis (Bateman and Mason 1984; Daniloff, Schuckers, and Feth 1980; Dickson and Maue-Dickson 1982; Kahane and Folkins 1984; Kaplan 1971; Palmer 1984; Perkins and Kent 1986; Titze 1994; Zemlin 1988). We also cannot provide an elaborate description of each voice disorder type; this information is available to the student in several sources (Aronson 1985; Boone and McFarlane 1994; Greene 1980; Luchsinger and Arnold 1965; Stemple 1984).

Our major focus will be on the actual planning, preparation, and execution of voice diagnoses. Diagnosis is intended to assess the parameters of the voice, determine the etiology and/or perpetuating factors, and outline a logical course of intervention, if warranted.

The diagnostic process begins with a careful scrutiny of the original statement of the problem as provided by the referral source. Four perspectives guide our evaluation of this information: Who? What? Why? and When?

Who Makes the Referral?

It is important to know who presents the original complaint about the client's voice. We have found that the "best" source from a motivational standpoint is the client, but any individual who might have a significant impact upon the client may be a satisfactory referral source. If the client does not consider the voice to be a problem, treatment may not be in order or, if it is, this denial may necessitate counseling and educating as precursors to the actual voice treatment.

In the schools, it is often the classroom teacher who notices a vocal difference in a student and makes a referral to the SLP. Awareness training may be necessary in the early sessions here too. It should be pointed out, however, that without prior training, such as listening experiences during in-service programs, classroom teachers are not particularly good at recognizing and referring students with voice disorders. Several investigations have studied the classroom teacher's efficacy in referral of children with voice disorders (Diehl and Stinnett 1959; James and Cooper 1966).

What Problem Is Reported?

The description of the problem in the presenting complaint is important not only because it helps us to understand the difficulty better, but also because it allows us to see the problem through the eyes and ears of another. When the statement comes from the person with whom we will be working, we listen not only to the actual words spoken, but also to the way in which they are presented. One of the best sources of information about the impact of the problem upon the individual is the way in which it is described. If possible, preinterview questionnaires should be completed and returned by mail to the clinician prior to the evaluation session. The submitted material is helpful in guiding the diagnostic inquiry. Questions asked on preinterview forms are important to probe further during the case history intake. Preinterview questionnaires invariably ask for a description of the voice problem: when it started and what might have caused it. Health, occupation, and family information is also typically garnered. Weinberg (1983) provides a detailed questionnaire that is a useful preinterview tool.

Why Was the Referral Made?

The reason for referral to the voice clinician may vary from something as simple as an impending trip ("I just have to sound better than this by the first of August") to fears of serious medical problems. In evaluating the reasons for referral, it is important to keep in mind that contacting a speech clinician is often seen as psychologically safer than going to medical doctors or psychologists. This points up the importance of secondary referrals.

When Was the Referral Made?

Three things are of concern here. First, it is important to know when in the sequence of development of the problem the referral was made. Is this a long-standing problem that has only recently become serious, or is it a relatively new phenomenon that has been detected early? Second, what is this person's age and maturational level? Certain vocal changes are to be expected before puberty (Curry 1949) and would be considered normal, but a similar vocal quality at a later maturity level may be abnormal. Third, does this problem appear in cycles? For example, the client may suffer from this vocal change only during "hay fever" season. The time of year of the referral may provide some important diagnostic information.

Referral by the Speech Pathologist

Laryngologists often refer clients to SLPs for behavioral vocal intervention. Equally often, persons with voice problems seek the help of SLPs without first seeing a doctor. In most cases of phonatory voice disorders, some type of referral for medical or psychological evaluation will be necessary. We must remember that SLPs diagnose the voice and its characteristics, whereas medical doctors—particularly laryngologists—diagnose the vocal mechanism per se. It is not within the province of the SLP to diagnose nodules, inflammation, cancer, or the like; the SLP does assess the parameters of the voice that may or may not reflect such structural changes. Voice disorders may be caused by life-threatening situations such as carcinoma of the larynx or something as simple as vocal misuse. The importance of medical referral, then, is obvious. Structural changes such as ulcers, polyps, tumors, or nodules may be detected by the laryngologist through laryngeal examination (and confirmed by tissue biopsy). Auditory symptoms such as hoarseness or harshness of the voice and/or sensory complaints (e.g., laryngeal pain, lumps, and the like) should prompt the clinician to make the referral. Hoarseness lasting beyond fourteen days, particularly in persons over the age of forty, should be referred on a suspicion of being a serious, life-threatening condition until proven otherwise (Pracy et al. 1977). The need for a medical diagnosis cannot be underestimated because of the life/health implications for the client, the legal implications for the practicing clinician, and the requirement of third-party reimbursement agencies that services provided be "medically necessary."

It is widely accepted that the speech pathologist and the laryngologist should ideally cultivate a close working relationship when dealing with voice cases (Aronson 1985; Boone 1982, 1993). Each professional can provide significant information to the other, and *voice treatment* that attempts to alter one or more parameters of the voice, such as pitch, should not begin without a laryngological examination. A *vocal hygiene* program, which does not alter the voice but teaches care of it, can begin with many clients prior to laryngoscopic examination. Thus, waiting for medical examination in cases of vocal abuse should not be used as a reason to postpone enrollment in an intervention program.

During an examination by a medical specialist, indirect laryngoscopy will be accomplished via a mirror or fiberoptiscope. In cases of infants or preschool children, for whom indirect procedures are difficult, the laryngologist may use direct laryngoscopy under anesthesia. Other sophisticated methods are available for observing the condition and function of the vocal folds and will be discussed later in the chapter. The SLP will be interested in the findings of the laryngeal examinations for several reasons and may wish to personally view the folds to better understand the reported findings and diagnosis.

First, the examination can document any physical alteration to the vocal mechanism (e.g., nodules, polyps) that may account for vocal differences.

Second, the speech pathologist will want to have the extent of any vocal fold pathology documented as baseline information if voice therapy is indicated so that alterations in the client's voice over time, as the result of treatment, might be correlated with concomitant organic changes that show in future laryngological examinations. Forms containing drawings of the vocal apparatus have been recommended so that the physician can make notes indicating the size and location of abnormalities (Boone 1982, 1993; Stone, Hurlbutt, and Coulthard 1978; Weinberg 1983). This could become part of the client's record and be used for comparisons over time with other examinations.

A third reason the speech pathologist will be interested in the laryngeal examination is that surgical intervention may be recommended as the treatment of choice for a particular patient. A dialogue between the clinician and the doctor may be necessary to discuss this decision and to discuss recommendations regarding the appropriateness of follow-up voice therapy.

Finally, the absence of organic deviations on the laryngoscopic examination may suggest more functional bases for the client's disorder. Such knowledge would have direct implications for the direction of voice treatment and may also indicate that other referrals by the speech pathologist (e.g., to a psychologist) are in order.

A general medical evaluation or specific neurological or endocrinological examination may be indicated in certain cases. When dysfunction of the peripheral or central nervous system appears to be a possible contributing factor to the voice disorder, as in dysarthria (see Chapter 9), referral is indicated.

During a routine screening of all college students entering the teacher education and certification program, Susan came to our attention. Susan's voice was weak, and she had difficulty projecting it louder or trying to shout when requested to do so. On questioning, it was revealed that her voice tires easily throughout the day and a slight hoarseness is typical. This prompted us to inquire further—trying to unravel the mystery of Susan's voice problem and wondering about a possible endocrinological basis. Suspicions of a hyperactive thyroid gland became stronger when Susan complained of nervousness and irritability, generalized muscle weakness, and fatigue—making it difficult for her to complete her aerobics routine at the local gym (one day her legs trembled and were so weak she could not rise from a squat), excessive sweating, weight loss—which she was happy about even though she still ate lots of food, suffered from insomnia, and had irregular menstrual periods. Her once-radiant skin had turned sallow in recent months. Referral to a physician was made and hyperthyroidism (Grave's disease) was diagnosed.

The Case History Interview

There are many excellent sources for guidance in taking an adequate case history with an emphasis on voice disorders, and many of these sources provide forms for the clinician's use (Aronson 1985; Boone and McFarlane 1994; Fox and Blechman 1975; Greene 1980; Johnson, Darley, and Spriestersbach 1963; Moncur and Brackett 1974; Murphy 1964; Wilson 1987). Table 10.1 lists sample case history questions that we routinely ask during a client interview. Table 10.2 may be used as a checklist on which clients may indicate any coexisting sensory symptoms (Cooper 1973; Pindzola 1987). In the following section, we will elaborate on those case history topics most relevant to vocal diagnosis and subsequent intervention.

Family Data
Information regarding the parental occupation, number of siblings, history of family adjustment, other voice problems within the family, and general health pattern

TABLE 10.1 Sample Questions to Ask in the Case History Intake

1. In your own words, describe the problem.
2. When did the voice problem begin?
3. Did the problem begin suddenly or develop slowly?
4. What conditions surrounded the onset of the voice problem (colds, illness, surgery, personal problems, etc.)?
5. When is your voice better? When is it worse?
6. Describe the daily use of your voice (typical weekday behaviors and job demands on the voice; typical weekend activities).
7. Are there specific situations when abuse occurs? (Inquire about the frequency of common misuses and abuses such as excessive crying, throat clearing, coughing, smoking, screaming, etc.)
8. Describe your general health (sinus problems; allergies; illnesses; injuries to head, neck or scrotum; endocrine disorders; heart disease; surgery; use of medications; fatiguability; smoking/drinking habits; etc.).
9. What has your doctor told you about your voice?

TABLE 10.2   Checklist of Sensory Symptoms

Mark (X) all symptoms associated with the voice problem.

_____ 1.   Frequent throat clearing
_____ 2.   Frequent coughing
_____ 3.   Vocal fatigue that progresses with use of the voice
_____ 4.   Irritation or pain in the voice box or throat
_____ 5.   Strain or bulging of neck muscles
_____ 6.   Swelling of veins and/or arteries in the neck
_____ 7.   Feeling of a foreign substance or "lump" in throat
_____ 8.   Ear irritation, tickling, or earache
_____ 9.   Frequent sore throats
_____ 10.   A tickling, soreness, or burning sensation in the throat
_____ 11.   Scratchy or dry throat
_____ 12.   Tension and/or tightness in the throat
_____ 13.   A feeling that talking is an effort
_____ 14.   Pain or difficulty swallowing
_____ 15.   Pain or burning sensation at the base of the tongue

of the family tells us a great deal about the young client's social and physical milieu. Generally, the following characteristics may be considered potentially remarkable and should be explored further: (1) too much or too little structure and organization to the home; (2) premium placed on verbal competition; (3) interparental friction; (4) unusual sibling competition; (5) history of voice disorders; (6) poor parental adjustment; (7) history of extended recurrent health problems; and (8) general level of concern for physical and health problems. For the adult client, we are interested in many of the same issues, particularly occupation, number of persons living in the home, and health problems or communication disorders among those living in the home.

> *Barbara was a 32-year-old mother of twins. Both four-year-old boys were described as rambunctious, and Barbara was the archetypical housewife. She also cared for her mother-in-law who was hard-of-hearing, a bit senile, and lived in the same home. Barbara just could not understand why she had developed bilateral vocal nodules and why the doctor insisted on her enrolling in voice therapy. Clearly, family information of this type suggests etiological factors of vocal abuse and provides behavioral change as a direction for treatment.*

Onset of the Problem
In many instances, the beginning of the voice problem will have great diagnostic significance. It is important to investigate not only the nature of the onset, but also the circumstances surrounding it. Physical or psychological trauma may have equally instant effects upon voice production. In some cases, extended questioning may be necessary because it is common for clients to repress uncomfortable incidents

of the past. Aronson (1985) indicates that a sudden onset within hours suggests the high probability of a conversion vocal disorder or a neurological origin (such as stroke), whereas many other types of vocal disturbances develop gradually (mass and approximation lesions, degenerative disease, etc.).

Although the abrupt onset of a vocal disorder is traumatic and startling, most voice disorders are of insidious origin. Many people cannot pinpoint the exact date of the onset and tend to indicate when people first noticed or remarked about their voices. Since a gradual onset is not necessarily specific to organic or functional etiologies, the examiner must look to other data for final answers. Probably more important than the rate of development is information on coincident factors such as the client's general health and emotional state.

Course of Development

A careful description of the developmental stages of the voice disturbance may provide helpful diagnostic information. The course of the development of the voice disorder may be found to parallel a chronic medical problem, cumulating vocational stress, certain periods of physical maturation, changes in family relationships, or developing financial crises. We want to know how the problem has changed since its onset, and we want to know about any circumstances surrounding variability of the voice disturbance. For instance, were there changes in the voice disorder during its development that might be correlated with changes in personal habits (e.g., smoking, use of alcohol), work conditions (e.g., excessive noise, stress), or medical conditions (e.g., sinus, allergy). The clinician will want to keep in mind that once a voice disorder has been firmly established, only a minimal amount of tension, misuse, or abuse will be necessary to perpetuate the problem.

Description of Daily Vocal Performance and Problem Variability

While the course-of-development questions seek a historical perspective, we need information on factors that influence the voice at the time of the evaluation. For instance, we might ask the client to describe his/her daily routine and relate it to talking. Does the problem become worse through the day? Does it become better as the day progresses? Boone and McFarlane (1994) suggest having the patient identify any situations that seem to be consistently related to good and poor vocal performance. It is especially important in cases of childhood vocal pathology to obtain an accurate picture of the youngster's typical use of voice and instances of misuse or abuse (Wilson 1987).

Social Adjustment

Assessment of the personality characteristics of the individual may assist the diagnostician in interpreting other information. Formal personality testing is not within the jurisdiction of the speech pathologist, but each clinician is expected to be perceptive and sensitive to clues about the client's basic adjustment of life. The notion that the voice is closely related to the individual's self-concept and reveals inner conflict has been carefully examined by several researchers. Moses (1954) and Rousey and Moriarty (1965) present interesting views of the interaction of the personality and voice production. Classification of voice characteristics with specific personality types has not provided overwhelming evidence of definite relationships; but the personality and the voice interact in a complex fashion, and this results in many symptomatic characteristics.

Vocation

We are interested in the vocation of our voice client for two reasons. First, we must determine if the occupation demands a great deal of talking and if that talking is under adverse conditions. Not all teachers develop "teacher's nodules," however, and the vocation must be judged in relation to the person. Several writers have postulated that there is a personality type that develops vocal nodules (Green 1989; Jackson 1941; Withers 1961). We have found many of these people to be tense, energetic, high strung, and verbally aggressive. Place this type of person in an occupational setting that demands a great deal of speaking under tension, and a bit of poor judgment in choosing adaptive procedures, and the chances of finding an individual with vocal nodules could be greatly enhanced.

A second factor in our evaluation of the vocation of an individual is to assess the possibility of changing aspects of the client's job routine or behavior at work if the vocation has a deleterious effect on the voice disorder.

We worked with a college professor who taught several large lecture classes to groups of over 150 students. His vocal abuse and misuse during these presentations had resulted in small nodules for which voice therapy was recommended. In an effort to be audible, dynamic, and authoritative, he had been speaking loudly, with a lower pitch, and excessive tension. We explored the possibility of his using a lavalier microphone in the large lecture rooms, and this effectively eliminated an abusive situation that was vocationally related.

Health

Realizing that the voice is influenced by many physiological systems, a complete medical history and examination are necessary in many instances. A history of the general health and physical development of the client should be obtained, along with information about specific illnesses, surgeries, and medications. The clinician should also obtain data concerning the general energy level and health-related habits such as smoking, drinking, and drug usage. Luchsinger and Arnold (1965) present a particularly comprehensive discussion of vocal disorders of organic etiology. Referral of a client to a physician may uncover a medical problem of which vocal quality is a symptom:

Sherry was identified in the speech and hearing screening program. Her voice was described as breathy, low in pitch and volume, expressionless, and varying in degrees of nasality. The more she talked, the more noticeable these symptoms became. Shouting while counting was particularly difficult for her, and articulatory slurring became evident at the higher numbers. Sherry complained of excessive fatigue by the end of the day and frequently found chewing steak dinners more of a chore than a pleasure. Subsequent medical referral indicated specific muscle weakness and a medical diagnosis of myasthenia gravis. It should be noted that the speech clinician's alertness to the accumulation of medical danger signs in addition to the speech characteristics resulted in a proper referral and subsequent identification of the problem.

Informal Evaluation: A Listening and Rating Process

The first step in voice analysis is simply listening to the client in an analytical manner. Obviously, this listening process is largely judgmental. Much of what we do in a routine voice assessment is perceptual and subjective. The "craft" of vocal evaluations is augmented with informal tasks, ratings scales, and the like. Often we consider what we do in the diagnostic session as constituting a formal evaluation, but we must recognize the informal, perceptual basis of our techniques and observations. In recent years, instrumentation to objectify our perceptual methods has become more readily available in medical and research settings. However, the evaluation remains, for most clinicians, a listening process. As such, rating scales, profiles, checklists, and assessment outlines are the order of the day.

A checklist, such as the simple one shown in Table 10.3, may guide the clinician in a cursory appraisal of the various characteristics of the voice. Many voice assessment tools (rating scales, profiles, checklists, open-ended observation forms, and the like) are available; Table 10.4 list some of the more commonly used resources. Let us highlight a few of them here.

Profiles and assessment instruments typically include scales that rate a variety of vocal aspects in terms of severity of deviation from the norm. The Buffalo III Voice Profile (Wilson 1987) rates on a five-point scale laryngeal tone, pitch, loudness, nasal resonance, oral resonance, breath supply, muscles, voice abuse, rate, speech anxiety, and speech intelligibility and provides for an overall voice rating. The Voice Profile System by Wilson and Rice (1977) has received wide acceptance. It rates the laryngeal cavity, resonating cavity, intensity, vocal range, and overall severity using numbered scales. Ratings of these types should be a helpful starting point in the voice evaluation; the clinician who notes disturbance in any parameter of vocal production can move on to more specific analysis techniques that illuminate further the affected aspect of the voice.

A detailed analysis of vocal parameters is typical in clinical practice. The critical listening, previously described, combined with estimates or measurements of the voice, using little or no specialized equipment is perhaps a blending of the informal-formal dichotomy. An assessment tool illustrative of this type of appraisal is the Voice Assessment Protocol for Children and Adults (Pindzola 1987). The protocol facilitates quick interpretations of vocal parameter normalcy by use of a Likert scale, or grid-marking system. Five parameters of the voice are assessed: pitch, loudness, quality, breath features, and rate/rhythm. Analysis of a client is best done by using a conversational speech sample supplemented with phoneme prolongation tasks, singing the scale, diadochokinetic testing, reading, and similar tasks of one's choos-

TABLE 10.3 Checklist of Vocal Characteristics

Pitch
 1   2   3   4   5   6   7

Description		Severity						
—Too high		1	2	3	4	5	6	7
—Too low		1	2	3	4	5	6	7
—Invariant		1	2	3	4	5	6	7
—Pitch breaks		1	2	3	4	5	6	7
—Diplophonia		1	2	3	4	5	6	7
—Repetitive pattern		1	2	3	4	5	6	7

Loudness
 1   2   3   4   5   6   7

Description		Severity						
—Excessive		1	2	3	4	5	6	7
—Inadequate		1	2	3	4	5	6	7
—Uncontrolled variation		1	2	3	4	5	6	7
—Repetitive pattern		1	2	3	4	5	6	7
Invariant		1	2	3	4	5	6	7
—Tremulous		1	2	3	4	5	6	7

Quality
 1   2   3   4   5   6   7

Description		Severity						
—Hoarseness		1	2	3	4	5	6	7
—Harshness		1	2	3	4	5	6	7
—Breathiness		1	2	3	4	5	6	7
—Hypernasal		1	2	3	4	5	6	7
—Hyponasal		1	2	3	4	5	6	7
—Other (describe)		1	2	3	4	5	6	7

Judgment of Vocal Tension

 —Aphonia/whisper
 —Breathy phonation
 —Normal
 —Hypertension
 —Hypertension/intermittent phonation

Overall Judgment of Voice
 1   2   3   4   5   6   7

Note: 1 = normal; 7 = severely disordered

ing. A high-quality tape recording of the voice is suggested. Perceptual judgments are adequate, or the clinician may choose to supplement estimations with instrumental measurements, such as a piano or other musical instrument, pitch pipe, sound spectrography, loudness indicators, and the like.

TABLE 10.4   An Annotated Listing of Some of the Available Rating Scales and Evaluation Materials

Remediation of Vocal Hoarseness
(Blonigen 1980)
Although primarily a treatment guide, this booklet will prove useful in the appraisal stage where abuses and misuses must be identified.

The Boone Voice Program for Children (2nd ed.)
(Boone 1993)
Screening, evaluation, and referral instructions are included in a manual with this remediation kit. Also provided are the necessary forms and stimulus materials.

The Boone Voice Program for Adults
(Boone 1982)
Both diagnosis and remediation procedures for vocal disorders are contained in this kit.

Voice Patient Case History
(Fox and Blechman 1975)
A detailed listing of case history questions is presented. Testing of vocal function is also described and presented in a concise format. Pitch, loudness, quality, time, and breathing are tested.

General Voice Quality Examination,

Supplementary Examination for Harshness,

Supplementary Examination for Breathiness,

Supplementary Examination for Nasality
(Johnson, Darley, and Spriestersbach 1963)
The detailed examination form is dominated by case history questions and clinical observations. Three supplementary forms provide for detailed observations of vocal quality. The effects of phonetic context, loudness, pitch, rate, and other factors are investigated.

Voice Assessment Protocol for Children and Adults
(Pindzola 1987)
This protocol directs and quantifies clinical observations of voice. The following vocal parameters are assessed: pitch, loudness, quality, breath features, and rate.

Symptomatic Voice Therapy
(Polow and Kaplan 1980)
This detailed notebook describes the differential diagnosis, possible etiologies, management decisions, and therapy techniques for disorders of pitch, loudness, phonation, and resonance.

Systematic Assessment of Voice (SAV)
(Shipley 1990)
This is a comprehensive inventory of tasks, strategies, and guidelines for assessing functional and organic voice problems in children and adults. It contains reproducible lists of words, phrases, sentences, passages for oral reading, case history forms, letters to parents, and so forth.

Voice Profile System
(Wilson and Rice 1977)
This Programmed Approach to Voice Therapy includes two methods of treatment for voice disorders in children and adults (tension increase and tension decrease). It also contains a profiling system useful for vocal assessment. Sample recordings (on cassette) accompany the program with training instructions for severity judgments.

Continued

TABLE 10.4 *Continued*

Buffalo III Voice Profile

Buffalo III Voice Screening Profile

Buffalo III Group Behavior Profile

Buffalo III Voice Abuse Profile

Buffalo III Speech Anxiety Profile

Buffalo III Voice Recording Profile

Buffalo III Voice Diagnostic Profile
   (Wilson 1987)
      The Buffalo system consists of ten profiles for various purposes (seven pertinent here)
      with the "Voice Profile" being a general, overall rating scale.

Let us now turn our attention to a discussion of the vocal parameters and how they are routinely assessed. As in evaluating other communication disorders, the clinician must realize that the type of sample obtained affects how "ecologically valid" it is. For instance, in the case of a child with vocal nodules who is suspected of being a vocal abuser, it would be ideal to observe the youngster in a play situation with others, during school activities, and in the home environment. Most often, a variety of sampling activities is used in the evaluation, ranging from conversation, counting, coughing, singing the scale, and prolonging isolated speech sounds. The point here is that the clinician should be aware that a broad sampling of vocal performance is needed in order to make correct judgments on any parameter of the voice.

Pitch Assessment

Clinicians routinely evaluate various pitch characteristics of the client's voice. Pitch is a perceptual phenomenon that correlates with the valving rate of the vocal folds. Rightly or wrongly, clinicians interchange the terms *pitch* and *frequency* when talking about a client's voice. *Pitch determination* of the speaking fundamental frequency, also known as habitual pitch, can be accomplished with musical-matching methods or by instrumental analysis (e.g., Visi-Pitch, Computerized Speech Lab from Kay Elemetrics). The client's speaking fundamental frequency can then be compared to normative data, based on age and sex. Table 10.5 shows average fundamental frequencies for a representative sample of ages, synthesized from the literature (Hollien and Shipp 1972; Kelley 1977; Wilson 1987).

Pitch determination methods can also be used to locate a client's optimal pitch. *Optimal pitch* is a controversial concept that supposes each person has an optimal or natural pitch range at which he/she *should* be speaking. If we accept the premise of optimal performance, then, when optimal pitch does not match habitual pitch, habitual pitch may need to be raised or lowered in treatment. The determination of optimal pitch is by no means precise. In addition, it should be emphasized that optimal pitch is not a single note, but a range of notes where the vocal mechanism

TABLE 10.5   Average Fundamental
              Frequencies for Selected Ages

Age	Sex	Mean Fundamental
1–2	either	445 Hz
3	either	390 Hz
6	either	320 Hz
10	male	235 Hz
15	male	165 Hz
20–29	male	120 Hz
50–59	male	118 Hz
60–69	male	112 Hz
80–89	male	146 Hz
10	female	265 Hz
15	female	220 Hz
20–29	female	227 Hz
50–59	female	214 Hz
60–69	female	209 Hz
80–89	female	197 Hz

appears to function best with the least muscular tension. Various vegetative (natural, involuntary, and nonspeech sounds) and range singing techniques have been proposed for eliciting optimal pitches from clients; once elicited and recorded, the value of the optimal pitch can be determined musically or instrumentally. The following sources can be consulted regarding procedures for determining optimal pitch: Boone and McFarlane (1994), Fairbanks (1960), Murphy (1964), Moncur and Brackett (1974), Polow and Kaplan (1980), and Pindzola (1987). Table 10.6 summarizes some of the more commonly used methods for eliciting a client's optimal pitch. Later in the chapter, we will discuss how these techniques are useful as probes or facilitators of voicing abilities.

The normal voice is characterized by *pitch variability,* also known as *intonation* or *inflection.* The voice is abnormal when there is a lack of pitch variability or when pitch fluctuations are excessive. Dysarthrias may be characterized by monopitch where a limited range of notes are used monotonously (Darley, Aronson, and Brown 1975). Monopitch and restricted pitch ranges are also associated with superior laryngeal nerve paralysis (Luchsinger and Arnold 1965), additive lesions (Boone and McFarlane 1994), and other disorders. Excessive pitch variability or prosodic excess may be heard in the dysarthrias, particularly spastic, ataxic and hyperkinetic forms (Darley, Aronson, and Brown 1975). Hearing-impaired and deaf speakers also often utilize excessive pitch fluctuations (Martony 1968).

Diplophonia refers to the presence of two or more simultaneous pitches or tones in the voice and may be caused by separate or unequal vibratory sources. Possible causes include a paralyzed vocal fold vibrating at a rate different from the healthy one, a vibration of a growth or lesion, simultaneous adduction of the ventricular folds and true folds, and even an innocuous saliva globule.

Pitch breaks most often occur in a person using an inappropriately low-pitched voice. Intermittently, the pitch will suddenly break upward toward a more opti-

TABLE 10.6   Some Techniques for Determining Optimal Pitch

Resonance-Swell Method

Have client hum at the same intensity up the scale, and note whether his voice becomes louder or swells in a given range of pitches. Client and/or clinician should listen for this swell in loudness.

Loud-Audible Sigh

Client should take a deep breath and produce /a/ as a loud sigh. Listen most carefully for the pitch at the onset of the sigh because one tends to lower the pitch during the sound. Optimal is said to be the onset tone.

Yawn-Sigh

The client should yawn and sigh audibly in a relaxed manner. Yawning opens the throat and minimizes the constriction around the larynx.

Vegetative Techniques

Listen to the natural, spontaneous laugh, cough, throat clearing, or grunt of the client. These vegetative forms of phonation may be representative of optimal pitch.

Inflection Methods

Have the client say "um hum" using a rising inflection with lips closed, as though he/she were spontaneously and sincerely agreeing with what was just said. In addition, the clinician could have the client say "hello" in a natural, spontaneous, and sincere way. An automatic affirmative utterance often approximates optimal pitch. A related method is to have the client say "hello" with rising inflection, as though asking a question. The slight inflection may reveal a more optimal voice.

Pushing or Pulling Techniques

The client should attempt to phonate /a/ of optimal quality while pushing down or pulling up on his/her chair. This method may be particularly useful for clients with disordered closure of the vocal folds.

Pitch Range Methods

The type of phonation may be do-re-mi or ah-ah-ah or one-two-three, and so on. The client phonates her entire vocal range from the lowest sound that can be produced to the highest, excluding falsetto. One third of this range should represent optimal pitch. An alternate, and popular, method is to have the client phonate his/her entire vocal range from the lowest note to the highest, including falsetto. The total range is then divided by one fourth to locate the optimal. For example, calculate the number of full-step notes in the client's range and then locate the note that is one fourth of the way from the bottom.

mal level. Any condition that adds to the mass or size of the vocal folds may alter their vibratory characteristics. Pitch breaks may be one symptom of additive lesions such as, but not limited to, nodules, polyps, and tumors.

To summarize our discussion of pitch, the clinician must observe the client and seek answers to the following questions: What is the client's habitual pitch (speaking fundamental frequency), and is this pitch appropriate for the person's age, sex, and body stature? What is an optimal level for the client to use? Is a normal amount of pitch variability present in the speaking voice, or is the voice monotoned or widely varying and sing-songed in pattern? Are pitch breaks present? Is diplophonia present?

Loudness Assessment

Perceptual judgments of vocal loudness are sufficient for appraisal purposes. Instrumentation is available for measuring intensity and may prove useful in providing feedback to the client during intervention. Of interest during the assessment is whether the *loudness level* is appropriate for the speaking situation. In normal conversational speech, some three feet from the speaker, the average sound intensity is 65 dB (range 55–75 dB) (Van Bergeijk, Pierce, and David 1960). Typical loudness levels may be abnormal in various pathologies. Adults with dysarthria may speak too softly (as in Parkinsonism) or with a booming voice (as in some spasticities and dystonias) (Darley, Aronson, and Brown 1975). Lack of vocal loudness is characteristic of paralyzed cords and psychogenic disorders. Vocal abuse cases often speak with excessive effort and loudness, at least in some situations; the end result however may be hypofunctional loudness.

The clinician should also note if the typical loudness level can be maintained comfortably, without trailing off, or whether there is a *degree of effort*. Listen for loudness that trails off at the end of a sentence, which may be typical in vocal fold paralysis, dysarthrias, or obstructive lesions (Darley, Aronson, and Brown 1975; Wilson and Rice 1977). *Phonation breaks* or momentary skips of loudness are abnormal and may indicate difficulty maintaining vocal fold adduction and vibration.

A certain amount of *loudness variability* is normal and is reflected in the stress patterns of the language. In addition to critically listening to conversational speech, we often ask the client to read "with feeling" sentences such as the following:

> *Get out of here, get out of here!*
> *I don't know, I said I don't know!*
> *I need more money, Dad, I'm broke!*
> *Where did she go? I can't find her.*
> *Will you cut that out!*

Other vocal variety drills are available in the drillbooks of Fairbanks (1960) and Hanley and Thurman (1970). We have observed that lack of loudness variability may take two differing forms of monoloudness; excess and equal stress patterns are typical of many dysarthrias (Darley, Aronson, and Brown 1975) whereas the monoloud but weak and "bland" voice is typically seen in affective disorders (Leff and Abberton 1981; Weintraub, Mesulam, and Kramer 1981) and some forms of dysarthria (Darley, Aronson, and Brown 1975).

The clinician may wish to have the client demonstrate his/her *loudness range*, from soft to maximal levels. Whispering and shouting can be requested. One method is to ask the client to count, beginning softly and increasing loudness with higher and higher numbers. Restricted loudness range is often seen in clients with respiratory involvement, particularly the dysarthrias (Darley, Aronson, and Brown 1975).

Loudness abuses may be situation-oriented. For instance, conversational levels may be appropriate but frequent loud talking or screaming (as in lectures, sermons, playground activities, etc.) may be perpetuating a vocal disorder. Questions asked in the interview should probe the client's daily uses of the voice with the purpose of discovering situational abuses.

After appraising the client's voice, the clinician should then have answers to the following questions about loudness: Is the loudness level that is used appropriate for the speaking situation? Can the level be maintained comfortably without undue strain? Can the level be maintained throughout the entire utterance or does it begin to trail off? Are loudness breaks present? Is the loudness variable in order to reflect stress and emphasis patterns of English or is the client monoloud? Can loudness vary from minimal (whispered) to maximal (shouted) levels? What, if any, situations are frequently encountered in which loudness abuse occurs?

Quality Assessment

The descriptive terminology used with disorders of vocal quality reflects the perceptual nature of the judgments. It can be argued that the clinician's ear is the best tool for describing the quality of a voice—and many clinicians use just that. However, rather sophisticated equipment is also available to study, categorize, and "objectify" acoustical parameters of the voice. For example, Isshiki, Yanigahara, and Morimoto (1966) provide some spectrographic guidelines for classifying four severity levels of hoarseness. Technology is available to measure periodicity of vocal fold vibrations, changes in amplitude (shimmer), changes in frequency (jitter), and opening-closing characteristics. (The Computerized Speech Lab from Kay Elemetrics has many software options for voice measures.) Still, deciding whether a voice is breathy, harsh, or hoarse is done most efficiently by critical listening.

Vocal quality is affected by the manner of vocal fold vibration. Many terms of vocal quality appear in the literature. Most disorders are classified as "breathy," "harsh," or "hoarse"; hoarseness is the most prevalent. Designations such as "strident" and "husky" are used less frequently.

The breathy voice is characterized by an audible escape of air through partially closed folds. The lack of firm adduction may be due to obstruction by a mass or lesion, a paralyzed cord, or muscular incompetence.

The voice displaying effort and force is the harsh voice. Harshness is usually perceived in a phonatory milieu of hard glottal attacks, low pitch, intensity problems, and overadduction of the vocal folds. Equivalent terms are "roughness" and "unpleasantness," although "strident," "course," "grating," "rasping," "rough," "metallic," and "guttural" have been used as synonyms for "harshness" (Murphy 1964).

The hoarse voice incorporates the features of both breathiness and harshness. As such, turbulent air flow, rough/aperiodic vibrations, low pitch, and neck muscle strain may be evident. Hoarseness is a common symptom of many vocal pathologies and should be recognizable by all SLPs. In particular, the public school clinician should be familiar with the auditory symptoms of hoarseness as a warning sign of vocal abuse and related lesions in children. The clinician must make medical referrals as appropriate. In addition, the clinician must educate teachers through in-service programs to recognize voice disturbances in students so that teacher referrals to the SLP will be accomplished.

The perception of vocal quality also is affected by *glottal approximation.* The hard glottal attack refers to an abrupt impact or strong initiation of speech. Extra effort is used to start the vibrations of tightly adducted folds. Presumably, then, prior to phonation there is too much tension in laryngeal muscles. Conversely, soft attack is an abnormally weak glottal approximation. Breathiness usually precedes this phonation. The astute clinician is listening for symptoms of an inappropriate glottal approximation.

Quality can also be affected by resonance imbalances; however, these problems will be discussed in Chapter 12.

Assessment of Breath Features

Breathing variables affect laryngeal function in general, and vocal loudness and rate of speech in particular. Several features of the respiratory system and breath management are typically assessed in a voice evaluation. The clinician may first want to observe the *predominant region* used for breath support. The diaphragm is the principle muscle of inhalation and various thoracic muscles assist when needed in expanding the lung-thoracic unit (Zemlin 1988). Diaphragmatic breathing involves descent of the diaphragm and expansion of the abdomen during inhalation. Although quite normal—and a preferred way of breathing for both song and speech—it is difficult if not impossible to observe in a clothed, seated client. Expansion of the chest, not the shoulders, in a slight heaving motion is more observable; this type of thoracic breathing is used by many people. Clavicular breathing, in contrast, is characterized by shoulder elevation, upper thoracic tension (in the area of the clavicle or collar bone), and neck muscle strain. Clavicular breathing is an inefficient method of lung expansion for inhalation as it involves too much effort for too little breath. The clinician should try to observe the region predominately used for breathing by clients; many hyperfunctional voice cases employ this inefficient form of breathing.

The maximum amount of air that can be exhaled following maximal inhalation is called *vital capacity.* The relationship of vital capacity to speech production is somewhat a matter of conjecture at this point. Vital capacity is apparently related to several factors, such as body size, physical condition, and sex (Gray and Wise 1959; Van Riper and Irwin 1958). There is little or no research to vindicate those who have worked to increase the vital capacity of their voice clients. On the other hand, it is logical to assume that an individual with an extremely small amount of available air would find it difficult to sustain phonation and might resort to increased laryngeal tension and forcing to maintain normal or near-normal phrasing. It is probably not so much the volume of air as it is the individual's ability to control the air flow (Hardy 1961).

Equipment, such as the spirometer, is necessary to measure vital capacity. Clinically, however, we have found that a vital capacity insufficient for normal speech purposes was so obvious from normal observation that further formal testing was not necessary. Vital capacity measurements may be of particular concern in cases of emphysema, later stages of Parkinson's disease, and cerebral palsy in children. Related to lung volume are indications of the client's tidal volume, inspiratory reserve volume, expiratory reserve volume, and air flow rates, which some authorities recommend measuring clinically (Boone and McFarlane 1994; Hirano 1981).

Inhalation for speech should be quick and quiet. The clinician should listen for *associated noises* such as gasps and vocalizations during inhalation as the client speaks. Rating scales may also prompt the clinician to judge their conspicuousness or severity. *Inhalatory stridor* refers to noticeable phonatory sounds during inhalation and may be common in cases of vocal fold paralysis and dysarthrias (Darley, Aronson, and Brown 1975).

When respiratory support is inadequate for normal speech, clients may breathe more frequently. In addition, fewer words (or syllables) may be spoken per breath group. These two factors contribute to the perception of "choppy" speech. The clinician should assess *words per breath;* a patient who can only utter six or so words per air charge is displaying poor breath support. Occasionally, a patient may say an excessive number of words per breath group. Research as to what is excessive is, however, lacking. Perhaps upward of twelve or thirteen words per breath group is typical of normal speakers. Increased speaking rates and loss of intelligibility may be the negative by-products of too many words per breath.

Of interest in a voice evaluation is the maximum duration that a client can sustain sound plus air. *Maximum phonation time* (MPT) is typically measured with a stopwatch as the client prolongs certain voiced phonemes, such as /a/ or /z/. A similar measure is that of *maximum exhalation time* (MET), where a voiceless phoneme such as /s/ is used. The clinician should provide several trials, instruct the client to use a deep breath, and record the longest sustained attempt. Wilson (1987) presents data on average maximum phonation times for /a/, /i/, and /u/ for ages three to twenty-nine years. Hirano (1981) also provides normal MPT values for adults. Condensing this information, we find the following rules of thumb to be clinically useful: Elementary school-age children (six- to ten-years-old) should be able to prolong /a/ for at least 9 seconds, regardless of sex; adult males average 25 to 35 seconds MPT; and adult females average 15 to 25 seconds MPT. Coleman, Michel, and Lynn (1987) caution against using normative data collected from healthy, young and middle-aged adults when evaluating geriatric clients. They encourage collection of local norms by practicing clinicians. Values for maximum exhalation time (MET) that they report as clinically useful are 35 seconds for clients who are trained singers or actors; 20 seconds for a typical young adult; and 12 seconds for persons over age sixty-five.

Related to the measures of MPT and MET is the clinical procedure of computing the *S/Z ratio*. The S/Z ratio as proposed by Eckel and Boone (1981) and Tait, Michel, and Carpenter (1980) is a quick screening device used to determine how much of a voice problem may be related to respiration control and how much may be the result of laryngeal problems. Clients who have laryngeal pathology will have less control of the air stream during the production of a prolonged /z/. Using a stopwatch, two trials are given for the prolongation of both the voiceless /s/ and the voiced /z/ phonemes. The best or longest /s/ and the longest /z/ are used in calculating the S/Z ratio. If the S/Z ratio is greater than 1.2 for a child or 1.4 for an adult, a laryngeal pathology may exist (Eckel and Boone 1981).

Assessment of Rate and Rhythm

Although traditionally not part of vocal evaluations, the *rate* at which a client talks should be assessed as rate can affect or be affected by other variables of speech and the voice. Often excessive rates are related to poor breathing features and improper phrase groupings. The client may try to say too many words on one breath, giving the perception of an excessive rate of speech, as in Parkinsonism. The converse may also occur. Frequent air intakes may give the perception of choppiness—the client may only be able to say a few words, then breathe, then say a few more words, then breathe, and so forth. The result is not only a choppy *rhythm* but an overall slowness of speech owing to the increased pause time. Rate changes may also interfere with intelligibility, as is so typical of the dysarthrias (Yorkston, Beukelman, and Bell 1988).

Rate is typically expressed as words per minute or syllables per minute. It can be quite cumbersome to measure an entire speech sample for the determination of rate. Therefore, we offer the following efficient and clinically useful estimation method (tape-recording for later playback is recommended): Count the number of words in a 60-second sample of "connected" speech. If no connected 60-second samples are available on the tape recording, then count the number of words in whatever connected sample is available and mathematically calculate words per minute. For example, if a 20-second speech sample contains 50 words, then, on the average, the person is talking at 150 words per minute (60 seconds divided by 20 seconds = 3, and 3 times 50 words = 150 wpm). An alternative method, useful for determining rate of speech during reading, has been suggested by Fox and Blechman (1975). Give the client a reading passage with prenumbered words. Allow the client to read aloud for one minute, as timed with a stopwatch, and note how many of the words were read.

Conversational speech rates typical of young children have only recently been published. Ryan (1984) found that normal-speaking children (ages two-years, ten-months to five-years, two-months) converse at 195 syllables per minute or 157 words per minute. A slightly slower rate was reported by Pindzola and colleagues in that normal three-, four-, and five-year-olds average 148 syllables per minute of talking with a range between 109 and 183 syllables (Miller and Pindzola 1985; Pindzola, Jenkins, and Lokken 1989). During an oral reading task, normal adult speakers speak at a mean rate of 167 words per minute (Darley 1940), yet conversational rates may be higher at 195 words per minute (Walker 1979). Since rate norms were collected from young, healthy adults, caution is advised in assessing speech rates of geriatrics. Preliminary studies suggest that older adults speak slower than younger adults. Persons over age sixty-five average about 141–144 words per minute or 186–289 syllables per minute (Duchin and Mysak 1987; Leeper et al. 1990). At the present time, we do not know what constitutes "too fast" or "too slow" a speech rate, and so the clinician's judgment of normalcy is important. Rate determinations may be most necessary with neurological voice disorders (Darley, Aronson, and Brown 1975; Yorkston, Beukelman, and Bell 1988).

Objective and Sophisticated Measures

Great strides have been made in the last decade to advance our knowledge of voice science. Technological advances have permitted us to study laryngeal function, and much of this technology is now ready for clinical application. Ludlow and Hart (1982) concluded from a conference involving voice scientists, speech pathologists, and laryngologists that fiberoptic, electromyographic, air flow, acoustic, and laryngographic techniques are useful in the assessment of neurologic dysfunction, vocal fold lesions, morphologic changes of the folds, and abnormal phonatory function. The serious reader should consult the work of Titze (1994).

Hirano (1981) has done much to standardize the clinical examination of the voice and feels that proper instrumentation is essential to a thorough assessment. The following section of this chapter will outline equipment-dependent techniques and provide a framework for interpretation of the data generated from such instrumentation.

Electromyography

Electromyography, or EMG, permits direct assessment of the laryngeal muscles. Hirano (1981) describes the necessary apparatus and electrode insertion techniques. Electromyography has not been used routinely in this country except in major research centers with medical affiliations. Yet, EMG is important to the diagnosis of vocal fold paralysis; true paralysis may be differentiated from other forms of vocal fold immobility. In addition, EMG can indicate the degree and extent of paralysis, which may suggest recovery potential in that the presence of action potentials induced by voluntary activity indicates a favorable prognosis. It can also be useful in shaping the course of surgical procedures, as in lateral fixation of a fold for cases of bilateral paralysis.

Aerodynamic Tests

Aerodynamic tests can assess the aerodynamic properties of phonation, including subglottal pressure, supraglottal pressure, glottal impedance, and the volume velocity of the air flow at the glottis. Hirano (1981) states that the values of these four parameters vary during the opening and closing maneuvers of the glottis and may be difficult to measure. For example, the determination of subglottal pressure necessitates an invasive approach (such as a tracheal puncture), and glottal resistance must be mathematically calculated since it cannot be measured directly. The measure of *mean flow rate* (MFR), however, is often done as an office procedure.

The MFR of a sustained vowel, such as /a/, spoken at a natural pitch and loudness level, has been used clinically to evaluate phonatory function. The patient sustains the vowel for a maximum period of time while wearing a mask fitted tightly to the face or using a mouth piece with the nose clamped. The mask or mouth piece is coupled to a spirometer, pneumotachograph, or hot-wire anemometer. The MFR is obtained by dividing the total volume of air used during phonation by the duration of phonation.

As reviewed by Hirano (1981), numerous studies suggest that normal values of the MFR range from 40 to 200 ml/sec in adult males and females. The work of Shigemori (1977) suggests that similar values hold true for children. Values for MFR greater than 200 ml/sec or less than 40 ml/sec obtained at habitual pitch and loudness levels should be regarded as abnormal.

The MFR is greater than normal in cases of recurrent laryngeal nerve paralysis. Values for MFR in cases of nodules, polyps, polypoid swelling (Reinke's edema), and neoplastic tumors also exceed the normal range but are not as marked as with recurrent laryngeal nerve paralysis. In contrast, MFR values are typically within normal limits for the conditions of laryngitis, contact granuloma, and spastic dysphonia. Hirano (1981) concludes that MFR is not only diagnostically important but may be used to monitor treatment as well.

Another aerodynamic measure that may be calculated is that of *phonation quotient*. Hirano (1981) calculates the phonation quotient (PQ) by dividing the vital capacity (VC) by the maximum phonation time (MPT):

$$PQ = \frac{VC}{MPT}$$

He also reports that the phonation quotient has a high positive relationship to the MFR and therefore is a reasonable, clinical substitute for MFR when no equipment for air flow measurement is available. Normal values of the PQ in adults and children are typically between 120 to 190 ml/sec. High phonation quotients are associated with recurrent laryngeal nerve paralysis and additive lesions of the folds, such as nodules, polyps, polypoid swelling, and neoplasms.

Subglottal pressure measures are also aerodynamic, yet invasive, tests. To measure air pressures below the vocal folds, a tracheal puncture needle, transglottal catheter, or esophageal balloon may be used. Clinicians working in nonmedical settings do not typically measure subglottal pressure in their clients. Normal values of subglottal pressure during habitual phonation are typically 5 to 10 cm H_2O but these values change with variations in vocal intensity and fundamental frequency (Hirano 1981). Subglottal pressure values are abnormally high in laryngeal carcinoma, recurrent nerve paralysis, laryngocele, and perhaps even in functional dysphonias.

Examination of Vocal Fold Vibration

By observing the vibrating vocal folds, clinicians and researchers can better understand both healthy and pathological laryngeal characteristics. Special equipment is needed to view movements occurring 100 to 300 times per second, as is typical during conversational speech. Stroboscopy and glottography are clinically useful methods; other, more elaborate research methodologies are also available. The serious student will want to consult Hirano (1981) for a detailed account of examination techniques and the numerous behaviors that can be assessed by such vibration studies (e.g., horizontal excursion of the vocal fold edge, glottal width, glottal area, frequency of vibration, symmetry of movements, closure phase information).

Acoustic Measures

Acoustic measures, according to Perkins (1985), are the most frequently employed, and perhaps preferred, objective or formal techniques for assessing the voice. This is because acoustic measures are nonintrusive; easily gathered, analyzed, and quantified; and applicable to a wide range of normal and abnormal laryngeal conditions. The serious student will want to consult the works of Davis (1979, 1982) regarding the applications of acoustic measures to the assessment of voice. Research has shown that acoustic measures are useful in both the detection of laryngeal pathologies and the assessment of voice quality. Perkins (1985) states:

> *Pathology that affects vocal fold mass, elasticity, stiffness, or length will affect fundamental frequency. Paralysis of respiratory or laryngeal musculature will reduce sufficiency of subglottal pressure and, accordingly, of vocal intensity. The traditional early warning sign of laryngeal pathology, hoarseness, is heard as a deviant quality but can also involve fundamental frequency and intensity. A tumor or paralysis of one cord that produces asymmetric mass, stiffness, or elasticity will cause asymmetric cord vibration with consequent breathiness, reduced intensity, pitch perturbation (jitter) and amplitude perturbation (shimmer). (82)*

The measures of jitter and shimmer are becoming more commonplace because of their utility in early detection of pathology, even when the laryngologist sees no obvious lesion or tissue change. Speech pathologists working in concert with laryngologists will be called upon to obtain measures of jitter and shimmer on their patients. There are several methods of computation for jitter and shimmer values; the serious student is urged to study this topic further.

The sound spectrogram has long been a favorite piece of equipment for the voice scientist and clinician. Isshiki, Yanigahara, and Morimoto (1966) proposed that narrowband analyses can provide measures of hoarseness. They described four types:

- Type 1 shows the slightest degree of hoarseness where the distinct harmonic component is mixed with the noise component which is limited within the formant region of the vowels; vowels to use are /u, o, a, e, i/.

- Type 2 shows a slight noise component in the high frequency region (3000–5000 Hz). The noise components predominate over the harmonics, most noticeable for the vowels /e/ and /i/.
- Type 3 shows only noise in the second formant of /i/ and /e/; there is also a further intensification of noise above 3000 Hz.
- Type 4 is characterized by noise in the second formant of /e/, /i/, and /a/ and in the first formant of /a/, /o/, and /u/. In these formant regions, the harmonic components are hardly noticeable.

The clinician can use the typing system of Isshiki, Yanigahara, and Morimoto for baseline, objective documentation of a patient's hoarseness. Spectrographic reassessments and retyping could be used as a barometer of improvement through treatment.

Informal Assessment Probes

We have now explained both the perceptual-informal and the technological-formal methods of voice appraisal. Clearly, most SLPs operate in work settings with limited instrumentation available. Over the years, then, clinicians have developed effective behavioral techniques for assessing, probing, treating, and reassessing laryngeal voice disorders. Indeed, the process of voice therapy is behavioral; that is, we as clinicians use strategies, techniques, devices, and even psychological "tricks" to change or alter a client's voice. Of course this presupposes that the changes are somehow better for the client—the voice sounds better, less effort is expended in its production, further damage is not being inflicted on the vocal mechanism, and so forth. But just completing a voice evaluation, where deviant vocal parameters have been analyzed, in and of itself does not suggest how to proceed clinically. As clinicians, we want to know what we can do to make the client's voice "better." Here we enter the world of trial therapy and the use of facilitating techniques to probe the client's potential to alter his/her voice for the better. Let us now highlight some of these probe techniques in hopes that clinicians will try out the client's ability to modify and improve parameters of the voice during the initial diagnostic evaluation. By doing so, the clinician will be able to accomplish two important things: a meaningful prognosis and a direction for intervention.

Patients with hypofunctional voice problems often show improved phonatory abilities by increasing glottal tension. Indeed, Wilson and Rice (1977) have developed a clinical approach termed *tension increase therapy*. The clinician should probe which maneuvers, if any, are successful in improving the voice. Do any of the so-called optimal pitch techniques help, such as grunting, pushing, pulling, throat clearing, or coughing (see Table 10.6)? An intentional hard glottal attack, even if accompanied by increased tension in the arms and trunk while pushing forcefully, may facilitate approximation of the vocal folds. Used this way, these may be thought of as hypertonic techniques rather than as techniques to achieve optimal pitch. Table 10.7 presents a useful sampling of techniques that may facilitate, or improve, voice production. The works of the following authorities should be consulted for more

TABLE 10.7 Some Facilitating Techniques for the Improvement of Voice

To improve adduction and phonatory abilities:
  Gutzmann lateral compression of thyroid lamina
  Head turning or tilting
  Pushing or pulling concomitant with voicing
  Hard glottal attacks

To alter pitch and/or quality:
  Gutzmann frontal compression of thyroid prominence
  Any/all of the optimal pitch techniques (Table 10.6)
  Change in loudness
  Change in speech rate
  Soft glottal attacks
  Relaxation of musculature/reduction of tension
  Alteration of respiratory patterns

in-depth discussions of facilitating techniques: Boone and McFarlane (1994); Johnson, Darley, and Spriestersbach (1963); Moncur and Brackett (1974); Prater and Swift (1984); and Van Riper and Irwin (1958).

Two case examples may illustrate how the use of hypertonic probe techniques in the evaluation affected treatment recommendations.

Mrs. Hernandez was involved in a rather messy divorce settlement after 22 years of marriage. Over the past few months, she has experienced periodic losses of voice—sometimes during heated conversations but occasionally for an afternoon or an entire day. Mrs. Hernandez indicated that the voice was reduced to a whisper during these episodes and was not hoarse as with laryngitis. The current episode of voice loss, and the reason she was seeing a speech-language pathologist, had lasted over a week. The clinician was not able to get Mrs. Hernandez to speak above a whisper in the evaluation; she showed no potential to talk, sing, or shout. The clinician was able to elicit, rather quickly, a cough and a throat-clearing maneuver that contained true phonated sound. A diagnosis of hysterical aphonia was made and, because of the rehabilitation potential displayed for phonation, treatment was recommended immediately. After three sessions of behavioral shaping, beginning with vegetative eliciting techniques, the client was speaking normally. Referral was then made for psychological support services.

Mrs. Osborne, age 42, presented with unilateral vocal fold paralysis subsequent to thyroid surgery. The laryngologist referred the patient for voice improvement therapy. Teflon injection was contraindicated as it would further compromise the reduced glottal airway. The patient presented with stridor during physical exertion; the speaking voice was hoarse and of limited loudness. Hoarseness diminished and loudness improved when the speech-language pathologist exerted medial pressure against the thyroid lamina on the side of the paralyzed fold (a rendition of the Gutzmann medial compression technique). Other hypertonic facilitating techniques were helpful, as well, in improving Mrs. Osborne's voicing abilities. With medical management contraindicated, the clinician felt compensatory strategies involving increased muscular effort and glottal attack were appropriate and realistic. Treatment was recommended along these lines.

Vocal quality improvements can also be brought about by changes in the manner of speaking. Adjustments in the respiratory, phonatory, and articulatory processes impact on the overall perception of the voice. We provide one case example here.

Greg was a college student referred to us by the university infirmary. Greg had gone to see the doctor with general complaints of not feeling well, simply in an effort to get a medical excuse for missing a class exam for which he had not studied. The doctor could find nothing wrong with Greg but was concerned by his "gravel-sounding, hoarse voice." Indirect laryngoscopy revealed normal structures and referral was made to our speech clinic. Greg's voice was pitched abnormally low and the quality was indeed abnormal. The aberrant quality was the more conspicuous problem. He indicated that his voice always sounded like this and gave him no trouble other than fatigue after any day of heavy talking. Part of our evaluation session was spent with "trial and error" attempts to change Greg's voice. Some things we tried had no effect, others made him sound more harsh, and a few techniques seemed to bring out a "better" voice. In particular, raising Greg's pitch slightly decreased the harshness. The higher pitch, he assured us, felt comfortable. We hypothesized that Greg was using an inappropriately low and harsh voice, perhaps to project a more masculine image, and that the functional disorder would remediate quite well. Treatment was recommended to improve the harsh quality by raising pitch.

Prognosis

Prognosis has several aspects. First, there is the question of spontaneous remission of the presenting symptoms. Will this individual display an improvement in voice without intervening therapy? Second, how much improvement can be expected following the prescribed clinical program? That is, to what degree is the voice therapy, as projected, going to be effective? Third, how permanent are the gains shown in therapy going to be? Is the vocal improvement such that continuous therapy will be necessary to maintain optimal voice performance? (Medicare and most third-party reimbursement agencies will not fund "maintenance therapy.") Finally, would some other clinical procedure be of greater benefit to the client?

A variety of factors have potential prognostic value in voice cases. Some of the variables are directly observable and subject to quantification; others are much more subjective. The factors appear to fall into three broad categories: characteristics of the disorder, the person, and the environment. Those factors include:

1. *Duration of the problems.* Generally disorders of long standing have greater resistance to clinical treatment.

2. *Etiological factors.* Two factors are relevant here. First, is the cause of the problem identifiable? Second, is the cause of the problem alterable? And if so, is the type of habilitating service required available?

3. *Degree of secondary psychological components.* Generally, the greater the degree of psychological disturbance, the poorer the prognosis.

4. *Variability and general flexibility of the voice.* Generally, the more the client is able to alter his/her vocal behavior, the better the prognosis. This underscores the importance of probing for vocal change with facilitating techniques during the initial session.

5. *Auditory and imitative skills.* The better the client is at hearing differences in quality, pitch, and loudness, coupled with the ability to imitate these differences, the more favorable the prognosis.

6. *Impact or degree of disability.* The greater the impact of the voice difference upon the individual, the better the chances for cooperation and motivation. Generally, too, if the family of the client is supportive, the outlook is more favorable.

7. *Structural integrity of the vocal mechanism.* Clearly, the more the speech mechanism is disrupted anatomically or neurologically, the more limited the prognosis will be.

Conclusion

The evaluation of voice disorders is a challenge to the speech pathologist. It requires the ability to deal with older adults as well as young children. The clinician must often work closely with medical personnel and other allied health workers, which necessitates knowing procedures and terminologies that are peripheral to speech-language pathology. The clinician must also remain abreast of current technological developments in electronics, surgery, and medical technology. Finally, the clinician must keep interpersonal clinical skills finely honed so that psychological aspects of vocal disorders can be detected and dealt with through treatment or referral. Beginning students are encouraged to read widely about voice disorders, seek out clients with vocal problems, and gain as much clinical experience as they can in this interesting area.

Bibliography

Aronson, A. (1985). *Clinical Voice Disorders.* 2nd ed. New York: Thieme-Stratton.

Bateman, H. E., and Mason, R. M. (1984). *Applied Anatomy and Physiology of the Speech and Hearing Mechanism.* Springfield, IL: Charles C. Thomas.

Blonigen, J. A. (1980). *Remediation of Vocal Hoarseness.* Hingham, MA: Teaching Resources Corporation.

Boone, D. (1982). *The Boone Voice Program for Adults.* Austin, TX: Pro-Ed.

Boone, D. (1993). *The Boone Voice Program for Children.* 2nd ed. Austin, TX: Pro-Ed.

Boone, D., and McFarlane, S. C. (1994). *The Voice and Voice Therapy.* 5th ed. Englewood Cliffs, NJ: Prentice Hall.

Coleman, R. F., Michel, J., and Lynn, P. (1987). "Use and Misuse of Instrumental Analysis in Clinical

Voice Practice." Paper presented at annual convention of the American Speech-Language-Hearing Association, New Orleans, LA.

Colton, R. H. and Casper, J. K. (1990). *Understanding Voice Problems: A Physiological Perspective for Diagnosis and Treatment*. Baltimore, MD: Williams and Wilkins.

Cooper, M. (1973). *Modern Techniques of Vocal Rehabilitation*. Springfield, IL: Charles C. Thomas.

Curry, E. (1949). "Hoarseness and Voice Change in Male Adolescents." *Journal of Speech and Hearing Disorders* 14:23–24.

Curtis, J. (1968). "Acoustics of Speech Production and Nasalization." In *Cleft Palate and Communication*, ed. D. Spriestersbach and D. Sherman (New York: Academic Press).

Daniloff, R., Schuckers, G., and Feth, L. (1980). *The Physiology of Speech and Hearing: An Introduction*. Englewood Cliffs, NJ: Prentice Hall.

Darley, F. L. (1940). "A Normative Study of Oral Reading Rate." M. A. Thesis, University of Iowa.

Darley, F. L., Aronson, A. E., and Brown, J. R. (1975). *Motor Speech Disorders*. Philadelphia, PA: W. B. Saunders.

Davis, S. (1979). "Acoustic Characteristics of Normal and Pathological Voices." In *Speech and Language: Research and Theory*, ed. N. Lass (New York: Academic Press).

Davis S. (1982). "Acoustic Characteristics of Normal and Pathological Voices." In *Proceedings of the Conference on the Assessment of Vocal Pathology: ASHA Reports* 11:97–115.

Deal, R., McClain, B., and Sudderth, J. (1976). "Identification, Evaluation, Therapy and Follow-up for Children with Vocal Nodules in a Public School Setting." *Journal of Speech and Hearing Disorders* 41:390–397.

DeJarnette, G., and Holland, R. W. (1993). "Voice and Voice Disorders." In *Communication Disorders in Multicultural Populations*, ed. D. E. Battle (Boston, MA: Andover Medical Publishers).

Dickson, D., and Maue-Dickson, W. (1982). *Anatomical and Physiological Bases of Speech*. Boston: Little, Brown.

Diehl, C., and Stinnett, C. (1959). "Efficiency of Teacher Referrals in a School Speech Testing Program." *Journal of Speech and Hearing Disorders* 24:34–36.

Dobres, R., Lee, L., Stemple, J. C., Kummer, A. W., Kretschmer, L. W. (1990). "Description of Laryngeal Pathologies in Children Evaluated by Otolaryngologists." *Journal of Speech and Hearing Disorders* 55:526–532.

Duchin, S. W., and Mysak, E. D. (1987). "Disfluency and Rate Characteristics of Young Adult, Middle-Aged, and Older Males." *Journal of Communication Disorders* 20:245–257.

Eckel, F., and Boone, D. (1981). "The S/Z Ratio as an Indicator of Laryngeal Pathology." *Journal of Speech and Hearing Disorders* 46:147–150.

Fairbanks, G. (1960). *Voice and Articulation Drillbook*. 2nd ed. New York: Harper and Row.

Fox, D. R., and Blechman, M. (1975). *Clinical Management of Voice Disorders*. Lincoln, NE: Cliffs Notes.

Gray, G., and Wise, C. (1959). *The Bases of Speech*. 3rd ed. New York: Harper and Row.

Green, G. (1989). "Psycho-Behavioral Characteristics of Children with Vocal Nodules: WPBIC Ratings." *Journal of Speech and Hearing Disorders* 54:306–312

Greene, M. (1980). *The Voice and Its Disorders*. Philadelphia, PA: Lippincott.

Hanley, T., and Thurman, W. (1970). *Developing Vocal Skills*. New York: Holt, Rinehart, and Winston.

Hardy, J. (1961). "Intraoral Breath Pressure in Cerebral Palsy." *Journal of Speech and Hearing Disorders* 26:309–319.

Hirano, M. (1981). *Clinical Examination of Voice*. Vienna, Austria: Springer-Verlag

Hollien, H., and Shipp, T. (1972). "Speaking Fundamental Frequency and Chronological Age in Males." *Journal of Speech and Hearing Research* 15:155–159.

Isshiki, N., Yanigahara, N., and Morimoto, H. (1966). "Approach to the Objective Diagnosis of Hoarseness." *Folia Phoniatrica* 18:393–400.

Jackson, C. (1941). "Vocal Nodules." *American Laryngological Association* 63:185.

James, H., and Cooper, E. (1966). "Accuracy of Teacher Referral of Speech-Handicapped Children." *Exceptional Child* 30:29–33.

Johnson, W., Darley, F., and Spriestersbach, D. (1963). *Diagnostic Methods in Speech Pathology*. New York: Harper and Row.

Kahane, J., and Folkins, J. (1984). *Atlas of Speech and Hearing Anatomy*. Columbus, OH: Charles E. Merrill.

Kaplan, H. (1971). *Anatomy and Physiology of Speech*. New York: McGraw-Hill.

Kelley, A. (1977). "F₀ Measurements of Female Voices from 20–90 Years of Age." Unpublished manuscript, University of North Carolina at Greensboro. Cited in Aronson, A. (1980), *Clinical Voice Disorders: An Interdisciplinary Approach* (New Yorg: Thieme-Stratton), pp. 52–53.

Leeper, L. H., Culatta, R. A., Pindzola, R. H., and Ceska, S. (1990). "Elderly Speakers' Rate/Fluency: What We Know, What It Means." Paper presented at annual convention of the American Speech-Language-Hearing Association, Seattle, WA.

Leff, J., and Abberton, E. (1981). "Voice Pitch Measurements in Schizophrenia and Depression." *Psychological Medicine* 11:849–852.

Luchsinger, R., and Arnold, G. (1965). *Voice-Speech-Language*. Belmont, CA: Wadsworth.

Ludlow, C., and Hart, M. (1982). Preface. *Proceedings of the Conference on the Assessment of Vocal Pathology. ASHA Reports* 11:v.

Martony, J. (1968). "On the Correlation of the Voice Pitch Level for Severely Hard-of-Hearing Subjects." *American Annals of the Deaf* 113:195–202.

Miller, M. K., and Pindzola, R. H. (1985). "The Development of Speaking Rates in Preschool Children." Paper presented at the annual convention of the American Speech-Language-Hearing Association, Washington, DC.

Moncur, J., and Brackett, I. (1974). *Modifying Vocal Behavior*. New York: Harper and Row.

Moses, P. (1954). *The Voice of Neurosis*. New York: Grune and Stratton.

Murphy, A. (1964). *Functional Voice Disorders*. Englewood Cliffs, NJ: Prentice Hall.

Palmer, J. (1984). *Anatomy for Speech and Hearing*. New York: Harper and Row.

Perkins, W. H. (1985). "Assessment and Treatment of Voice Disorders: State of the Art." In *Speech Disorders in Adults: Recent Advances*, ed. J. M. Costello (San Diego, CA: College-Hill).

Perkins, W. H., and Kent, R. D. (1986). *Functional Anatomy of Speech, Language, and Hearing: A Primer*. San Diego, CA: College-Hill.

Pindzola, R. H. (1987). *A Voice Assessment Protocol for Children and Adults*. Austin, TX: Pro-Ed.

Pindzola, R. H., Jenkins, M. M., and Lokken, K. J. (1989). "Speaking Rates of Young Children."

Language, Speech, and Hearing Services in Schools 20:133–138.

Polow, N. G., and Kaplan, E. D. (1980). *Symptomatic Voice Therapy*. Austin, TX: Pro-Ed.

Powers, M. (1971). "Functional Disorders of Articulation: Symptomatology and Etiology." In *Handbook of Speech Pathology and Audiology*, ed. L. Travis Englewood Cliffs, NJ: Prentice Hall.

Pracy, R., Siegler, J., Stell, P. M., and Rogers, J. (1977). *Ear, Nose and Throat Surgery and Nursing*. New York: John Wiley.

Prater, R. J., and Swift, R. W. (1984). *Manual of Voice Therapy*. Boston: Little, Brown.

Rousey, C., and Moriarty, A. (1965). *Diagnostic Implications of Speech Sounds*. Springfield, IL: Charles C. Thomas.

Ryan, B. P. (1984). "Stuttering in Preschool Children: A Comparison and Longitudinal Study." Paper presented at the annual convention of the American Speech-Language-Hearing Association, San Francisco, CA.

Shearer, W. M. (1972). "Diagnosis and Treatment of Voice Disorders in School Children." *Journal of Speech and Hearing Disorders* 37:215–221.

Shigemori, Y. (1977). "Some Tests Related to the Air Usage during Phonation: Clinical Investigations." *Otologia* 23:138–166.

Shipley, K. G. (1990). *Systematic Assessment of Voice (SAV)*. Oceanside, CA: Academic Communication Associates.

Silverman, E., and Zimmer, C. (1975). "Incidence of Chronic Hoarseness among School-Age Children." *Journal of Speech and Hearing Disorders* 40:211–215.

Stemple, J. (1984). *Clinical Voice Pathology: Theory and Management*. Columbus, OH: Charles E. Merrill.

Stone, E., Hurlbutt, N., and Coulthard, S. (1978). "Role and Laryngological Consultation in the Intervention of Dysphonia." *Language, Speech and Hearing Services in Schools* 9:35–42.

Tait, N., Michel, J., and Carpenter, M. (1980). "Maximum Duration of Sustained /s/ and /z/ in Children." *Journal of Speech and Hearing Disorders* 45:239–246.

Titze, I. (1994). *Principles of Voice Production*. Englewood Cliffs, NJ: Prentice Hall.

Van Bergeijk, W. A., Pierce, J. R., and David, E. E. (1960). *Waves and the Ear*. Garden City, NY: Anchor, Doubleday.

Van Riper, C., and Irwin, J. (1958). *Voice and Articulation.* Englewood Cliffs, NJ: Prentice Hall.

Walker, V. G. (1979). "Speech Durations of Young Adults during Speaking and Reading." Unpublished doctoral dissertation, The Florida State University, Tallahassee, FL.

Weinberg, B. (1983). "Phonatory Based Voice Disorders." In *Diagnosis in Speech-Language Pathology*, ed. I. Meitus and B. Weinberg (Baltimore, MD: University Park Press).

Weintraub, S., Mesulam, M., and Kramer, L. (1981). "Disturbances in Prosody: A Right Hemisphere Contribution to Language." *Archives of Neurology*, 38:742–744.

Wendahl, R., and Page, L. (1967). "Glottal Wave Periods in CVC Environments." *Journal of the Acoustical Society of America* 42:1208.

Wilson, D. K. (1987). *Voice Problems in Children.* 3rd ed. Baltimore, MD: Williams and Wilkins.

Wilson, F., and Rice, M. (1977). *A Programmed Approach to Voice Therapy.* Austin, TX: Learning Concepts.

Withers, B. (1961). "Vocal Nodules." *Eye, Ear, Nose and Throat Monthly* 40:35–38.

Yorkston, K. M., Beukelman, D. R., and Bell, K. R. (1988). *Clinical Management of Dysarthric Speakers.* Boston, MA: College-Hill.

Zemlin, W. (1988). *Speech and Hearing Science.* 3rd ed. Englewood Cliffs, NJ: Prentice Hall.

Chapter 11

Assessment and Reassessment of the Laryngectomee

Laryngeal excision is done primarily to preserve the life of the patient, most often because of the presence of cancer. However, the surgeon, in removing the malignant tumor and a healthy margin of tissue, is also conscious of the need to provide as great a chance for continued vocal function as is possible. Surgery may include excision of the total larynx, half of the larynx, one vocal fold and part of the other, removal of the anterior section of the thyroid cartilage and both vocal folds, or various other combinations. In cases of early detection, subtotal laryngectomies are becoming more routine, and the surgeon is often able to reconstruct a serviceable larynx and preserve voice. It is important that the SLP know exactly what procedures were undertaken since the rehabilitation program will vary relative to the type of surgery and the condition of the remaining structures. This chapter, however, will focus on the assessment process following total laryngectomy.

Differential health-related conditions (smoking, drinking, nutritional factors) and environmental exposures no doubt affect the incidence of respiratory tract carcinomas in multicultural populations. According to the National Cancer Institute (1985), the incidence of cancer of the larynx among U.S. minority groups is greatest among African Americans, followed by Hawaiians, Hispanics, Japanese, Chinese, Filipinos, and then Native Americans. The clinician should be cognizant of cultural differences when assessing and rehabilitating laryngectomized persons.

The assessment of a person who has undergone a total laryngectomy is inherently different than the initial assessment of persons with other communication disorders. We do not approach the initial session to solve the problem/no problem issue. When we get a referral to see a laryngectomee, we immediately know that the ability to speak has been lost—there is a problem and the diagnosis is obvious—we also know that some form of intervention will be necessary to reestablish a means of communication for the patient. What needs to be assessed is the current status of the patient (physically, psychologically, and the like), the potential for rehabilitation, and the direction (or directions) that the intervention program should take. Questions floating through the clinician's mind are likely to include: Is the patient psychologically ready to begin rehabilitation in earnest? What is the physical health of the patient like, both in general and as relates to the laryngeal surgery? Are there cultural, educational, or intellectual limitations that may affect the short- and long-term courses of treatment? And, most important, for which avenues of communication does the patient show potential or preference (e.g. gestures, artificial devices, esophageal speech, tracheoesophageal speech)?

From this overview, it should be clear that the evaluation process involves the collection of background information, current status indicators, and trial therapy, among other things. There really are no formal "tests" to administer, and so the clinician's insights, judgments, and competencies with trial therapy techniques are crucial. The evaluation session is truly the initial treatment session as well.

In this chapter, then, we will discuss the process of informally evaluating a newly laryngectomized patient. Since standardized tests do not exist, it could be said that formal diagnostic procedures also do not exist. We will include, however, the screening-testing procedures used to evaluate a patient's candidacy for tracheoesophageal puncture techniques. In addition, we will discuss the ongoing assessment of a patient enrolled in the various alaryngeal speech rehabilitation programs. Once the patient is talking, it is important to subjectively and objectively appraise the quality of the speech. Research has provided us with many yardsticks with which to measure the progress of our patients. Many reevaluation materials are available for this purpose.

The Counseling Process

The evaluation will seek to determine a patient's rehabilitation potential and to provide information necessary to shape the direction of treatment. But the evaluation process also has the goal of providing information, support, and emotional release for the patient and the patient's family. The clinician must wear many hats. In this section, let us explore the clinician's role in the preoperative visit, family and spouse counseling, arranging or assisting with the visit by another laryngectomee, and postoperative counseling of the patient.

The Preoperative Visit

Ideally, the surgeon requests that a preoperative visit be made by the SLP. When the physician informs the patient of the cancer, a thousand thoughts must surge through the patient's mind: Will I die? Will I be disfigured? Will my family be able to look at me? Will I talk again? Will I lose my job? Private thoughts, such as these, may happen so forcefully and quickly that the patient does not absorb much of what else the physician says. We often see patients with only a small understanding of the surgery and its many consequences for daily living. Explanations offered by the physician, then, can be supplemented at a later meeting by the speech pathologist. A preoperative visit is an ideal time to meet the patient, who can still talk, ask questions, express feelings and fears, and so forth. The clinician must be emotionally and professionally capable of dealing with the issues of this meeting. It can be a time when grown men cry, when women react with such anger as to order you out of their room, when denial is apparent, and/or when the patient needs desperately to hear some words of hope and optimism.

One goal of the first meeting, then, is to provide emotional release and support. The clinician must remember in the preoperative visit that the patient is facing a trauma unparalleled in his/her lifetime. Fears of death, loss of communication, loss of job, and social and marital adjustments plague such patients. The first confrontation is no social chat and may well demand all of the professional proficiency the clinician can muster. Occasionally, the clinician might find that the patient is not capable of dealing rationally with the topic immediately before surgery and, in these cases, it may be preferable to postpone detailed discussion until after recovery.

Another major goal of the first meeting is to provide some information about the operation and the implications for speech. After consultation with the physician, every attempt should be made to present a clear discussion of the anatomical changes. Charts and diagrams are helpful. We often give the patient some booklets or pamphlets, available from the International Association of Laryngectomees (IAL) of the American Cancer Society (contact the IAL for a list of available materials). The one entitled *Helping Words for the Laryngectomee* (IAL 1964) contains a positive emotional message, some information of interest, as well as sketches of the vocal tract before and after total laryngectomy. We make sure the patient understands, among other things, that the vocal folds will be removed (consequently no speech will be possible) and that a stoma will be cut permanently into the neck for a breathing passage. We mention these two items here because so many patients have been misinformed and fully expect to be able to talk or whisper and that the "hole in their neck" is only temporary.

While we are explaining the stoma to the patient, using language that can be easily comprehended, we stress the notion that "breathing for breathing and breathing for speech" will be different in the future (unless tracheoesophageal puncture is planned). We find that planting this idea early will help later in teaching esophageal speech and minimizing associated noise.

We explain that many communication avenues exist. At this time, we decide on an appropriate short-term method (e.g., writing, gesturing, pointing to pictures), depending on literacy, vision, and manual dexterity abilities or limitations. We arrange for the hospital, family, speech services, social services, or other department or agency to make the necessary supplies available immediately after surgery (e.g., paper/pencil, wipe-off writing boards, picture communication boards, synthetic speech devices, and so forth). We also introduce other methods that the patient may learn to use, such as esophageal speech and speech with an artificial larynx. The introduction must offer the optimism that he/she may actually speak again but care must be taken not to overwhelm the patient with too many details at this point.

A brief explanation of the methods and some of the novel terminology may be all that is appropriate at this time. Showing and demonstrating an artificial larynx, playing a tape of an esophageal speaker, and/or showing a film about alaryngeal rehabilitation (available from IAL) certainly can be done in this initial meeting, but we typically do not. These aids seem more fitting for a subsequent session. Other authorities do recommend presurgery speech instruction, such as initiating esophageal air charging and vibration. The works of Green (1980) and Gardner (1971) can be consulted in this regard.

Family-Spouse Counseling

Providing adequate information to the family can have far-reaching clinical implications. The spouse and immediate family also must understand the anatomy of the operation. Often, clinicians stress what the laryngectomee will be unable to do; and although this information is important, it is also important to stress to the family what the patient will be able to do. We generally attempt to have a frank discussion with the spouse about the typical reactions of the family. If a problem can be identified before it develops, it may be easier to control. The tendency to dominate the silent mate (or parent) must be controlled, as must the inclinations to infantilize, overindulge, and pity. Often we have to warn the family not to shout at the patient—they may think that someone who cannot talk also does not hear well. Some families readily admit to a feeling of repulsion because of the physical changes; this can be easily conveyed to the patient. The silent mate is sometimes excluded from conversation and decision making in the family. The clinician must be sensitive to the fact that the spouse will have significant concerns. The fear of death, reduced income, new responsibilities, social changes, and alterations in the marital (and sexual) relationship may be topics for discussion. One of the primary purposes of the clinician's visit with the family members is to let them know that their feelings are understood. It is expected that the clinician will be warm, sincere, and insightful, but we resist the temptation to dictate any specific attitude beyond this because each patient will require a somewhat different approach. Some need to be dealt with gently, others straightforwardly and frankly. Find the level and type of interaction your patient and his/her family respond to best and use it.

Materials available from the IAL are useful in spouse-family counseling. Many different pamphlets can provide the family with information and inspiration. We also like to arrange a viewing of one or more films; the patient should attend with the family. The IAL film list should be consulted for something appropriate. *To Speak Again* is well suited for families and new patients still in the hospital; we also like *A Second Voice*, which is an overview of the total rehabilitation of the laryngectomee. At a subsequent spouse-family session, after the surgery but ideally before the patient is discharged home, we like to show a film about first aid. *Check the Neck* or *Three Critical Minutes: Emergency Air for Neck-Breathers* are available from the IAL. The IAL also has pamphlets describing "mouth-to-neck" resuscitation techniques that we like to provide families. Family counseling, then, seeks to ensure that the family is emotionally and physically ready to assist in the rehabilitation program and care of their loved one.

Laryngectomee Visitation

It is ideal when the surgeon and/or the SLP can arrange for the patient to be visited by a laryngectomee either before or after the surgery. The laryngectomee visitor, by his/her sheer presence, offers the patient hope: He/she sees a person who survived cancer, survived the operation, learned to talk, perhaps returned to work, and generally has gotten back into life. The laryngectomee can offer to the patient sincere understanding of the emotional turmoil—he/she has been down that road—and may be the best paraprofessional to offer advice and empathy. The laryngectomee visitor is also a model of alaryngeal speech. The patient hears first-hand what practiced esophageal speech and/or artificial larynx speech sound like. Visitors are also great at explaining the importance of personal drive and daily practice. They come prepared with self-help items, information, and advice; the visitor's kit may include such things as stoma covers (hand-made crocheted bibs), emergency decals, and IAL reading materials.

Visits by laryngectomees are becoming less casual and more organized. The American Cancer Society offers a *Laryngectomee Visitor Program Manual* (1985) as a training program for these paraprofessionals. The SLP should become familiar with visitor guidelines. Opportunities abound for mutual cooperation. If available, the patient should be recruited into the community's Lost Cord Club, a self-help group sponsored by the IAL.

Postoperative Counseling

If preoperative referrals were not made, the postoperative meetings will offer the opportunity for emotional release, support, and information sharing. All that we have described in the previous sessions needs to be accomplished now. If preoperative visits were done, then postoperatively the speech clinician is ready to move forward with the rehabilitation program, which involves a balance between treating and reassessing the patient's emotional, physical, and speech status.

The first few postoperative days may be the emotional low point for the patient. Frequent and brief visits may provide the support needed. The speech pathologist should also ensure that the patient has a means of communicating. Earlier we mentioned planning for written messages, picture communication boards, and the like. Patients with limited reading and writing abilities may benefit from the book of pictures depicting daily needs entitled *Communication for the Laryngectomized* (Bradley and Ormond 1970). The clinician, with physician knowledge, may introduce artificial larynx devices for immediate speech. The interested student is urged to consult any of the many excellent sources describing the available devices, their types, and how to begin training a patient in their use. In addition to the usual voice disorders textbooks, we would like to suggest the specialized book by Salmon and Goldstein (1978).

The use of artificial larynx devices early in the rehabilitation has long been debated because of their supposed deleterious effects on the subsequent learning of esophageal speech. Current thinking seems to be supportive of colearning both methods of esophageal and artificial larynx speech. What we wish to stress in this section on postoperative work is that artificial devices do offer a means of immediate speech. Let us also summarize some of our experiences with the use of the devices immediately after surgery. We tend not to get a good seal between the stoma cup of the pneumatic devices and the protruding steel or plastic tracheostomy tube. Electric neck-type devices may work, and a variety of placement sites may be tried, but generally neck tenderness is such that the patient seems not to like using the device. Electric intraoral devices, or neck-type devices adapted temporarily for intraoral use, seem to be best in those first few days or weeks following surgery. We acknowledge that intraoral tubes adversely affect intelligibility and overall speech acceptability, and so we strive to switch the patient over to a neck-type device when possible (Moffet and Pindzola 1988; Pindzola and Moffet 1988).

After a certain amount of counseling and information sharing, the speech-language pathologist may wish to administer the *Inventory for the Assessment of Laryngectomy Rehabilitation* (La Borwit 1981). The purpose of this inventory is to assess the patient's functional knowledge of his/her overall condition. The more functional information a laryngectomee possesses, the greater will be the capacity to act upon that information and achieve rehabilitation goals. As stated by La Borwit (1981):

> *Scores serve as an index of the level of rehabilitation likely to be attained. Results of scores and the specific responses . . . can expedite the therapeutic process by denoting to the clinician the type and quantity of information (or misinformation) upon which the patient may be relying. Awareness of these responses on the clinician's part can facilitate such decision making as the need for counseling intervention, utilization of artificial larynges or other devices, a modification of clinical teaching or reiteration of necessary concepts, influencing family support, and consultation with the physician.* (2)

Using a multiple-choice format, seventy-two questions are posed in seven categories: speech, family, vocation, attitudes, anatomy, first aid, and support groups.

Efforts to begin esophageal speech training await clearance by the physician. Some physicians refer for treatment once the patient is moved out of intensive care, perhaps two or three days postoperatively. Others wait for removal of the nasogastric feeding tube and resumption of chewing and swallowing, typically four to fourteen days postoperatively. Prior to the go-ahead for initiating esophageal speech training, the physician's orders for a speech consult include the pre- and/or postoperative counseling (emotional support and information sharing), establishment of a temporary means of communication, and the evaluation proper.

One final comment as to what we do for the patient and family postoperatively. We provide or assist the family in ordering detailed reading material. The pamphlets, given earlier, surely have served a useful purpose, but the patient may further benefit from books such as *Self-Help for the Laryngectomee* (Lauder 1996) or *Looking Forward: A Guidebook for the Laryngectomee* (Keith et al. 1984).

Background and Current Status Information

The evaluation of the newly laryngectomized patient truly began with the first preoperative meeting and has continued through all subsequent contacts. Where the patient is psychologically, physiologically, and intellectually is important to know, and these places keep changing. Dynamic assessments, rather than static evaluations, are the order of the day. Yet, as in traditional evaluations of a patient, we need to collect background as well as current status information. We begin by reading the patient's hospital chart with particular emphasis on the initial (admitting) medical report, the surgical report, the daily notes by the nursing staff, and the family history critique provided by the social worker.

In determining the potential for speech, a thorough case history is helpful with laryngectomized patients. Three facets are particularly crucial. It is important to know the extent of the surgery, the degree of involvement of related structures such as the tongue or pharynx, general health of the patient, and medical prognosis. The second critical area is the individual's vocation and interests. We find it most helpful to plan our clinical work about the patient's preferred activities. It is also important to know if the person will be able to continue in those vocations and hobbies that involve communication. A third variable related to the patient's potential for learning esophageal speech is attitude and motivation. Some patients are depressed, discouraged, and unmotivated, while others evidence a high level of interest in recovering their communication abilities. This is a subjective judgment on the clinician's part, but it is one of those intangible variables that certainly relates to the potential of the patient to speak again.

Knepflar (1960, 1962) has compiled an extensive list of the necessary medical and background information helpful in planning a rehabilitation program. Case history forms have also been published by Johnson (1960), Snidecor (1962), Travis (1971), and Kelly (1983). Table 11.1 lists questions that guide us in the thorough collection of information on a patient. In addition to shaping the treatment program, such information provides prognostic insights.

A necessary part of the evaluation concerns the current status of the patient's oral-motor abilities. Chapter 9 provided details on an oral examination; suffice it to say that we thoroughly evaluate the tongue, lip, and jaw mobility. Articulation may be affected if surgery involved the hyoid bone, which is an anatomical connection for many muscles of the tongue, mandible, and pharynx. In addition, it is not uncommon that surgical alterations were necessary to contain concomitant oral, lingual, or lymph node cancers. Some information about the previous articulation, speech, and language patterns of the patient is also helpful. For example,

TABLE 11.1   Laryngectomee Case History Outline

1. *Surgical Factors*
   Date of surgery
   Extent of surgery
   Postoperative complications
   Irradiation/other treatment procedures

2. *Physical-Mental Factors*
   General physical condition
   Upper respiratory health
   Status of oral structures
   Hearing acuity
   Other physical factors or conditions
   Cognitive-mental clarity
   Educational background

3. *Emotional Factors*
   Level of negative emotion—depression
   Level of motivation
   Degree of dependency on spouse/family
   Other personality traits or problems

4. *Social Factors*
   Home/family situation
   Occupational aspects
   Hobbies/pastimes
   Smoking and drinking habits
   Social network/sociability
   Family attitudes and acceptance

we have had poor success with alaryngeal speech intelligibility in cases where, premorbidly, the patient was edentulous and seldom wore dentures.

An assessment of the patient's hearing acuity also is desirable. Since a high percentage of laryngectomees are above the age of fifty-five, it is common to find a presbycusic hearing loss. A moderate-to-severe hearing loss may hinder the learning process and, of necessity, shape the direction of the rehabilitation program. Artificial larynx speech, which is typically about 7 dB more intense than normal speech, may prove to be the treatment of choice for cases with significant hearing loss; in contrast, esophageal speech averages 6 to 10 dB below normal speech levels (Goldstein and Rothman 1976; Hyman 1955; Robbins, Fisher, and Blom 1984).

Case Example. *Mr. Wayne Johnson, a sixty-one-year-old white male, was admitted with a six-month history of hoarseness. Examination by otolaryngologist revealed a hard mass in the neck at the angle of the jaw (at the area of the middle one third of the left anterior lymphatic chain), and dysplasia involving the left aryepiglottic fold, false fold, and true fold. Biopsy confirmed locations with the finding of squamous cell carcinoma. A left radical neck dissection and total laryngectomy were performed.*

Background information, contained in the report from social services, included mention that Mr. Johnson was a salesman and lived in an affluent resort community on a lake and golf course. He and his wife golfed several times a week and enjoyed all water sports, including skiing.

The speech pathologist, after reading the medical chart, began to wonder about the quality of life for Mr. Johnson following laryngectomy. Being a salesman, communication and meeting the public are necessary parts of his job. Will he return to work? Will he experience a loss of earnings from lost commissions (the public might not buy from an unusual-sounding person)? Will the company "urge" him to take early retirement? Could the company shift his duties from sales force to office work? To be sure, questions such as these were not only going through the mind of the speech pathologist but also of the patient and his wife. The clinician felt that an impending return to work would be a strong motivator for Mr. Johnson to speak. The clinician also had thoughts concerning his avocations and knew future counseling would have to deal with these issues. Mr. Johnson almost certainly would play golf again, but with a reduction in general strength, head-neck rotation abilities, and a less effective golf swing because of the radical neck dissection. The lake lifestyle posed particular dangers. Stoma breathers generally are advised to stay clear of water. Skiing is out for Mr. Johnson, as is swimming; riding in a motor boat carries a certain risk (accidents do happen). Will Mr. Johnson adjust to these restrictions? He could wade in the water and even try to snorkel with a special breathing device for laryngectomees, but clearly his lifestyle is in for a drastic change. Of prime importance, however, is the containment of cancer, his survival, and a return of the ability to communicate.

The Process of Getting Started

The scope of this book does not allow for a discussion of alaryngeal treatment options nor the training methods used. Many excellent texts on laryngectomee rehabilitation are available to the serious student. Typically, the postoperative evaluation session is also the "let's get started in treatment" session. The ease or difficulties encountered in the initial learning attempts with an artificial larynx, or in trying to inject air and get sound back out, or in diverting lung air through a prosthesis are diagnostically important.

Artificial Larynx Attempts

A patient should not just be given an artificial larynx; instructions on its use and training in its use are essential. With a neck-type device, help the patient seek out its best placement. How quickly will the patient learn to return the vibrating head precisely to that spot—five trials or fifty? Are other feedback cues necessary to learn this skill? If so, things such as tactile stroking of the spot by the clinician be-fore each attempt at placement may prove beneficial. In addition, marking an "X" on the skin with a washable marker and having the patient practice placement drills in front of a mirror may be just what is needed. Explain and demonstrate the noisy effects of poor contact of the vibrating head with the skin. How efficiently will the patient absorb this knowledge and learn to consistently place the device in the correct spot with *firm* contact? Advise the patient to exaggerate articulation movements, especially in opening the mouth and moving the tongue. Will the patient quickly adjust to such pantomiming actions or persist in trying to "breathe for speech" only to have a noisy exhalation out the stoma? Explain and demonstrate the on–off mechanism and the precise timing needed to coordinate phrasing. How agile or clumsy will the patient be in manipulating the switch concurrent with phrases? Slow learners make one or more mistakes here: having the device continuously on and not stopping at grammatical junctures, turning the device off and on excessively and creating choppy speech, or turning the device on or off in a poorly timed fashion at the beginning and ending of utterances. The result is that sounds or syllables are chopped off or buzzing noises occur when speech is not being mouthed.

In training the use of artificial devices with intraoral tubes, how quickly can the patient learn proper placement? Efficient and accurate placement are necessary for speech spontaneity and intelligibility. The tube's orientation must minimize inter-ference with articulation and saliva buildup and must radiate the tone well.

The point here is that during the early training in the use of an artificial lar-ynx device, the clinician should constantly be evaluating the learning skills of the patient. Some patients can speed quickly through your teaching units and others will progress with painful slowness. Observations, such as those just presented, therefore, shape the prognosis and course of treatment.

Esophageal Speech Attempts

Regardless of the technique being taught, be it inhalation or any of the variants of the injection method, the essence of learning esophageal speech involves getting "air in and sound out." As baseline data, the clinician can rate the client's esophageal production abilities. Some fortunate patients will be successful in eruc-tating simple words or sounds in the first session, others may occasionally get out a "burp," and still others may remain mute—unable to get any sound out and needing much practice in performing air intake maneuvers appropriately. A scale, such as that suggested by Wepman et al. (1953), may be useful for a baseline rat-ing. The following are Wepman's seven self-explanatory points:

1. Automatic esophageal speech
2. Esophageal sound produced at will with continuity; word grouping
3. Esophageal sound produced at will; single-word speech
4. Voluntary sound production most of the time; vowel sounds
5. Voluntary sound production part of the time; no speech

6. Involuntary esophageal sound production; no speech
7. No esophageal sound production; no speech

Certainly, the baseline data for most patients would be a Wepman score of 7 or 6. This same scale can be used periodically to reassess and document the progress of the patient in producing esophageal sound and speech.

Of interest in these early sessions is the learning skill and potential displayed by the patient following adequate instruction and demonstration. Early eructation abilities suggest a favorable prognosis for acquiring esophageal speech and perhaps a speedy trek through the treatment stages.

Early Speech Attempts with a Tracheoesophageal Prosthesis

The evaluation may proceed differently with patients planning to have a tracheoesophageal puncture (TEP), also known as tracheoesophageal fistulization. Since this is a relatively new, but ever more popular procedure, we will first provide some background.

The surgeon places a hole (puncture or fistula) in the membranous wall between the trachea and the esophagus, thus providing a route or connection between these two structures. A prosthesis placed in this opening will allow for pulmonary air to be routed into the top of the esophagus under certain conditions. Breathing is still done through the stoma. Aspiration of saliva, liquids, and foods is minimized by the one-way directionality of the prosthetic device. The conditions that allow for diverting exhaled air into the esophagus, rather than out the stoma, are digital occlusion of the prosthesis opening, located in the stoma, or the use of a valving device to reroute the airstream.

Upon muscular effort, air diverted into the esophagus will be compressed, and forced through the top of the closed esophagus, thereby setting the pharyngoesophageal segment into vibration. This segment is the sound source or pseudoglottis; articulation of the sound is accomplished in the usual manner in the upper vocal tract. In essence, tracheoesophageal speech (TE speech) is esophageal in nature, yet supported by the pulmonary system. Tracheoesophageal speech obviates the need to learn esophageal speech via injection or inhalation methods and is therefore easily mastered. Furthermore, the use of lung air provides acoustic and perceptual advantages over traditional esophageal speech.

Hospitalization for healed laryngectomees who come back for only the TEP procedure is brief; some surgical procedures can even be done on an outpatient basis or as an office procedure. Punctures also can be done on newly laryngectomized patients; still, many surgeons prefer the patient to convalesce for a period of weeks or months before puncture. Screening for candidacy, fitting of the device, and instructing in the care and use of the device often is done solely by the speech pathologist, sometimes in concert with the nurse and doctor. Fluent conversational speech typically is acquired rapidly. The SLP, then, has a brief but vital role to play in the rehabilitation of TEP patients.

The success of any method depends, in part, on the proper selection of candidates for that method. Patient selection criteria and contraindications for tracheoesophageal puncture include the following (Singer and Blom 1980):

1. Motivation to undergo the procedure and sustained motivation to care for the prosthesis on a daily basis.
2. Absence of physical or mental limitations to the daily care and fitting (insertion) of the prosthesis. In particular, the patient should have adequate vision and eye-hand coordination to place the prosthetic device while in front of a mirror. Manual dexterity (e.g., absence of arthritis) is necessary for the handling of the prosthesis and all associated materials (particularly if a tracheostoma valve is also used).
3. Good general health. Weak, feeble persons do not do well with TEP; however, conditions such as chronic pulmonary disease, diabetes, and alcoholism do not necessarily rule out candidacy.
4. Concern for hygiene in cleansing of the device, in neck tissue care (adhesives used with the valve can be irritating to sensitive skin), and in touching/handling all materials.
5. Adequate stoma characteristics. In particular, the stoma must not be retracted behind the manubrium. Size of the opening should be a minimum of 1 cm across the axis, but for some procedures 2 cm are needed. An excessively large stoma can be corrected somewhat by tape.
6. Recovery from postsurgical radiation treatment, if any.
7. Absence of chronic tracheitis or ulceration.
8. Absence of a history of unplanned fistulas, pharyngoesophageal stricture (spasm), or flap reconstruction. The presence of any of these conditions, however, does not necessarily rule out TEP candidacy but suggests the need for a more detailed assessment. A barium esophagram may yield findings suggesting that dilation may be necessary to maintain an adequate opening for airflow and voice.

In this regard we need to explain that the primary reason for failure with tracheoesophageal speech is spasms of the pharyngoesophageal segment. Spasms make the vibration and production of sound difficult, if not impossible. The spasms usually can be relaxed by surgically cutting some of the muscle fibers in the pseudoglottis. The need for this surgical procedure, called a myotomy, can be predicted with a simple screening test. The pathologist, or surgeon, or both perform an air insufflation procedure, where air is introduced into the esophagus and the patient is asked to phonate. Good phonation, of course, indicates that the patient's pharyngoesophageal segment is capable of vibration, and therefore a myotomy would not be needed. Such a patient is considered an excellent candidate for TEP. Getting a patient started in the use of tracheoesophageal speech is a complex issue. We will attempt to subdivide the tasks and provide an overview of each.

Prosthesis Fitting

The speech pathologist is often responsible for fitting the patient with a prosthesis of proper size. Brands differ in size, features, and design to optimize individual patient fit. The Blom-Singer Voice Prosthesis and the Blom-Singer Low Pressure Voice Prosthesis (both marketed by American V. Mueller) are available in the following sizes: 1.8 cm, 2.2 cm, 2.6 cm, 3.0 cm, 3.3 cm, and 3.6 cm. The Bivona Duckbill Voice Prosthesis is available in the following lengths: 2.2 cm, 2.6 cm, 3.0 cm, 3.3 cm, 3.6 cm, 4.0 cm, and 4.3 cm. The Bivona Low Resistance Voice Prosthesis is available in the same lengths, except for 4.3 cm.

Following typical TEP surgery, a catheter is left in place for 24 to 72 hours to prevent closure of the puncture site. After that, a prosthesis should be fitted and voice will be possible. The speech pathologist should recheck the patient in four to five weeks and refit the prosthesis, if necessary. Occasionally, after the edema subsides, a shorter prosthesis is more appropriate. The majority of patients seem to need the 2.2-, 2.6-, or 3.0-cm size.

The process of fitting the prosthesis is as follows: Instruct the patient not to swallow. Remove the catheter that has been in place since the surgery. Insert the Dummy Prosthesis Depth Gauge (from Bivona, Inc.) or the Fistula Measurement Probe (from American V. Mueller) through the stoma and into the puncture; feel it "pop" into place. Pull out slightly until the retention collar is firmly against the puncture opening and read the distance on the imprinted probe. This indicates the length of prosthesis needed.

An alternative to using a depth gauge or measurement probe is to use the stick end of a long cotton-tipped applicator. Insert the stick through the stoma, exploring carefully to find the puncture opening. Then, mark the depth on the stick with a pencil and withdraw it. The distance on the stick may now be measured with a ruler. Yet another alternative, for those experienced in fitting, is to shine a light in the stoma and "eyeball" the distance to the puncture site.

Once the size of the needed prosthesis has been determined, insert one, applying double-faced tape on the flanges, if necessary (depending on design). Once in place, have the patient drink some water to make sure there is no leakage around or through the prosthesis. Demonstrate digital occlusion for the patient and instruct him/her to try to talk on exhalation while the stoma/prosthesis opening is occluded with the clinician's thumb or finger. If voice is not produced, assess the reason(s) why (see next section). If successful, continue talking practice. Later, allow the patient to do his/her own digital occlusion.

During the fitting process and placement of the prosthesis, do not be alarmed by blood-tinged mucous. Also, it is important that either a catheter, a prosthesis, or some sort of dummy device be inserted in the puncture at all times (even during sleep) to prevent its closure. The patient must remember this as well.

Voice Failure Assessment

If the patient is unable to produce voice, the speech pathologist should try to determine whether the problem lies with the prosthetic device or with the patient.

The speech pathologist should try troubleshooting with and without the prosthesis in place.

Common problems of voice failure, owing to patient factors, include the following: (1) The patient may be using excessive finger pressure against the stoma. (2) The patient may be using inadequate expiratory pressure. A weak, feeble patient is a poor candidate for TE speech because of the energy necessary to overcome the air resistance of the plastic devices. Alternately, perhaps the patient simply needs to be instructed to use more effort and more air in speech attempts. Other devices (styles and brands) may be tried as well; each model differs in its air-flow resistance. An ultra-low resistance model may work for the patient. (3) Salivary secretions may have accumulated, blocking the pharynx. In this case, the speech will sound "gurgly." Expectoration should solve the problem. (4) A most likely reason for the absence of voice is the presence of pharyngoesophageal spasm. Perhaps the air insufflation pretest was not done prior to TEP. At any rate, do the insufflation test to see if voice is possible with the prosthesis removed. A myotomy may be necessary to counteract the spasms.

Voice failure may be due to problems with the prosthetic device. These problems are often easily identified and rectified. In these cases, the patient would have voice without the prosthesis (with stoma digital occlusion or with the air insufflation test), but no voice with a faulty prosthesis in place. (1) The patient may be unable to produce voice because the prosthesis is inserted upside down. Remove and reinsert the prosthesis. (2) The valve slit may be stuck together on devices with a slit (duckbill) design. (3) Incorrect prosthesis length could be the reason for lack of voice. A device that is too long, particularly a device with a slit design that would be so impeded, may be touching the posterior wall of the esophagus. Refitting the patient with a shorter device and/or changing to a different design (nonslit, flap-door) is in order. A prosthesis that is too short would not have the tip residing in the lumen of the esophageal tube. A slit-designed tip would be impeded from passing its air into the esophagus. Try rotating the placement a bit. A longer prosthesis may be necessary. (4) Occlusion of the port may block air flow and hence voice. Clearing of saliva (or other matter) is in order.

If the patient has used TE speech for a period of time and begins to experience a change in the voice, or loss of it, troubleshooting to find and eliminate the cause is necessary. We recommend the work of Bosone (1986) for troubleshooting ideas.

Tracheostoma Valve

Talking with the voice prosthesis requires digital occlusion (finger or thumb). This may be an unnecessary inconvenience for users of the Blom-Singer (American V. Mueller) or Bivona brands of prostheses. After a few weeks' experience with the voice prosthesis, the patient may be a candidate for using a Blom-Singer Tracheostoma Valve (marketed through American V. Mueller), the Bivona Tracheostoma Valve, or the Bivona Tracheostoma Valve II. More and more often, the patient is trained with a valve at the same time the prosthesis is introduced. The valve is fitted into the stomal opening; naturally, the patient still wears the voice prosthesis. Again, these are tasks that are within the purview of the SLP responsible for assessing and rehabilitating the laryngectomee.

Tracheostoma Valve Contraindications

The valve fits into a flexible circular housing which is attached to the skin area surrounding the stoma with nonirritating adhesive. When positioned over the stoma the valve diaphragm remains in a fully open position during quiet breathing and routine physical activity. For speech, a slight increase in exhalation causes the valve diaphragm to close and divert air into the esophagus. The valve automatically reopens when exhalation decreases at the completion of an utterance.

A tracheostoma valve must be maintained by the patient; it is easily disassembled for cleaning. The diaphragm can be replaced by the patient without return to the manufacturer.

Four contraindications to using a valve seem to exist: (1) Patients with high phonatory pressure may blow the seal often. (2) A very recessed or irregular stoma may not accommodate the valve. (3) Patients with excessive tracheal discharge may occlude or dangerously hinder the operation of the valve. (4) Inadequate pharyngoesophageal segments preclude usable speech, even with a valve.

Valve Fitting

The diaphragm is available in several thicknesses or sensitivities. Bivona, Inc., markets four valve diaphragms: ultra light, light, medium, and firm. American V. Mueller markets three diaphragm thicknesses: ultra light, light, and medium. Select the diaphragm thickness that does not inadvertently close on the patient during routine physical exertion or heavier-than-usual exhalation. Conversely, do not select one too thick as to require excessive exhalation for the generation of voice. A practical method for fitting involves the "stair-step" test. Have the patient try out a diaphragm sensitivity while going up and down some stairs. The speech pathologist and patient should carefully watch for valve closure as breathing deepens during this exertion. If the valve closes, remove it and try the next-thicker size. Repeat the stair-step test until the proper diaphragm size has been determined. Some patients may wish to purchase two diaphragms: one for general use and a thicker one for use while dancing, exercising, and the like.

Patients should be instructed not to sleep with the tracheostoma valve in place. In addition, patients may find it helpful to remove the valve from its housing when they feel an urge to cough or forcefully exhale. This prevents blowing the seal and the necessity of cleaning and reapplying the adhesive. The Tracheostoma Valve II, by Bivona, contains a spring action valve (rather than the usual butterfly valve) with a cough relief valve that is said to eliminate blowout from a cough or instance of high airway pressure production.

To summarize the placement procedure, the prosthesis is first inserted. Next, the valve housing is glued over it and to the neck/stoma skin with an adhesive. The valve assembly is then placed into the housing.

Voice Treatment Sessions

Treatment begins with prosthesis fitting, usually done by the speech pathologist, as described previously. Once fitted, demonstrate digital occlusion for the patient. Instruct the patient to try to talk (on exhalation) while the prosthesis opening is digitally occluded. If voice is not produced, assess reasons that it is not. If successful, continue talking practice. Later, allow the patient to do his/her own finger occlusion. It is simple, yet the coordination needs to be practiced.

Concomitant with speech practice, the patient should be trained in the placement of the prosthesis and the valve, if applicable. Instructions as to taping and/or gluing should be detailed for some types of devices, allowing for much supervised practice. Care and cleaning of the devices should be taught as well. Usually by the third session, the patient is independent in talking with the prosthesis and in its placement, adhesion, and daily care.

We would like to offer a few observations about these first few sessions. One aspect of treatment may involve the unlearning of esophageal speech techniques in the patient who spoke esophageally prior to TEP. The two forms of speech are incompatible. Patients using esophageal speech must break whatever habits they have developed and return to what amounts to their prelaryngectomy form of speaking with lung air. This is usually easily achieved; yet, patients may require the speech pathologist to guide and monitor their unlearning or deconditioning of the esophageal speech habit.

Train the patient to use the proper amount of finger pressure on the prosthesis opening at the stoma. There is a tendency to first push too forcefully at first. Similarly, patients may need the speech pathologist to assist in learning the minimal amount of expiratory pressure needed to drive the system. Some begin learning TE speech with a valve, using an excessive amount of air pressure. This can result in "blowing a seal" or loosening of the valve housing. If the housing develops a broken seal, it becomes difficult to close the valve and utilize the prosthesis for voice production. Instead, the air leak becomes audible and speech breakdown occurs. When this happens, the patient must manually hold the housing down while speaking, until there is an opportunity to reapply the housing. This is less of a problem with low-resistance prostheses. Regular prostheses have a higher resistance to opening and to air flowing through them. A greater air pressure build-up is required of the speaker with the danger of straining the glued seal of the housing.

In addition to learning the minimal amount of pressure needed on which to speak, the patient must learn proper ways to adhere the device to prevent blowout. Applying the proper amount of glue is important, as is getting the taped collar onto the housing without wrinkles in it, and applying it to the neck evenly. This is highly individualistic and must be learned by each patient with the help of the speech pathologist and sheer practice.

Treatment should focus on articulatory intelligibility, such as distinguishing between voiced/voiceless cognates (e.g., face/vase) and between easily confused sounds (e.g., ship/chip), as done in traditional esophageal speech rehabilitation.

Ongoing Assessments: A Dynamic Process

Assessing the proficiency of alaryngeal speech and refining that speech in treatment sessions are two intertwined processes. The direction that treatment should take is directly related to how well the patient is doing in the various components of speech. Ideally, the patient's status changes for the better on a daily or weekly basis, making frequent reassessments a necessity. Dynamic, ongoing assessments, then, suggest to the clinician (1) what to work on, (2) how much therapeutic time needs to be devoted to certain tasks, and (3) what tasks or steps in the program may be skipped or bypassed. This last item points out that reassessments serve as probes as to what the patient can already do without training, as well as measures of achievement.

Assessing Artificial Larynx Speech

Rothman (1978) consolidated much of the research information concerning acoustic characteristics of artificial larynx speech and perceptual ratings of what comprises "good" and "poor" users. Information of this kind is useful in setting goals toward which patients can strive. That is, we want our patients to acquire characteristics typical of "good" speakers. The information also serves as a useful barometer of patient progress. The clinician should frequently reassess the patient to see the current level of achievement and how that compares to the norms.

Information of this type collected by Rothman (1978) and others (Fleming, Simpson, and Weaver 1983; Gandour and Weinberg 1983; Moffet and Pindzola 1988; Pindzola and Moffet 1988; Weiss, Yeni-Komshian, and Heinz 1979; Williams and Watson 1985) seems to cluster into six categories. We will summarize them here.

Frequency Range
"Good" speakers using neck-type devices acquire a variety of techniques to alter the frequency output, such as "riding" the device on the neck using different pressures. They exhibit a frequency range, or pitch variability, between 13 and 20 Hz, with an average range or fluctuation of 16 Hz. In contrast, "poor" speakers range from 6 to 15 Hz with a mean of 11 Hz.

Speech Rate
Speech rate is the best variable to differentiate "good" from "poor" users of artificial larynges (Rothman 1978). "Good" users speak test sentences faster than "poor" users. Research also indicates that a mean rate of speech with an electric larynx is 125 words per minute (Moffet and Pindzola 1988).

Intensity Variations
Intensity variations, which contribute to perceptions of linguistic stress or emphasis, are greater in "good" speakers. "Poor" users tend toward monoloudness.

Extraneous Noise

"Poor" users frequently fail to achieve firm coupling of the vibrating head with their neck tissues. "Good" users do not generate leaked, extraneous noises.

Inappropriate Pauses

Instances when the electric device is shut down during utterances occur more frequently with "poor" users. "Good" speakers are adept at timing and phrasing.

Consonantal Differentiation

"Good" users employ buccal air and precise timing of device activation to more effectively produce stops, fricatives, and affricates. Voiced/voiceless distinctions are also achieved by careful manipulation of buccal air and/or by varying the coupling pressure of the device with the neck tissue. "Poor" users have yet to master the nuances of consonant production with artificial larynges.

Assessing Esophageal Speech

Once a patient has begun learning esophageal speech, some measure of their current performance level is necessary. Most authorities would agree that a clinician with critical listening ability is the most effective means for evaluating esophageal productions. It is perhaps best to judge the overall effectiveness of the patient's speech and then focus on more-specific parameters. The clinician can rate the patient's esophageal speech production on one of many scales available for this purpose (Barton and Hejna 1963; Berlin 1963; Robe et al. 1956; Shipp 1967; Snidecor 1969; Wepman et al. 1953). We will discuss several assessment instruments here.

Earlier we mentioned the Wepman et al. (1953) seven-point scale for establishing baseline esophageal proficiency. In addition to a baseline rating, the clinician should periodically rescore the patient to document improvement. Little to no time is necessary to do this rating.

A patient's learning curve should continuously shape the clinician's prognostic statement and modify the treatment program and pace. Berlin (1963) described four skills and their clinical measurement for use in assessing the acquisition efficiency of patients' learning esophageal speech. Berlin's classic criteria recently have been resurrected and modified by Dabul (1981). Table 11.2 displays information from Berlin and Dabul regarding the four skills, their elicitation procedures, patient criteria, and comparative acquisition data from "good" and "poor" speakers.

Rigrodsky and Lerman (1971) suggest the following treatment outline for acquiring competent esophageal speech: Learn an air intake method; practice esophageal speech on basic sounds, short words, polysyllabic words and phrases, then sentences and connected speech; improve articulation, phrasing, inflection, pitch, and loudness. A similar progression was suggested by Snidecor (1971). The final level in Snidecor's six-level program calls for practice on articulation, stress, pitch, quality, loudness, and time in a conversational situation.

We mention these two treatment programs as being typical; both stress that getting the patient talking does not mean discharge from treatment is at hand.

TABLE 11.2   Four Classic Skills in the Acquisition of Esophageal Speech

1. Consistency: Ability to phonate reliably on demand

   Patient makes a single inflation and phonates /a/. Allow 20 trials. Clinician scores each attempt with plus or minus scoring. Compute final score as a percentage of correct attempts. Goal is 100 percent.

   Good speakers phonated 100 percent of the time on demand after 10 to 14 days of daily speech treatment. Poor speakers averaged 68 percent after 20 days of treatment.

2. Latency: Short latency between inflation and vocalization

   Patient phonates as quickly as possible after inflation. Have the patient signal the clinician at the start of inflation; clinician engages a stopwatch. Clinician stops the watch at vocal onset. Allow 10 trials and compute an average latency time. Goal is 0.5 seconds or less.

   Good speakers maintained latency of 0.2 to 0.6 seconds by the 20th day of treatment; poor speakers 1.3 seconds.

3. Duration: Duration of phonation of /a/

   Patient makes a single inflation and a single phonation of /a/, sustaining it as long as possible. Allow 10 trials and compute an average duration. Goal is 1 to 2 seconds.

   Good speakers sustained the vowel for 2.2 to 3.6 seconds by the 24th day of treatment.

4. Syllables: Sustaining phonation during articulation of /da/

   Patient makes a single inflation and repeats the syllable /da/ as many times as possible. Allow 5 trials and compute an average number of syllables spoken. Goal is 5 to 7 syllables.

   Good speakers phonated 8 to 10 syllables after 25 days of treatment; poor speakers averaged 2.3.

Rather, patient and clinician must strive to perfect the esophageal speech—there is almost always room for improvement. The clinician's responsibility, then, includes frequent monitoring of the patient's conversational speech for adequacy in the more sophisticated areas of speech, such as rate, pitch, and loudness variability, consonantal differentiation, and the like. Many assessment checklists, whether published or not, seem to be in the possession of most speech pathologists. A good many have been acquired through convention presentations, Lost Cord Clubs, or college courses.

The Alaryngeal Speech Proficiency Evaluation (Knepflar 1962) has the clinician rate ten areas of speech using a five-point scale of proficiency. "Highly proficient, normal or near normal" is a rating of one while "generally inadequate for basic communicative needs" is a five. The ten areas assessed are loudness, pitch, quality, inflection, rate/rhythm/fluency, articulation proficiency, linguistic proficiency, acoustic distractions, visual distractions, and overall proficiency.

The factors on which we rate our patients are shown in Table 11.3. These eleven factors are taken from the literature on characteristics of esophageal speech, in particular, the differences between "superior" users of esophageal speech and "poor" users. Such information can be used in setting treatment goals for patients. The information is also useful as a yardstick for measuring progress over time. The early

TABLE 11.3 Factors on Which to Rate Esophageal Speech

1. Pitch Level

   Estimate or measure fundamental frequency.

   Is a higher pitch possible and comfortable?

2. Inflection or Pitch Variability

   Rate degree of inflection: absent/monotoned; present, needs improvement; present, typical of good user.

3. Quality

   Note degree of tension or strain.

   Is degree of roughness excessive or typical?

   Other comments.

4. Excess Noise

   Note presence or absence of noticeable klunking.

   Note presence or absence of stoma noise.

   Note conditions that improve or worsen the excess noises.

5. Visual Distractors

   Note and comment on types observed.

6. Rate of Speech

   Measure rate as words per minute or syllables per minute.

   Comment on perceptual impact (e.g., choppiness).

7. Words per Charge

   Average words (or syllables) per air charge.

   Compare between reading and conversation.

8. Latency of Air Charge

   Measure average time between start of air maneuver and onset of voice.

   How easily is the air charging accomplished (relaxed vs. effortful)?

9. Latency of Phrasal Pauses

   Does patient pause at linguistically appropriate junctures?

   For how long?

   Compare durations between items 8 and 9.

10. Articulatory Intelligibility

    Comment on perceptual confusions noted (e.g., ship-chip).

    Rate intelligibility:
    Poor
    Requires careful listening and topic knowledge
    Generally good but errors noted
    Good to excellent

11. Intensity and Intensity Variability

    Comment on ability to display stress and emphasis on key words.

    Rate overall loudness:
    Adequate in quiet environment
    Adequate against normal background noise
    Adequate in noisy situations

research of Snidecor and Curry (1959, 1960), among others, is acknowledged in our overview of the characteristics of esophageal speech as they relate to our clinical ratings.

Pitch Level
According to Martin (1979), an average male esophageal speaker will have a fundamental frequency of about 65 Hz, which is about half that of a normal speaking male. Weinberg and Bennett (1972) reported esophageal speech in males to average 58 Hz, and in females to average 87 Hz. Perceptual ratings seem to suggest that esophageal speech is more acceptable at higher, rather than lower, fundamental frequencies.

Inflection
Pitch variation is difficult to achieve with the pseudoglottis. Rate of frequency movement varies over a range of 7.9 tones per second in esophageal speakers as compared to normal values of 17.7 tones per second. Kelly (1983) notes that listeners will perceive a change in pitch through control of loudness, rate, length of time spent on a word, and the use of pauses. For example, an esophageal speaker should use a greater volume to raise the pitch but less intensity to lower the pitch.

Quality
Speech quality is not normal and never will be; a certain amount of hoarseness or roughness is typical. Strain and tension, however, adversely affect the quality of the speech produced. The clinician should take note of the ease with which the patient can charge air into the esophagus.

Excess Noise
Esophageal speakers exhibit some problems unique to their disorder. All distracting noises should be diagnosed early because they are more easily eradicated before a great deal of practice occurs. Excess noise can be associated with air intake or it can occur at the level of the stoma. When a patient injects air too rapidly into the esophagus, a "klunking" sound can occur. Some patients exhibit multiple "klunks" when they attempt more than one inflation before phonation. Another distracting behavior is stoma noise, or stoma blast, which is caused by the patient's forcing exhalations through the stoma at the time he/she is phonating esophageally. The patient has not adequately learned that "breathing for breathing and breathing for speech" are two separate functions. Sometimes the stoma noise masks the esophageal speech to the point of affecting intelligibility.

Visual Mannerisms
Other, nonvocal aspects of communication can be distracting to the listener. Facial grimaces, including eye squinting, and head movements often occur when a patient is trying to learn an air intake method such as injection. The clinician should note these types of behaviors in patients and seek to eliminate them early in the treatment program before they become habituated.

Rate of Speech

Perceptual studies suggest that rate of speech is the most important aspect that differentiates superior from poor esophageal speech. According to Snidecor and Curry (1960), superior esophageal speakers average 113 words per minute, with a range of 85 to 129 words per minute. This also is a rate that can be achieved by "good" patients, and we should point out that this rate is approximately 80 percent as fast as for normal (laryngeal) speakers, who average about 166 words per minute. Rate of speech declines as a function of air charging. The more frequently a patient charges, the slower the overall rate becomes. Superior esophageal speakers charge air less often than do poor speakers. Although the clinician should encourage proficiency at charging and increasing speech rates, we should point out that undue emphasis on increasing speech rates may be at the expense of loudness and suitable phrasing.

Words per Charge

In the study by Snidecor and Curry (1960), superior esophageal speakers used thirty air charges to read a paragraph that took normal speakers eleven breaths to complete. Esophageal speakers, therefore, recharged air three times more often. Superior esophageal speakers utilized their charge for 1 to 1½ seconds during which they averaged 2.8 to 6.3 words. This is compared to normal speakers who utilized a breath for 4.19 seconds and spoke 12.5 words. A satisfactory number of syllables on a single insufflation is eleven to twelve. During connected speech, four to nine syllables may be more typical.

Latency of Air Charge

Superior esophageal speakers gulp air at a rate of 0.42 to 0.80 seconds. Some patients can even get as low as 0.17, which is as fast as normal speakers. A good rule of thumb for setting treatment goals is a latency of 0.5 seconds or less. It is easier for patients to take air in quickly than it is to take in large amounts of air. In addition, we should point out that a 0.5-second charge is more rapid than the time most normal speakers pause for a phrasal juncture.

Latency of Phrasal Pauses

Phrase-limiting pauses are longer than the pauses for air charging—approximately 1.41 times longer. Both normal and esophageal speakers pause for phrases, but the superior esophageal speaker pauses longer than the normal person in order that such pauses contrast with air charge pauses. In other words, practiced esophageal speakers have learned to use silent times differentially, thus aiding the listener in linguistic comprehension. For example, a patient who charges air in 0.5 seconds would use a phrase-limiting pause of 0.7 seconds ($0.5 \times 1.41 = 0.7$).

Articulatory Intelligibility

Removal of the larynx and hyoid bone disrupts the muscular connections of the tongue and so articulatory mobility may be affected. Most patients, however, compensate quite well. The surgery also shortens the effective length of the vocal tract, altering format frequencies, and perhaps affecting vowel intelligibility. The pseudo-glottis is not equipped for abductor-adductor coordinations, and so the voicing of cognate phonemes is often a problem, and the glottal fricative /h/ is impossible for a laryngectomee to produce. Clearly, then, articulation and speech intelligibility are of concern to the SLP.

Treatment should involve practice with strategies to differentiate similar pho-nemes and periodic assessments of how well the patient is doing are in order. For example, can a listener distinguish between "jip–chip–ship"? We feel strongly that intelligibility testing should be done in a regular fashion and treatment exercises be assigned for any deficiencies noted. Kelly (1983) recommends daily intelligibil-ity testing by a family member. Kelly also suggests a four-step process:

1. Speaker and listener stand close together. Stimuli can involve lists of sounds, words, phrases, or sentences.
2. Speaker and listener stand across the room from each other.
3. Listener looks away while speaker is speaking.
4. Speaker stands four to six feet away from the listener and turns with back to the listener.

Intensity

Intensity is approximately 6 to 10 dB softer in esophageal speech than in normal speech (Hyman 1955). The intensity range is also more restricted: esophageal speakers exhibit a range of about 20 dB and normal speakers 45 dB. Lack of loud-ness is often an early concern for patients. We like to discourage this concern as at-tempts to speak louder may be counterproductive. In trying to talk louder, patients adopt patterns of strain and effort, develop more noticeable klunking noises, and have longer injection latencies as they try to take in more air. We explain that loud-ness will improve over time. When appropriate, we also teach techniques for pro-jecting louder, such things as digital pressure on the throat or using a handkerchief tied about the neck (Snidecor 1971). We monitor loudness subjectively in our pa-tients, although objective measures could be made.

We would also like to mention that assessment checklists can be useful for the patient to complete, as well as for the clinician. Self-ratings provide an opportunity for the patient to "take stock" of his/her progress and often serve as motivating de-vices. Table 11.4 displays an Esophageal Communication Checklist that we ac-quired at a Greater Atlanta Voice Masters Meeting in 1976. The author is unknown to us. We have often found this self-administered checklist useful to the patient.

Since TE speech is produced with exhaled lung air, we need not concern our-selves with latency of air charging, klunking noises, or stoma blasts. Yet, using lung air does not mean that TE speech will be equivalent to normal, laryngeal speech. More air will be expended in TE speech because of the resistance of the prosthetic device and routing passage. Hence, duration of sustained phonation and number of words spoken per breath will be shorter than normal. Lung air will permit variety in pitch

TABLE 11.4   Self-Administered Esophageal Checklist

NOTE: The following list comprises a few areas that contribute to effective esophageal communication. Others can and should be added. It is hoped that these will provide some assistance in helping you evaluate your esophageal speech and communication.

Distractors   Yes   No

1. Eyes
   a. I close my eyes as I try to produce esophageal tone.   ____   ____
   b. I blink my eyes as I speak.   ____   ____
   c. I look away from my listener as I speak.   ____   ____
2. Shoulders
   a. I move my shoulders as I try to produce speech.   ____   ____
3. Hands
   a. I move my hands as I try to speak.   ____   ____
4. Arms
   a. I move my arms as I try to speak.   ____   ____
5. Chin
   a. I move my chin, bob it up and down as I take in air for esophageal speech.   ____   ____
6. Mouth
   a. I twist or stretch my mouth as I try to speak.   ____   ____
7. I have watched myself in the mirror as I speak.   ____   ____
8. I look "ill at ease" or "tense" when I speak.   ____   ____
9. I sometimes lose saliva from my mouth as I speak.   ____   ____
10. I sometimes fail to cover my stoma when I cough or sneeze.   ____   ____
11. I make audible noises as I breathe when I speak.   ____   ____
    (I hear noises as I breathe in and out.)

Other Noises

1. I use the air in my mouth to make sounds such as "p" and "t," by moving the air in my mouth with my tongue against the roof of my mouth or by moving my cheeks or lips against my teeth (buccal speech).   ____   ____
2. I use the air in my mouth to produce a "Donald Duck" type of speech. The sounds come from the back of my mouth and sound "slushy" and are short (pharyngeal speech).   ____   ____
3. I make "clunking" noises in my throat just before I produce an esophageal tone.   ____   ____
4. I breathe heavily as I produce the esophageal tone, to "get it out," and I hear a rush of air coming out of my stoma. It sometimes covers up the esophageal speech sounds I've produced.   ____   ____

Phonation

1. I produce belches but do not have control over them when they come. They are produced by the air that has gone to my stomach and is coming up without my control (gastric speech).   ____   ____
2. I produce short esophageal speech sounds most of the time when I try to produce the sounds.   ____   ____

TABLE 11.4   *Continued*

	Yes	No
3. I can produce 1–2 syllable-length words using esophageal phonation (e.g.,"pop," "popcorn").	___	___
4. I can produce 3–4 syllable-length words using esophageal phonation (e.g.,"policeman," "constitution").	___	___
5. I can produce words of 5 syllables or more using esophageal speech (e.g., "hospitalization").	___	___
6. I can, after producing a word or short phrase, get another charge of air and produce the next word very rapidly without a long pause.	___	___
7. I can judge how much air I have in my esophagus so that I do not complete each word and phrase without running out of phonation or tone.	___	___
8. I can be heard in most speaking situations where there is not an unusual amount of noise.	___	___
9. I can vary the loudness of my esophageal speech.	___	___
10. I can change the pitch of my esophageal speech by 1 tone.	___	___
11. I can change the pitch of my esophageal speech by 2 or more tones.	___	___
12. I can clearly articulate the final sounds of words in my speech.	___	___
13. I do not overarticulate the sounds of words making my speech sound stilted or formal.	___	___
14. I can produce all the consonants and vowels of speech clearly.	___	___
15. I can produce all but "h."	___	___
16. I can produce all but "m," "n," and "ng."	___	___
17. I can clearly produce "p" and "b," "k," and "g" and "t" and "d" so that each sound is clearly distinctive from the other.	___	___
18. I pace my rate of speech so that each sound is clearly articulated.	___	___

Communication

	Yes	No
1. I check to see that the person I am speaking to truly understands what I have said.	___	___
2. If I am asked to repeat what I said, I rephrase what I have said.	___	___
3. I try to give my listener as much information as possible so I try to speak in full sentences as opposed to single words or short phrases.	___	___
4. I direct my listener to watch my mouth as I speak to give him/her further help in understanding what I have said.	___	___
5. I use an amplifier or artificial larynx		
a. If my listener has a hearing loss and cannot hear my esophageal voice.	___	___
b. If I'm tired and my esophageal voice is not adequate.	___	___
c. If I'm emotionally upset and I cannot adequately obtain a charge of air for esophageal speech.	___	___
d. If I am not feeling well physically and cannot produce esophageal speech readily.	___	___
e. If I'm speaking in a situation where there is a great deal of noise and I cannot produce adequate volume with my esophageal voice to be heard above the noise.	___	___
f. If I'm speaking or have used my esophageal voice for a long period of time.	___	___

and loudness but the pseudoglottis may tend to restrict it. The result of all this is that TE speech is generally superior to esophageal speech but inferior to normal speech on most measures (Pindzola and Cain 1989; Robbins, Fisher, and Blom 1984).

Many of the characteristics that clinicians use to rate esophageal speech can be used with the TE patient, but with some obvious exceptions, as previously noted. A prime area of dynamic assessment is that of articulatory intelligibility. Tracheoesophageal speakers need to constantly monitor and improve articulation proficiency with voiced/voiceless cognates and phonemes that pose perceptual confusion. Again we mention "jip–chip–ship" as an example of potential difficulties. The intelligibility testing by family members, as suggested by Kelly (1983) for esophageal speakers, would certainly be a useful clinical exercise for TE speakers as well.

Regarding specific data pertinent to the assessment of TE speech, we would like to mention the works of Robbins, Fisher, and Blom (1984) and Pindzola and Cain (1989). Both studies show good agreement in their data. Pindzola and Cain compared TE speakers, esophageal speakers, and normal speakers on certain criteria, including the following points:

1. Speech rate differed among the three groups of speakers. Normal talkers averaged 170 wpm, TE speakers averaged 152 wpm; and esophageal speakers averaged 94 wpm.
2. The fundamental frequency of the TE speakers was slightly lower than expected of normal males of the same age. TE speech averaged 108 Hz. Esophageal speech was much lower, with an average of 84 Hz. Lung air offers advantages here, even though the pharyngoesophageal segment acts as the pseudoglottis in both forms of alaryngeal speech.
3. The range of fundamental frequency, or pitch variability, was equivalent among the three groups. This indicates that both TE and esophageal speakers can achieve use of intonation with the pseudoglottis.
4. The number of words spoken per breath, or per air charge, showed the expected pattern: Normal speakers averaged 12 words per breath, TE speakers averaged 8 words per breath, and esophageal speakers averaged 3.5 words per air charge.

We would also like to remind the reader of the troubleshooting suggestions provided by Bosone (1986). Although most TE patients begin speaking immediately and need speech treatment only for a brief while, problems do arise. The speech pathologist will be called upon for reassessments and troubleshooting.

Prognosis

At the end of the evaluation sessions, we should have obtained pertinent case history data, and we should have provided information to the patient and the family about the anatomical changes and potential communication methods. We should also have a good idea about the patient's current method of communication and potential for treatment. As a review of much of what we have said in this chapter, we offer the following list of prognostic indicators for success.

1. The patient should have competent anatomical structures for the method or methods of speech chosen. The pharyngoesophageal segment must be adequate for development of esophageal or TE speech. The tendency for esophageal spasms (as pretested with air insufflation) is contraindicative for both forms of speech. Obesity and thick, scarred neck tissues may interfere with the use of neck-type artificial larynges.

2. The severity, extent, and type of surgery seem not to be related to the acquisition of speech. Yet, this assessment may be highly individualistic.

3. Patients should be of good general health. Feeble patients generally do not do well in learning esophageal or TE speech. These speech forms require energy to persist in the rehabilitation process. Artificial larynges, on the other hand, seem well suited for the more feeble patient.

4. The date of the surgery relative to the enrollment in the speech rehabilitation program is important. Gardner (1971) reviewed the literature and concluded that the chances for attaining adequate speech diminish with the passage of time since surgery. He was referring to esophageal speech, but the dictum probably holds true for all speech forms. The prognosis for speech after waiting one or two years postsurgery is extremely poor. By that time, other habits (such as total dependency on the spouse) have developed and are difficult to break.

5. Patients with a positive attitude and motivation to practice often throughout the day tend to be the successful ones, no matter which form of speech they are learning.

6. Those planning to return to work seem to have an extra ounce of motivation to master speech and to do so more quickly than those staying home or in an institution.

7. Patients who have family support at home, willing communication partners, and people willing to participate in the rehabilitation program and to help with daily practice generally do quite well.

8. Patients who are literate and willing to read and study materials about laryngectomy rehabilitation seem to make good progress. They make good use of workbooks, stimuli lists, and the like in daily practice.

9. Patients who were able to burp preoperatively or who quickly have acquired this ability postoperatively are good candidates for esophageal speech.

To conclude, then, we have shown the multitude of complex issues involved in the assessment, counseling, prognosing, and reassessment of persons with laryngectomies. The SLP must be well versed in the three main avenues of rehabilitation: artificial larynx, esophageal speech, and TE speech.

Bibliography

American Cancer Society (1985). *Laryngectomee Visitor Program Manual*. Available from IAL National Office, c/o American Cancer Society, 90 Park Avenue, New York, N.Y. 10016.

Barton, J., and Hejna, R. (1963). "Factors Associated with Success or Nonsuccess in Acquisition of Esophageal Speech." *Journal of the Speech and Hearing Association of Virginia* 4:19–20.

Berlin, C. (1963). "Clinical Measurement of Esophageal Speech I: Methodology and Curves of Skill Acquisition." *Journal of Speech and Hearing Disorders* 28:42–51.

Bosone, Z. T. (1986). "Trouble-shooting after Tracheoesophageal Fistulization for Voice Restoration." *Seminars in Speech and Language* 7, no. 1:43–51.

Bradley, R. C., and Ormond, T. F. (1970). *Communication for the Laryngectomized*. Chicago, IL: Interstate Printers.

Dabul, B. (1981). "Early assessment of progress in esophageal speech." Paper presented at the annual convention of the American Speech-Language-Hearing Association, Los Angeles, CA.

Fleming, S. M., Simpson, M. L., and Weaver, A. W. (1983). "A Comparison of Four Types of Laryngectomized Speech Rehabilitation." Paper presented at the annual convention of the American Speech-Language-Hearing Association, Washington, D.C.

Gandour, J., and Weinberg, B. (1983). "Perception of Intonational Contrasts in Alaryngeal Speech." *Journal of Speech and Hearing Research* 26:142–148.

Gardner, W. H. (1971). *Laryngectomee Speech and Rehabilitation*. Springfield, IL: Charles C. Thomas.

Greene, M. (1980). *The Voice and Its Disorders*. Philadelphia, PA: Lippincott.

Goldstein, L. P., and Rothman, H. B. (1976). "Analysis of speech produced with an artificial larynx." Paper presented at the annual convention of the American Speech and Hearing Association, Houston, TX.

Hyman, M. (1955). "An Experimental Study of Artificial Larynx and Esophageal Speech." *Journal of Speech and Hearing Disorders* 20:291–299.

Johnson, C. L. (1960). "A Survey of Laryngectomee Patients in Veteran's Administration Hospitals." *Archives of Otolaryngology* 72:768–773.

Keith, R. L., Shane, H., Coates, H., and Devine, K. (1984). *Looking Forward: A Guidebook for the Laryngectomee*. Rochester, MN: Mayo Foundation.

Kelly, L. S. (1983). *A Guide for Rehabilitation and Assessment of the Total Laryngectomee*. Tucson, AZ: Communication Skill Builders.

Knepflar, K. J. (1960). "Individualized Speech Therapy for Laryngectomized Patients." Paper presented at the annual convention of the American Speech and Hearing Association, Los Angeles, CA.

Knepflar, K. J. (1962). "Therapy Approaches for the Improvement and Refinement of Pseudovoice in Laryngectomized Speakers." Paper presented at the annual convention of the American Speech and Hearing Association, New York.

La Borwit, L. J. (1981). *Inventory for the assessment of laryngectomy rehabilitation*. Tigard, OR: C. C. Publications, Inc.

Lauder, E. (1989). *Self-Help for the Laryngectomee*. San Antonio, TX: E. Lauder Pub.

Martin, D. (1979). "Evaluating Esophageal Speech Development and Proficiency." In *Laryngectomee Rehabilitation*, ed. R. Keith and F. Darley (Houston, TX: College Hill).

Moffet, B., and Pindzola, R. (1988). "Acoustic Properties of Artificial Larynx Speech." *Journal of NSSLHA* 16:1–9.

National Cancer Institute (1985). *Cancer Rates and Risks*. 3rd ed. Washington, DC: National Institutes of Health.

Pindzola, R. H., and Cain, B. H. (1989). "Duration and Frequency Characteristics of Tracheoesophageal Speech." *Annals of Otology, Rhinology, and Laryngology* 98, no. 12:960–964.

Pindzola, R., and Moffet, B. (1988). "Comparison of Ratings of Four Artificial Larynges." *Journal of Communication Disorders* 21, 5:459–467.

Rigrodsky, S., and Lerman, J. (1971). *Therapy for the Laryngectomized Patient: A Speech Clinician's Manual*. New York: New York Teachers College Press.

Robbins, J., Fisher, H., and Blom, E. (1984). "A Comparative Acoustic Study of Normal, Esophageal, and Tracheoesophageal Speech Production." *Journal of Speech and Hearing Disorders* 49:202–210.

Robe, E. Y., Moore, P., Andrews, A. H., and Holinger, P. H. (1956). "A Study of the Role of Certain Factors in the Development of Speech after Laryngectomy. 1: Type of operation." *Laryngoscope* 66:173–186.

Rothman, H. B. (1978). "Analyzing Artificial Electronic Larynx Speech." In *The Artificial Larynx Handbook*, ed. S. J. Salmon and L. P. Goldstein (New York: Grune and Stratton).

Salmon, S. J., and Goldstein, L. P. (1978). *The Artificial Larynx Handbook*. New York: Grune and Stratton.

Shipp, T. (1967). "Frequency, Duration and Perceptual Measures in Relation to Judgments of Alaryngeal Speech Acceptability." *Journal of Speech and Hearing Research* 10:417–427.

Singer, M., and Blom, E. (1980). "An Endoscopic Technique for Restoration of Voice after Laryngectomy." Paper presented at the annual meeting of the American Laryngologic Association, Palm Beach, FL.

Snidecor, J. C. (1962). *Speech Rehabilitation of the Laryngectomized*. Springfield, IL: Charles C Thomas.

Snidecor, J. C. (1969). *Speech Rehabilitation of the Laryngectomized*. 2nd ed. Springfield, IL: Charles C Thomas.

Snidecor, J. C. (1971). "Speech without a Larynx." In *Handbook of Speech Pathology and Audiology*, ed. L. E. Travis (Englewood Cliffs, NJ: Prentice Hall).

Snidecor, J. C., and Curry, E. T. (1959). "Temporal and Pitch Aspects of Superior Esophageal Speech." *Annals of Otology, Rhinology and Laryngology* 68:1–14.

Snidecor, J. C., and Curry, E. T. (1960). "How Effectively Can the Laryngectomee Expect to Speak? *Laryngoscope* 70:62–67.

Travis, L. E. (Ed.). (1971). *Handbook of Speech Pathology and Audiology*. Englewood Cliffs, NJ: Prentice Hall.

Vallencien, B., Bouchiere, D. M., Gaches, L., and Cabirol, F. (1971). "Social and Familiar Readaptation of Laryngectomees." *Folia Phoniatrica* 23:365–370.

Weinberg, B., and Bennett, S. (1972). "Selected Acoustic Characteristics of Esophageal Speech Produced by Female Laryngectomees." *Journal of Speech and Hearing Research* 15:211–216.

Weiss, M. S., Yeni-Komshian, G. H., and Heinz, J. M. (1979). "Acoustical and Perceptual Characteristics of Speech Produced with an Electronic Artificial Larynx." *Journal of the Acoustical Society of America* 65:1298–1308.

Wepman, J. M., MacGahan, J. A., Rickard, J. C., and Shelton, N. W. (1953). "The Objective Measurement of Progressive Esophageal Speech Development." *Journal of Speech and Hearing Disorders* 18:247–251.

Williams, S. E., and Watson, J. B. (1985). "Differences in Speaking Proficiencies in Three Laryngectomee Groups." *Archives of Otolaryngology* 111:216–219.

$$Chapter\ 12$$

Assessment of Resonance Imbalance

Disorders of voice, particularly disorders of vocal quality, may be due to defective transmission of sound through the vocal tract. Sound generation at the level of the larynx occurs normally, and so these are not laryngeal disorders discussed in Chapter 10. Problems of resonance may be classified as hyponasality, hypernasality, nasal emission, cul-de-sac resonance, or thin/effeminate resonance. The assessment of resonance imbalance will be the focus of this chapter.

Categories of Abnormal Resonance

The *denasal* or *hyponasal* voice lacks the normal nasal resonance expected on /m/, /n/, and /ŋ/ in English. Often these articulatory distortions resemble /b/, /d/, and /g/, respectively. The vocalic elements may also take on the characteristics of "talking with a head cold." Hyponasality usually results from some blockage or obstruction in the nasopharynx or nasal cavity. This obstruction may stem from congestion, nasal polyps, or various structural deformities.

Hypernasality is an excessive amount of nasal resonance during the production of vowels and vocalic elements. The nasal cavity is not adequately separated from the oral cavity during speech. Such velopharyngeal incompetence, or VPI, may stem from neuromuscular deficits or structural defects. Congenital clefts of the hard or soft palate are obvious examples of structural defects frequently leading to hypernasality, and we will discuss these conditions later in the chapter. Not only can hypernasality result from clefts of the hard or soft palate, but also from submucous clefts, velums with inadequate length, or pharyngeal dimensions that are too large. A neuromuscular deficit, such as a paralyzed or paretic velum, or dysfunction of the pharyngeal constrictor muscles may be attributed to trauma-induced dysarthria or disease-related dysarthria. Diseases such as myasthenia gravis, muscular dystrophy, and poliomyelitis often affect velopharyngeal functioning.

Hypernasality may be pronounced or only slightly apparent; in addition, it can be continuous or intermittent. In mild intermittent cases, the excess nasality on vowels may be most noticeable in the context of nasal consonants. This represents assimilation nasality and indicates a velum that can function but moves too slowly during connected speech.

Nasal emission is an audible escape of air through the nares during the production of pressure consonants, such as plosives, fricatives, and affricates. Implicated in this condition is an incompetent velopharyngeal mechanism. Nasal emission is different from the resonance imbalance of hypernasality, although the two problems may co-occur. It has been argued that nasal emission is more of an articulatory problem than a vocal resonance disorder (Peterson 1975); however, we will discuss it here because of convention.

Cul-de-sac resonance typically occurs in the oropharynx, largely owing to posterior tongue retraction. This resonance imbalance is heard as a muffled and hollow-sounding voice with a pharyngeal focus. In addition, Peterson-Falzone (1982) states that cul-de-sac resonance can result from an anterior nasal obstruction and a posterior aperature (opening). Cul-de-sac resonance associated with tongue retraction often occurs on a functional basis, as well as in patients with deafness, flaccid and spastic dysarthria, athetoid cerebral palsy, or oral verbal apraxia (Boone and McFarlane 1988; Prater and Swift 1984).

Thin vocal resonance, also known as an *effeminate voice quality,* seems related to an anterior tongue posture. The habitually high and excessively anterior tongue position is almost always due to functional, not organic, reasons. Prater and Swift (1984) explain:

> The voice sounds very weak and lacking in resonance, particularly for the back vowels . . . patients . . . articulate with a minimal oral opening and with little range of movement of the jaw. Because of . . . anterior tongue carriage and . . . restricted oral movement for articulation, the general impression . . . is that this type of speaker is using immature, baby-like, effeminate speech. Often, the speaker's vocal pitch is also elevated slightly, which aids in this perception of vocal immaturity and effeminacy. (241)

Case History and General Voice Assessment

The evaluation of a resonance disorder is often an outgrowth of a general voice evaluation; the clinician may not know beforehand the specific nature of a patient's problem. Consequently, the evaluation session proceeds along the lines described in Chapter 10. Suffice it to say that, first, a case history interview is done. Routine information is gathered, but particular questions need to be asked concerning the patient's description of the voice problem and known or suspected causes of the disorder. Oronasopharyngeal injuries, structural defects, and surgeries need to be thoroughly discussed. Second, the oral peripheral examination is crucial to the evaluation of resonance disorders; and, third, all parameters of the voice must be assessed.

Any of the assessment instruments mentioned in Chapter 10 would be appropriate to use. A Voice Assessment Protocol for Children and Adults (Pindzola 1987) is useful in assessing a multitude of vocal parameters. It evaluates the resonance of the patient's voice on a severity continuum. The patient may be scored as exhibiting normal resonance balance, cul-de-sac resonance, hyponasality (slight or intermittent vs. moderate-to-severe), hypernasality on vocalic elements (slight, intermittent, or assimilative vs. moderate vs. severe), and nasal emission on pressure consonants (slight or intermittent vs. moderate-to-severe).

After a thorough, overall voice assessment, emphasis is given to the appraisal of the resonance imbalance. Specific techniques can be employed by the SLP.

Assessment Techniques and Probes for Resonance Imbalance

In this section, we would like to discuss techniques requiring little or no instrumentation that the SLP can and should do to assess the various resonance imbalances. Before concluding the evaluation, we feel very strongly that the clinician should experiment, or probe, to see what improvements, or changes in general, can be effected in the patient's voice. Some writers have discussed this as *stimulability*. Wilson (1987) maintains that the ability of a patient to produce a clear voice upon stimulation means that voice treatment has a good chance of being successful.

Hyponasality

Since denasality is often due to obstruction in the nasal cavity, an examination of the nasal region is in order during the oral peripheral part of the assessment. Additionally, during the case history intake, the patient may indicate knowledge of having a deviated septum, nasal polyp, enlarged adenoids, and the like. On the other hand, the basis of a patient's hyponasality may be neuromuscular in origin and may reflect improper timing of velar movements. Case history questions should probe for trauma- or disease-related etiologies.

To evaluate a patient for hyponasal voice quality, SLPs rely on critical listening. While the patient is conversing or reading a standard paragraph, the clinician acutely listens for denasality shadowing the vowel portions of speech and, in particular, listens for the articulatory distortions or substitutions of b/m, d/n, and g/ŋ. By using specially constructed phrases, sentences, or paragraphs that have a preponderance of nasal phonemes, the clinician has a heightened opportunity to perceive denasal resonance. Suggested stimuli include the following examples, some of which we have devised or borrowed from the literature (Bloomer and Wolski 1968; Lippmann 1981):

> *Mama made some lemon jam.*
> *I know a man on the moon.*

Many a man knew my meaning.
Mike needs more milk.
My mom makes money.
When may we know your name?
I'm naming one man among many.

Having the patient count aloud from 90 to 100 is contextually appropriate, as well. Shupe (1968) provides word pairs useful in detecting hyponasality: "bake"/"make," "rib"/"rim," "dine"/"nine," "mad"/"man," "wig"/"wing," "bag"/"bang." In hyponasality, nasal resonance would be lacking and so, for example, the "bake"/"make" pair would sound like "bake"/"bake."

Another clinical task that is helpful in revealing hyponasal speech is to have the patient read a list of words initiated with the /m/ phoneme. Bzoch (1979) suggests these ten words: "meat," "moat," "mit," "mool," "mate," "mut," "met," "Mert," "mat," and "might." While the patient is reading, or repeating, each word from the list twice, the clinician alternately compresses and releases the patient's nostrils. In normal velopharyngeal function, the resonance becomes hypernasal when the nares are occluded, but no resonance change is heard in true hyponasality. Bzoch counts the number of words with no change in resonance and uses this figure as an index of hyponasality.

Operating on this same principle is the humming technique. The inability of a patient to hum or to hum clearly is suggestive of hyponasality (Prater and Swift 1984).

> Case Example. *Carmen Perez has fluctuating hyponasality. The severity of her hyponasality changes on a daily basis but there is a more noticeable fluctuation with the seasons. Carmen's ear, nose, and throat doctor observed nasal cavity characteristics typical of allergic inflammation: tissue coloration changes and hypertrophy of the nasal turbinates secondary to edema. The planned course of treatment involved use of prescribed antihistimines and the option of undergoing a lengthy allergen tolerance program.*

Hypernasality

Judgments about resonance are truly judgments of a perceptual nature; a well-tuned clinical ear is essential—and adequate—for the SLP. Critical listening by the clinician while the patient converses and/or reads a passage can be supplemented by rating the severity of the hypernasality on a rating scale. Several are available, including those by Subtelny, Van Hattum, and Myers (1972) and Van Demark (1974). Let us highlight a few others.

Fletcher (1978) rates the severity of hypernasality from mild to very severe. His descriptive categories are

- Normal nasality. Speech has enough nasality to sound normal, but not so much as to call attention to it unless specifically listening for it.

- Mild nasality. Nasality is apparent as the person speaks. It is somewhat greater than that of most speakers but would probably cause little or no distraction if not listening for it.
- Moderately nasal. Nasality is obviously present and is moderately distracting to the listener.
- Severely nasal. Nasality is prominent, is a highly distracting feature in the speech, and makes listening to the message difficult.
- Very severely nasal. Nasality is so distracting that it dominates all aspects of speech and makes hearing the message extremely difficult.

Fletcher's rating system recognizes the perceptual nature of hypernasality and is based on listener impact.

The Voice Profile System (Wilson and Rice 1977) includes a rating of resonance. Using a scale with 1 being a normal balance between nasality and orality, the following ratings are suggested:

−2 = denasal voice
+2 = assimilation nasality
+3 = nasalization of some vowels and some shading of consonants
+4 = nasalization with frequent consonant distortion by nasal emission.

The difficulty with such a scale is the "patient-fit" problem with dichotomous categories. Audiotaped samples, however, are available for reliability training.

The Buffalo III Resonance Profile (Wilson 1987) is a twelve-item supplement to Wilson's more general Buffalo III Voice Profile and is used when a patient has been rated 2 or higher on the nasal or oral resonance items of that voice profile. The profile for resonance uses a five-point rating scale where 1 is normal and 5 is very severe. Twelve parameters are then so rated: hypernasal resonance, hyponasal resonance, oral resonance, cul-de-sac resonance, nasal emission, facial grimaces, language level, articulation, speech intelligibility, speech acceptability, velopharyngeal competency, and overall resonance rating.

The SLP can use a "listening tube" to heighten the perception of a patient's hypernasality, thus facilitating its recognition (Mason and Riski 1982). We have used a makeshift listening tube fashioned from the plastic headsets provided by the airlines for in-flight movies. Prater and Swift (1984) explain an alternate construction and the use of a listening tube:

> The listening tube consists of a glass or plastic olive-shaped tip that is attached to a 2 to 3 foot piece of rubber tubing. Before beginning hypernasality assessment procedures, the nasal olive should be inserted into the patient's nostril and the free end of the tubing should be inserted into the clinician's ear. With this device in place, even the slightest degrees of nasal emission or hypernasality can be easily detected in the patient's speech. (1984, pp. 55–56)

The SLP may try a simple procedure sometimes known as the "nasal flutter test" (Hess 1976; Weiss 1974). Have the patient repeat in an alternate fashion the vowels /ɑ/ and /i/ while the clinician alternately compresses and releases the patient's nostrils. It is presumed that if velopharyngeal closure is adequate, there will be no noticeable difference in vowel quality as the nostrils are pinched. Conversely, if the clinician hears an increase in the nasal resonance during the nose-occluded condition, velopharyngeal incompetence may be suspected. The resonance quality change has also been described as a flutterlike sound; hence, the name of the test procedure.

Bzoch (1979) recommends a similar nose-occluded–unoccluded test procedure using plosive-vowel-plosive syllables. Ten vowels are tested in a /b—t/ context: "beet," "bit," "bait," "bet," "bat," "bought," "boat," "boot," "but," "Bert." In a person with normal velopharyngeal closure, the nose-occluded and unoccluded conditions sound the same.

Shelton, Brooks, and Youngstrom (1965) maintain that articulation tests are good measures of velopharyngeal closure and consequently are used for the clinical assessment of nasal emission and hypernasality. Most tests involve both consonants and vowels. Table 12.1 describes some commonly used articulation tests. Lintz and Sherman (1961) state that consonant environments influence the amount of nasality perceived on vowels. From least influential to most influential are /z, v, d, g, f, s, t, k/. It would seem, therefore, that nasality on vowels should be studied in these consonantal environments.

The perception of hypernasality can be heightened by using context-controlled stimuli. Mason and Grandstaff (1971) maintain that having the patient count aloud from 60 to 100 is an insightful, yet simple, assessment procedure. We offer the following summary of the counting task, which is a useful indicator of velopharyngeal incompetence and the symptoms of hypernasality, nasal emission, and hyponasality.

1. The 60 series of numbers may reveal velopharyngeal incompetence and nasal emission due to the frequent occurrence of the /s/ pressure phoneme.
2. The 70 series may reveal assimilative hypernasality owing to the embedded /n/ phoneme.
3. The 80 series should reveal normal or near-normal articulation and resonance.
4. The 90 series should sound normal when produced by a patient with hypernasality because of the frequent production of nasal consonants. The patient with hyponasality may display the articulatory substitution of d/n.

Shupe (1968) recommends testing for sound confusions in cases of suspected velopharyngeal incompetence. Have the patient read or repeat word pairs, such as "bake"/"make," "rib"/"rim," "dine"/"nine," "mad"/"man," "wig"/"wing," "bag"/"bang." In a patient with VPI, both sounds are hypernasal, making the "bake"/"make" pair, for example, sound like "make"/"make."

Instrumentation is also available that purports to detect or measure hypernasality. Like Moll (1964), we maintain that hypernasality is a perceptual phenomenon and must be assessed perceptually. Attempts to measure hypernasality "objectively" are really attempts to measure velopharyngeal function, oral and

TABLE 12.1   Articulation Tests Useful in Assessing Velopharyngeal Function

P-B Articulation Screening Test for Preschoolers
(Van Demark and Swickard 1980)

This is a 25-item single-word test of two phonemes, /p/ and /b/. The authors claim that velopharyngeal inadequacy is indicated when errors occur on at least 50 percent of the sounds tested.

Error Pattern Screening Articulation Test
(Bzoch 1979; Bzoch, Kemker, and Wood 1984)

The 31 words are purported to be useful in identifying gross substitution errors in children aged 3 and 4. Plosives, fricatives, affricates, glides, nasals, and blends are tested. Scoring involves assigning an error value to each sound. Sounds are scored as correct, indistinct from nasal emission alone, distortion, simple substitution, gross substitution, or omission.

Bzoch Error Pattern Diagnostic Articulation Test
(Bzoch 1979)

The diagnostic test has four forms, each with a different set of 100 words. Tested are 67 consonants and 33 blends in the initial, medial, final positions of the words. This is the full-length version of the screening test previously listed and is constructed with the same properties.

Iowa Pressure Articulation Test (IPAT)
(Templin and Darley 1969)

This test consists of 43 words containing pressure consonants. The percentage of correct responses is said to reflect the severity of velopharyngeal incompetence.

The reading passage "The Picnic"
(Wilson 1987)

The 43 words from the IPAT are incorporated in the short paragraph called "The Picnic." Production of the test words therefore can be tested in reading, rather than the traditional single-word method.

Sentence articulation tests
(Fletcher 1978; Van Demark 1964, 1966)

These are two examples of informal tests at the sentence level, which may be more ecologically valid than single-word tests.

Articulation Protocol
(McCabe and Bradley 1973)

The protocol, with a 10–15 minute administration time, compares accuracy of articulated words in automatic speech, single words, sentences, reading, and conversation.

---

nasal air flows, and the like. Although these data certainly relate to judgments of hypernasality, they are not measures of hypernasality per se. We will discuss instrumentation used to measure aspects of velopharyngeal function later in this chapter when we discuss the cleft palate population.

Once the SLP has determined that the patient exhibits some degree of hypernasality, the evaluative session should turn to discovering what, if any, techniques and manipulations lessen the perception of nasality. Together, the patient and clinician should experiment to find "what works," and in doing so they are arriving at a prognosis for change and are mapping the direction of future treatment, if warranted.

The variability of the hypernasality as it relates to phonetic context should be explored. Does the perception of hypernasality diminish or worsen in sentences loaded with high vowels? with low vowels? with numerous nasal consonants? with many pressure consonants?

Does the degree of hypernasality improve when the patient speaks with "open-mouth articulation" where there is exaggerated mouth opening and where speech sounds are enunciated with exaggerated movement? McDonald and Koepp-Baker (1951) discussed this technique as helpful in that air always takes the path of least resistance. By opening the anterior oral cavity wider, air will tend to flow outward rather than through the narrower, but opened, velopharyngeal port.

The SLP should also probe for possible improvements in hypernasality with changes in speaking rate, pitch, and loudness. These may be prime areas of manipulation in compensatory treatment programs. The literature reports that perceived hypernasality is lessened at higher pitch and intensity levels (Hess 1959; Rampp and Counihan 1970). The role of muscular fatigue can also be explored by having the patient determine whether there are times during the day that nasality is better or worse.

Case Example. *At the beginning of the second grade, Belinda Johnston was noticed by the SLP during school-wide screenings. The child's voice was hypernasal and nasal emission occurred inconsistently on words starting with /s/, /f/, and /p/. Belinda was failed on this brief screening and the SLP followed up on the case. In a telephone conversation with the mother, the clinician learned that Belinda had a tonsillectomy and adenoidectomy during the previous Easter break because of frequent ear infections and sore throats. The mother stated that Belinda's voice has sounded "unusual" only since the surgery, but she was told by the doctor that it would improve with time. The first-grade teacher confirmed that Belinda's voice sounded normal the previous year. As six months had elapsed since the surgery, the SLP and mother agreed to initiate appropriate school system procedures for a formal speech evaluation and subsequent intervention. In the evaluation, hypernasality was confirmed and its severity rated, as was the consistency and severity of nasal emission. The oral peripheral examination revealed several indicators of submucous clefting. There was a midline notching of the uvula (slight bifidity), an anteriorly placed velar dimple, midline translucency of the palate, and a highly vaulted hard palate. Velar movement occurred symmetrically, but contact with the posterior pharyngeal wall could not be observed with certainty. Air came out the nose when the clinician used the modified tongue–anchor technique, and Belinda was unable to blow up a balloon.*

The SLP wondered whether adenoidectomy should have been done on this child—the oral exam revealed several factors that would contraindicate a routine removal. (The adenoid's bulk compensated for the child's VPI.) The school SLP desired objective confirmation of the suspicions of VPI, available with sophisticated instrumentation, and expert opinions of the proper behavioral course of action, if any. Belinda was referred to the craniofacial team at a metropolitan hospital 100 miles away.

Case Example. *The SLP at a rehabilitation hospital received Delondo Hayes as a transfer patient from an acute care facility. Mr. Hayes was a 22-year-old automobile crash victim who had sustained brain stem and spinal cord injuries. The clinician noted in the initial speech consult that Mr. Hayes was partially paralyzed and used a wheelchair. His conversational speech was slow, slurred, and excessively hypernasal. In the oral examination, the speech pathologist also noted absence of gag reflex and weak lingual muscles. The patient was diagnosed with the motor speech disorder of flaccid dysarthria. Early treatment efforts would be directed at oral muscle mobility and precision of articulation. Slow speech rates would be accepted—indeed, encouraged as a means of achieving target articulatory placements, including velar gestures. The hypernasality would be monitored for four to six weeks of rehabilitation before considering further alternatives.*

Nasal Emission

Since nasal emission and hypernasality can both be due to inadequate velopharyngeal closure, it makes sense that they often co-occur; yet, we must keep in mind that the two problems are separate entities.

The assessment of nasal emission involves looking and listening. The expulsion of air through the nostrils may be so obvious as to flare the nares of the speaker. In contrast, in an attempt to decrease the outward flow of air, the person may constrict the nares. The clinician, then, looks for facial (nasal) grimaces.

Critical listening is crucial for the SLP to accurately diagnose the presence of nasal emission. Sometimes the emitted air is obviously noisy; in fact, *nasal snort* is a descriptive term encountered in this body of literature. At other times, the nasal emission is barely audible or detectable only with special techniques, as we shall see.

A frequent way to assess the presence of nasal emission is by administering a single-word articulation test. Although any articulation test will do, a few commercially available tests are designed to more thoroughly tap production of pressure plosives, fricatives, and affricates. Table 12.1 describes some of the more commonly used articulation tests. The results of the articulation test should answer the following questions posed by Morris and Smith (1962):

1. Does the speaker misarticulate fricatives, plosives, and affricates that have been demonstrated to require high intraoral breath pressure?
2. Do the misarticulations involve audible nasal emission?
3. Are there evidences of facial grimacing during the production of these consonants?
4. Does occluding the nostrils (preventing an air leakage) result in normal production of them?

We would add the following to the above list of questions for clinicians:

1. Regarding nasal emission, are voiced consonants less defective than their voiceless cognates? Typically, the required amount of oral air pressure is greater for voiceless phonemes (Moll 1968; Spriestersbach 1955).
2. Are single consonants less affected than blends (Moll 1968)?

3. Are consonants in the initial or final position in words articulated correctly more often than medial consonants are (Moll 1968)?
4. Does the patient use compensatory articulation patterns, such as glottal stop, pharyngeal stop, mid-dorsum palatal stop, pharyngeal fricative, posterior nasal fricative, and so forth (Trost 1981)?

In addition to, or in place of, a formal articulation test, the clinician may listen for nasal emission in specially designed words and sentences. Have the patient read or repeat stimuli loaded with pressure consonants, such as the following (Bzoch 1979; Hess 1971; Lippman 1981; Warren 1979):

Pick the peas.
Pappa piped up.
Polish the shoes.
Bessie stayed all summer.
We'd better buy a bigger dog.
Follow Sally, Charley.
People, baby, paper, Bobby, puppy, bubble, pepper, B. B., piper, bye bye.

Likewise, the clinician can listen carefully as the patient counts aloud. The numbers between 60 and 79 are especially evocative of nasal emission (Mason and Grandstaff 1971).

The SLP can use simple items to enhance the detection and monitoring of nasal air emission. A small mirror held under the patient's nostril will fog as air escapes. We have used a dental mirror with its convenient handle, a small lipstick mirror, and a special nonglass reflector manufactured by the Floxite Company (Niagara Falls, NY 14303). We prefer the latter for its sensitivity to fogging and its compact design with handle. Fog on the mirror during the patient's attempts at prolonging fricatives, repeating VCV syllables containing pressure consonants (such as /ipi ipi ipi/, /upu upu upu/), or saying the pressure-loaded sentences previously listed is strongly suggestive of velopharyngeal incompetence. These same procedures may be done with wisps of cotton on a wooden tongue depressor held beneath the nose when a mirror is not available. We find the cotton's sensitivity less reliable, though.

Bzoch (1979) describes an oral-nasal air paddle constructed from cardboard, and Bloch (1979) suggests the use of an airline music headset or a stethoscope to detect air flow. The listening tube, described previously, is also useful for assessing nasal emission (Mason and Riski 1982). A "scape-scope" (Shprintzen, McCall, and Skolnick 1975) can be constructed with a clear plastic cylinder, styrofoam piston, and tubing with a nasal olive. The same type of device is available commercially as the See-Scape (PRO-ED, Austin, TX 78758). We would like to mention that all devices used to detect and visualize the nasal emission of air are useful in treatment as well as in assessment.

After determining that a patient has nasal emission, the clinician should probe for techniques that diminish air escape. If none is found, behavioral treatment may be contraindicated, and physical management necessary. Here are some techniques the SLP can try.

Have the patient use light articulatory contacts on pressure consonants—the plosives, fricatives, and affricates. McDonald and Koepp-Baker (1951) suggest explaining this concept to young children by teaching "fish-talking." A complementary technique that may diminish nasal emission is that of open-mouth articulation, as was suggested for hypernasality.

Perhaps having the patient extend the vowel portions of speech will lessen the emphasis placed on pressure consonant articulation and so improve nasal emission. The fluency-enhancing techniques that involve vowel/syllable prolongations, found in many stuttering approaches, may prove useful with some patients. Reduced rates of speech may also be useful, especially in patients who show velar movement potential but suffer from sluggish timing maneuvers.

Van Demark (1971) described a stimulability evaluation for children with resonance problems. Each item missed on the Iowa Pressure Articulation Test (Templin and Darley 1969) is retested, using another picture. The SLP repeats the item twice, and the client responds immediately. Stimulation is then provided for the item in isolation, in nonsense syllables (all positions), and in words. Following this stimulation, the client is again shown the picture of the errored item and is made aware that the word contains the stimulated sound. The child should then attempt the word correctly, read the word, and produce a sentence with it.

Wilson (1987) and Rampp, Pannbacker, and Kinnebrew (1984) advocate use of the Miami Imitative Ability Test (Jacobs, Philips, and Harrison 1970) to determine the level of stimulability in patients with velopharyngeal incompetence. Twenty-four consonant sounds are used in the initial position, followed by a neutral vowel. The child is instructed to "watch and listen" as the clinician repeats each stimulus three times before attempting a production. The response is evaluated in two ways: the ability to imitate articulatory placement and the accuracy of the acoustic production. A three-point scoring system is used: 1 point if correct, ½ point if questionable, and 0 if incorrect.

> Case Example. *Philip Chang had a repaired cleft lip and palate. Owing to persistent velopharyngeal incompetence, the surgeon established an inferiorly based pharyngeal flap. (The interested reader should consult Randall et al. 1978 for information about flaps.) After the appropriate recuperative period, the doctor was still concerned about Philip's speech and ordered further tests. As part of a thorough evaluation, the SLP documented articulation errors of the type usually seen in cases of velopharyngeal incompetence. Stimulability probes, however, revealed some interesting changes. For example, Philip produced /t/ with nasal emission in place of /k/ on some test items, yet produced /k/ for /k/ on other items but with nasal emission. Glottal stops were noted in place of /g/ and sometimes for /k/. After stimulation, Philip was able to produce /k/ appropriately in phonetic contexts, without substituting. Furthermore, his /k/ productions were without nasal emission of air. A positive oral manometer ratio of 0.95 was obtained. The clinician interpreted Philip's stimulability as indication that velopharyngeal competence could be achieved, that old articulatory habits could be changed, and that phonetic placement training could be effective. Philip's prognosis for modifying his articulation toward normalcy was deemed good.*

Cul-de-sac Resonance

The hollow voice quality of this disorder is typically due to hyperfunction of the tongue. Speech is produced with the tongue posteriorly positioned in the oral cavity and oropharynx regions. The SLP should try to observe this posterior retraction when possible; having the patient phonate an open vowel, such as /a/, may facilitate viewing of the posterior tongue placement.

De facto diagnosis may come from probing for improvements in the cul-de-sac resonance. Experiment by having the patient read sentences or word lists loaded with phonemes that promote anterior tongue placement and inhibit lingual retraction. Prater and Swift (1984) suggest the following phonemes for developing clinical stimuli:

Tongue-tip: /t/, /d/, /s/, and /z/
Front vowels: /i/, /ɪ/, and /e/
Front consonants: /w/, /hw/, /p/, /b/, /f/, /v/, /θ/, and /l/.

It has been noted in the literature that hearing-impaired and deaf speakers often use too slow a rate of speech. The slow rate of speech seems attributable to altered syllable durations, which, in turn, adversely affects speech intelligibility and voice quality. Increasing the speaking rates of hearing-impaired persons may improve their perceived hypernasality or their cul-de-sac resonance and should be attempted by the SLP.

Thin Vocal Resonance

The thin, effeminate voice quality usually is related to anterior tongue carriage, and thus the oral resonance of vowels and consonants is affected. By moving the place of the primary articulatory constriction more forward in the oral cavity, energy loci are shifted to higher frequencies, and vocalic formats are likewise elevated (Minifie 1973). The perception of effeminancy may be increased by the patient's use of an elevated fundamental frequency and/or exaggerated use of the upper range for pitch inflections. Pitch, as well as quality, should be evaluated in these patients. As suggested in Chapter 10, A Voice Assessment Protocol for Children and Adults (Pindzola 1987), or a similar instrument, is a useful guide for appraising all parameters of a patient's voice. To assess thin resonance, have the patient read sentences or word lists containing many back vowels and back consonants (such as /k/ and /g/). Note whether there is an improvement in resonance with this probe technique.

Assessment Associated with Cleft Palate

In addition to the information presented on assessing hypernasality and nasal emission, we would like to elaborate on the diagnostic process used with patients who have clefts of the hard or soft palate. In the diagnosis of communication problems associated with cleft palate, the SLP is typically a member of a team. The craniofacial team is a well-accepted clinical entity, and in many communities represents the ultimate in interdisciplinary cooperation between SLPs, audiologists, psychologists, surgeons, otolaryngologists, prosthedontists, orthodontists, pedodontists, and educational personnel (Bzoch 1979; Wells 1971). The SLP is expected to inform the team members about the patient's communication abilities and disabilities, predict the effects of contemplated rehabilitative procedures, and serve as the primary agent for change in the patient's speech and language skills. The dramatic growth during the past three or four decades in the development of surgical and other rehabilitative procedures for the individual with a cleft has been encouraging.

Vanderas (1987) reviewed epidemiological studies of clefting across racial/ethnic groups. For minority groups in the United States, the highest incidence of cleft palate per 1000 population was among the Chinese (4.04), then American Indians (0.79), Japanese (0.82–2.41), and African Americans (0.8–1.67). Drawing on international data, the incidence for Filipinos/Hawaiians is 2.45 per 1000 population, and for Hispanics it ranges from 0.42 to 2.27, with Puerto Ricans showing a slightly greater incidence than Mexicans do. Vanderas also reviewed the incidence of different kinds of clefting (lip, palate, lip and palate) with most minority groups following the general population trend toward cleft lip with palate. A notable exception is that among African Americans a cleft palate only occurs more often.

Patients and families may obtain useful information from the American Cleft Palate–Craniofacial Association, 1218 Grandview Drive, Pittsburgh, PA 15211 (telephone [800] 24-CLEFT).

The SLP should endeavor to evaluate, or have evaluated at an appropriate facility, many aspects of velopharyngeal functioning. Table 12.2 lists areas and/or methods of appraisal. We will elaborate on many in the remainder of the chapter.

Case History

The routine case history data may need to be augmented for the cleft palate patient. Both general and special case history forms have been developed (Bloch

TABLE 12.2   Areas Typically Appraised in Suspected Cases of Velopharyngeal Incompetence

Case History

Articulation and Intelligibility—formal tests, informal stimuli

Resonance—perceptual scales, listening tubes, various other devices

Intraoral Examination

Endoscopy—with rigid or fiberoptic scopes

Radiographic Studies—cephalometry (still, lateral x-rays), videofluoroscopy, cinefluorography, tomography (laminagraphy), and/or computerized tomography (CT) scanning

Pressure-Flow Studies—oral manometer, nasometer, PERCI, ZIPPO

Others—accelerometry, electromyography, ultrasound

Stimulability Testing (Probes)

1979; Darley 1978; Peterson and Marquardt 1981; Rampp, Pannbacker, and Kinnebrew 1984; Saunders 1972; Westlake 1968).

Knowledge of the type and extent of cleft, as well as a description of the surgical, prosthodontic, orthodontic, and other rehabilitative procedures performed would be helpful. Some statement of the patient's current medical status and plans for future intervention procedures will also help direct the evaluative process. If the clinician is not a formal member of a craniofacial team, copies of reports from other professionals who have dealt with the patient should be obtained.

Critical Listening

Although the initial interaction between clinician and patient should be free and relatively unstructured, the clinician has a most demanding task. Once the patient is conversing in a spontaneous manner, the SLP must apply critical listening skills to assess the individual's total communicative effectiveness. This involves systematically shifting perceptual sets from one aspect of the patient's speech to another. The SLP should listen for the presence of a resonance imbalance (such as hypernasality, hyponasality, nasal emission, or a combination) and rate its severity. Although trained judges are able to identify nasality fairly adequately, the clinician may wish to tape-record the client and listen to several playbacks, or play the tape backward to isolate the nasality from articulation (Sherman 1954; Spriestersbach 1955). After noting the degree of resonance imbalance on some scaling device, the clinician should listen to the general articulatory pattern without recording actual errors. Is there an obvious preponderance of a particular type of error (such as glottal stops or pharyngeal fricatives)? Does the articulation appear to alter with differing communication situations, speech, or stress patterns? Next, listen to the language of the patient, particularly if it is a young child, and check for appropriate word choice, sentence complexity, and structure. The rate and rhythm of the patient's speech should be noted. Are there any other vocal quality differences (such as hoarseness)? Is there a facial grimace, constriction of the nares, or any other behavior which detracts from the individual's total communicative effectiveness?

Articulation Testing

After formulating a general impression of the patient's speech patterns, detailed phonology and articulation testing should be done. Standard articulation tests may be satisfactory for cleft palate individuals, but there are several considerations that may be best examined by "specialized" articulation tests and context-controlled stimuli. Certainly, all of the functional, perceptual, and sensory factors that affect the normal person could be active, but in cleft palate individuals there are added possibilities. Most important are the degree of velopharyngeal closure and the resultant air flow and intraoral pressure. The deviant geography of the oral cavity may contribute to this problem, which is also complicated by the fact that the oral structure may well have undergone several architectural changes within the first few years of life. The SLP must keep in mind that this individual has been trying to produce standard sounds with a nonstandard structure, and under these conditions unique compensatory adjustments may have been made. The patient may have increased the air flow in order to build up adequate oral pressure, or minimized it to lessen nasal escape; in the latter case, we say that the patient is producing weak pressure consonants (McWilliams and Philips 1979; Trost 1981).

Many patients with VPI adopt compensatory articulations, including glottal stop substitutions, pharyngeal fricatives, velar fricatives, and aspirant productions of vowels and consonants; other, unusual compensations may also be used (Rampp, Pannbacker, and Kinnebrew 1984; Trost 1981).

Glottal stop substitutions are produced by approximation of the glottis; they are generally used in the place of plosives and sometimes in the place of fricatives. Glottal stop substitutions are a difficult habit to break even after management of the palate and seem to be especially persistent for sounds in the medial position (Bzoch 1979; McWilliams and Philips 1979). Pharyngeal and velar fricatives are also attempts by the patient to valve air at a point in the vocal tract that is nearer the source of air pressure than the velopharyngeal valve (Morris 1979). The place of constriction is between the tongue and pharynx, or constriction of the pharynx, rather than more orally. Bzoch (1979) also reports that pharyngeal and velar fricatives persist longest for the /s/ and /z/ phonemes.

Trost (1981) described three types of compensatory articulation not typically reported in the literature: (1) The pharyngeal stop, used with /k/ and /g/, is produced with a posterior and inferior tongue placement. (2) The mid-dorsum palatal stop is a stop consonant substitution for /t/, /d/, /k/ or /g/. Posterior nasal fricatives are generally produced as substitutions for the /s/, /z/, /ʃ/ and /ʒ/ phonemes and may occur simultaneously with a fricative, affricate, or stop consonant.

Clinicians can gain listening and transcription experience with errors associated with clefting by using the Trost-Cardamone (1987) instructional videotape.

The clinician should keep in mind that it is entirely possible for the compensatory habits that developed before the final surgical adjustments to persist after competence of the velopharyngeal mechanism is established and the patient can make the correct articulatory movements. Stimulability probes therefore are important in determining the patient's prognosis for change. Articulation errors may also be related to an existing or prior hearing loss.

In addition to providing an inventory of the patient's sound productions, articulation testing can indicate the adequacy of velopharyngeal closure (Shelton, Brooks, and Youngstrom 1965). As we have said, certain sounds have a higher probability for error than others. The SLP should obtain a thorough sample of these sounds in articulation testing. Since articulation involves dynamic and overlapping movements, the clinician should be certain to get samples of the patient producing isolated sounds, syllables, words, and connected speech. In certain cases of assimilation nasality, it is necessary to evaluate specific phonetic contexts containing nasal and nonnasal sounds to determine if the patient can make the rapid velopharyngeal alterations. There are several formal test instruments that have been traditionally associated with cleft palate articulatory assessment. These were described in Table 12.1. The context-controlled stimuli mentioned earlier in this chapter would be useful for the clinician, as well.

In summary, the clinician analyzes speech samples, elicited productions and phonetic inventories for overall intelligibility and analysis of patterns, keeping in mind the main goal: To distinguish speech errors that may be due to faulty velopharyngeal or other structural deviations from speech errors that are compensatory or developmental. Trost-Cardamone and Bernthal (1993) provide a chart of guidelines for deciding on a direction for intervention based on these analyses.

Nasal Resonance

Resonatory voice disorders are frequently heard in individuals with clefts. The assessment process described earlier in this chapter, then, certainly applies to the diagnostic workup of a patient with a cleft palate. Any quality aberration is possible in persons with clefts of the palate but high probability disorders are hypernasality and nasal emission since both are related to inadequate velopharyngeal closure. It is worth mentioning that the clinician should attempt to determine to what extent the resonance imbalance is related to functional factors such as tension, fatigue, and learning or to organic factors such as neurological dysfunction or the structural defect of the cleft itself. We would like to restate that listener evaluation of a speaking voice is the best way for the clinician to judge the resonance parameter.

The Oral Peripheral Examination

Although velopharyngeal closure cannot be visualized in an oral examination, it is important to examine the orofacial region of patients who manifest resonation disorders. The examination is an initial step in determining the general relationships among all structures in the vocal tract. For instance, the clinician can get a gross picture of palatal shape, total and effective velar lengths, movement ability and symmetry of movement of the velum, and dimensions of the pharynx and can determine if any defects, such as fistulas of the palate, are present. If the SLP has any concerns regarding structure or function, the physician should be consulted.

Procedures for appraising the structure and function of the oral and peripheral regions are described in the literature (Bloch 1979; Dworkin and Culatta, 1980; Mason 1969; Mason and Grandstaff 1971; Mason and Simon 1977; Rampp, Pannbacker, and Kinnebrew 1984; St. Louis and Ruscello 1981). General information on conducting an oral peripheral examination is provided in Chapter 9. We offer a few special comments here.

Perhaps the most important thing for the SLP to do when VPI is suspected is to determine the effective length of the velum and the location of the velar dimple (Mason 1969; Mason and Grandstaff 1971). The effective velar length is that portion of the elevated velar tissue used in closure of the nasopharynx during phonation. The effected length can be estimated from intraoral inspection of the velar dimple during phonation relative to nasopharyngeal depth. The velar dimple on the oral surface of the velum is an indication of the point of maximum elevation on the nasal surface of the velum. It typically occurs at 80 percent of the total velar length. The more anteriorly the dimple is placed (say, at the 50 percent mark), the less the effective velar length, and the greater the degree of velopharyngeal incompetence.

Examination of the palate may reveal oronasal fistulas that are not always readily visible. What is the shape of the palatal vault? Is the coloration a healthy pink, or do there appear to be white or blue tinted regions? Is there a palatal translucency observed during the oral exam when, in a dark room, a flashlight is shined into a nostril? Upon palpation, does the bony substructure feel firm and have normal posterior edges? If there is a fistula, the degree to which it affects articulation or resonance may be determined by occluding the area with dental wax or chewing gum (Bloch 1979; Colburn 1982).

When overt clefting is present, the type and extent can be appraised. Many hospital-based craniofacial teams have devised specialized oral examination forms that contain diagrams of the lips and palate on which to mark the patient's features. Although many classification systems are still in use today (such as those proposed by Veau 1931; Davis and Ritchie 1922; Kernahan and Stark 1958; and the American Cleft Palate Association as reported by Harkins et al. 1962), the use of an individualized diagram not only documents the extent of the cleft but also facilitates communication among the team professionals.

Special Assessment Procedures for Velopharyngeal Function

As previously indicated, the oral peripheral examination does not allow for definitive judgments of velopharyngeal adequacy to be made. In addition, an articulation test, whether published or informal, is but an indirect measure of the client's velopharyngeal function (Shelton, Brooks, and Youngstrom 1965). Other techniques, many involving instrumentation, are available to directly or indirectly assess the velopharyngeal mechanism. We maintain that no single measure is adequate for appraisal of velopharyngeal function; and we also believe that articulation testing and resonance assessment *must* be part of any diagnostic process. Let us describe some of the other assessment procedures that are available for routine and/or sophisticated diagnostic sessions.

Fox and Johns (1970) describe a technique for measuring static closure whereby the patient is required to maintain intraoral pressure by puffing up the cheeks. If this procedure is accomplished, the patient is asked to protrude the tongue and then puff up the cheeks (to prevent lingual valving). The clinician holds the patient's nostrils while this exercise is done to aid in impounding pressure. If no air escapes when the nostrils are released, it is assumed that velopharyngeal closure is adequate.

As previously mentioned, informal and subjective measures of velopharyngeal leakage can be obtained by observing fog on a mirror held beneath the patient's nose, by seeing wisps of cotton move when so placed, by using listening tubes of various design, and by critically listening to controlled stimuli spoken in nose-occluded–unoccluded conditions.

The oral manometer is an affordable piece of equipment helpful in discriminating between persons with good and poor velopharyngeal closure. Procedures for use of the manometer and advantages of using an open bleed valve have been described elsewhere (Hardy 1965; Morris 1966; Shelton, Hahn, and Morris 1968). The patient either blows or sucks as forcefully as possible into/from a mouthpiece. The exhalation task yields a positive pressure reading from the manometer guages, while the inhalation task gives a negative reading. A ratio is obtained by comparing pressures achieved in the nostrils-open and nostrils-occluded conditions. A normal ratio of 1.00 is suggestive of velopharyngeal closure adequacy, particularly if an open bleed valve was used to inhibit compensatory maneuvers, such as tongue-palate valving. Ratios less than 1.00 may be indicative of VPI, hypernasal speech and reduced intelligibility in cleft palate patients; ratios less than 0.89 are particularly poor indicators (Subtelny and Subtelny, 1959; Van Demark 1966).

Air pressure and air flow techniques are based on the fact that VPI results in a decrement of intraoral air pressure and an increase in air flow through the nose. Consequently, pressure and flow measurements can be part of the total diagnostic workup; they are often used for research purposes. Pressure transducers, such as strain gauge transducers, are used to measure air pressures while air flow meters are used to measure volume rates of air flow. Types of flow meters include warm-wire anemometers, pneumotachographs, and thermistors. The pneumotachograph is perhaps the most commonly used and requires the use of a face mask to collect the air flow and direct it through a sensing screen (Rampp, Pannbacker, and Kinnebrew 1984). Air pressure and flow instrumentation is expensive and complex. McWilliams and Philips (1979) discuss the disadvantages of pressure-flow instrumentation and the limited information it actually provides about the velopharyngeal gap.

Warren (1979) designed an instrument called PERCI, which provides an oral and nasal air pressure ratio during the production of pressure (stop) consonants. A low oral/nasal pressure ratio is said to be indicative of velopharyngeal incompetence.

Fletcher (1970, 1976) developed the TONAR instrument, which measures the oral and nasal sound pressures. A ratio formed between the two measures, expressed as a percentage, is referred to as *nasalence*. Fletcher claims that nasalence is highly correlated with perceptual judgments of nasality. Normal oral/nasal ratios are said to be less than 10 percent, whereas patients with severe hypernasality have ratios in excess of 80 percent. TONAR is no longer available commercially, but Kay Elemetrics markets the Nasometer, a computer-based system that uses the TONAR method for clinical assessments. Peterson-Falzone (1994) suggests that use of a Nasometer is quite feasible with young children.

The Zemlin Index of Palatopharyngeal Opening, or ZIPPO, attempts to determine air flow leakage through the velopharyngeal port by measuring "vocal tract damping time" (Zemlin and Fant 1972). Disadvantages of this instrumentation have been discussed by Keuhn (1982); its usefulness in the evaluation of VPI has yet to be determined.

Referral for direct visualization of the velopharyngeal closure mechanism is, perhaps, in order when articulation and nasal resonance have been determined to be abnormal. Direct visualization involves radiographic, ultrasonic, and/or endoscopic methods. Let us say a brief word about each. The interested reader is referred to Moon (1993) for a discussion of imaging techniques.

Radiographic methods involve low doses of radiation to visualize the structures, including soft tissues. The SLP should work closely with the radiologist in selecting the most appropriate radiographic method and conditions of study. Knowledge of the literature is important in selecting which speech and nonspeech tasks to have the patient perform (Shelton, Hahn, and Morris 1968). Radiographic methods used in the assessment of velopharyngeal function were listed as part of Table 12.2. Several discussions of these methods are available in the literature (Bzoch 1970; Pigott 1980; Rampp, Pannbacker, and Kinnebrew 1984; Spriestersbach et al. 1973).

Ultrasound offers a noninvasive means of visualizing lateral pharyngeal wall movement during speech. This technique has been described by Kuehn (1982) and involves placing an ultrasonic transducer against the neck. Soft tissues and air in the pharyngeal cavities transmit the pulse differently, thus creating an image on the display screen. A number of difficulties exist in using ultrasound to study velopharyngeal function; these difficulties may be resolved in future research.

Direct visualization is easily accomplished through an invasive technique that uses viewing devices called endoscopes. Rigid forms of endoscopy useful in observing velopharyngeal closure are the oral panendoscope and the nasal endoscope. Flexible endoscopes use fiber-optic bundles. We again remind the reader that closure, or lack of it, is best viewed from above, and so the flexible fiberscope inserted through the nasal cavity is used quite often. Most, if not all, hospitals now have the necessary equipment. Cooperative patients can be examined while seated and performing speech and nonspeech tasks. Reviews of endoscopy can be found in the works of Karnell et al. (1983) and Osberg and Witzel (1981).

Other instrumental methods are available for research and clinician use. These include the use of accelerometers, or contact microphones, to measure the amplitude of nasal vibrations as an index of nasality in the patient's speech, electromyography to study muscle activity in velopharyngeal movement gestures, and photodetector assessment of velopharyngeal activity (Dalston 1982). Rampp, Pannbacker, and Kinnebrew (1984) provide a review of these methods, which are used primarily in the research arena.

The SLP may or may not have access to some of the instruments but should know that they are available. In this age of high technology it can be expected that access to such equipment from universities, medical centers, and clinics will become easier and more widespread.

Auditory Acuity and Language Ability

The high incidence of auditory acuity problems among children with cleft palate has been well documented (Heller 1979; Prather and Kos 1968). For this reason, it is absolutely essential that every patient have a hearing examination. These examinations should include both air and bone conduction testing and should be a part of every speech diagnosis.

The SLP will wish to see the child or infant as soon as possible. Typically, in major hospitals, once an infant is born with an orofacial anomaly, the work of a multidisciplinary team is set into motion. The SLP, as part of the team, will work closely with the parents—through counseling and training—to prevent future communication problems. During this early contact the parents can be informed about the need for normal speech and language stimulation, what to expect from their child regarding speech and language production, and the need for frequent audiometric testing. Some speech clinicians use established language stimulation programs as a preventative measure with these children.

Several researchers have documented the existence of a language deficit among children with cleft palate (Morris 1962; Nation 1970; Smith and McWilliams 1968). Likewise, those children who received proper stimulation in the early years often do not have language problems that persist into the school years. To be sure, then, the clinician should examine the child's language abilities and pay particular attention to expressive skills. The procedures discussed in Chapters 4 and 5 should be sufficient for this evaluation.

Prognosis Associated with Resonance Imbalance

Let us now return to our general discussion of resonance imbalance and list some of the prognostic indicators for the treatment of resonatory disorders. We freely admit that much is speculation or opinion or is simply based on assumptions of etiology. Research documenting clinical effectiveness is sorely needed.

1. Prater and Swift (1984) state that voice treatment for cul-de-sac resonance usually is not successful in patients with neurologic involvement of the articulators, which includes conditions such as oral apraxia, athetoid cerebral palsy, flaccid dysarthria, and spastic dysarthria. Patients with functional cul-de-sac resonance and, to a lesser extent, deaf speakers can benefit from intervention directed toward anterior positioning of the tongue.

2. Thin resonance, with its assumed functional etiology, is remediated easily only in patients motivated to change. Treatment efforts should be directed toward correcting tongue carriage. The clinician may benefit from knowledge of male-female communication differences when assisting a patient to reduce the effeminate aspects of speech. The emerging literature on communication treatment for transsexuals may be used as a resource, but appied in reverse for treating thin resonance. The works of Kline (1983) and Pryor and Scott (1983) can be consulted in this regard.

3. Hyponasality, when due to some nasal obstruction, necessiates physical management. Speech treatment alone is not likely to be beneficial.

4. The patient's motivation to change is paramount in predicting the outcome of voice treatment.

5. A favorable prognosis for treatment is indicated if the clinician was able to elicit a better voice from the patient during stimulability trials.

Pannbacker (1976) and Rampp, Pannbacker, and Kinnebrew (1984) reviewed the literature on indications and contraindications to speech treatment for individuals with cleft palate and concluded there is much misunderstanding and a paucity of research evidence supporting its effectiveness. We will cite some of the treatment indicators here. Much of what is listed applies to cases of hypernasality and nasal emission in the absence of clefting.

1. Speech treatment is contraindicated for patients with clearly inadequate velopharyngeal closure; physical management is warranted (Pannbacker 1976). As discussed in this chapter, evidence of velopharyngeal inadequacy should come from a variety of sources, including articulation testing showing consistent hypernasality and nasal emission, observation of nasal grimacing, radiographic evidence, and oral examination findings of an anteriorly displaced velar dimple and/or excessive nasopharyngeal dimensions.

2. Since home programs are essential in most therapeutic approaches, motivated and cooperative patients and their parents are a requirement for enrollment in a speech intervention program (Shprintzen, McCall, and Skolnick 1975).

3. Speech treatment is not warranted, or is low priority, when the patient needs language and communication improvement. Shelton, Hahn, and Morris (1968) stress the primacy of language treatment.

4. Pannbacker (1976) maintains that patients with boderline velopharyngeal closure "should not be subjected to the stress of speech therapy because of the chance that they may compensate laryngeally" (43). Speech treatment, then, is contraindicated if the patient presents with hoarseness. According to McWilliams, Bluestone, and Musgrave (1969),

> *Vocal cord nodules appear to be a danger signal and provide evidence that things are not quite as they should be higher in the tract; consideration should be given to secondary procedures designed to correct the velopharyngeal inadequacy which would appear to be related to the onset of vocal cord problems.* (2076)

5. Patients who demonstrated improvement during the assessment probes are good candidates for speech treatment. Especially favorable are reduced hypernasality when employing exaggerated, open-mouth articulation and a marked difference in velar activity when gagging and phonating (Mason and Grandstaff 1971).

6. Some patients with inadequate velopharyngeal closure cannot benefit from further physical management. The SLP may opt to provide compensatory treatment. The goal, then, is not normal-sounding speech, but the best speech of which the patient is capable. Tasks used in the assessment probes may be appropriate treatment techniques in that the perception of hypernasality is reduced by their use. These tasks include increased mouth opening, low and forward placement of the tongue, auditory training, exaggerated articulation movements, light and quick articulatory contacts, overall slowed rate of speech, and altered pitch and/or loudness levels.

Conclusion

The evaluation of disorders of resonance is a challenge to the SLP. The clinician must often work closely with medical personnel and other allied health workers, which necessitates knowing procedures and terminologies that are peripheral to speech-language pathology. The clinician also must remain abreast of current technological developments in electronics, surgery, and medical technology. Finally, the clinician must keep interpersonal clinical skills finely honed so that psychological aspects of vocal disorders can be detected and dealt with through treatment or referral.

Bibliography

Bloch, P. J. (1979). "Clinical Evaluation for the Cleft Palate Team Setting." In *Communicative Disorders Related to Cleft Lip and Palate*, ed. K. R. Bzoch (Boston, MA: Little, Brown).

Bloomer, H. H., and Wolski, W. (1968). "Office Examination of Palatopharyngeal Function." *Clinical Pediatrics* 7:611–618.

Boone, D. R., and McFarlane, S. (1988). *The Voice and Voice Therapy*. 3rd ed. Englewood Cliffs, NJ: Prentice Hall.

Bzoch, K. (1970). "Assessment: Radiographic Techniques." *ASHA Reports* 5:248–270.

Bzoch, K. (1979). *Communicative Disorders Related to Cleft Lip and Palate*. Boston, MA: Little, Brown and Company.

Bzoch, K. R., Kemker, F. J., and Wood, V. L. D. (1984). "The Prevention of Communicative Disorders in Cleft Palate Infants." In *Speech and Language: Advances in Basic Research and Practice*, ed. N. J. Lass (San Diego, CA: Academic Press).

Colburn, N. (1982). "Nonstrumental Assessment of Velopharyngeal Adequacy in Children." *Seminars in Speech, Language, Hearing* 3:212–221.

Dalston, R. (1982). "Photodector Assessment of Velopharyngeal Activity." *Cleft Palate Journal* 19:1–8.

Darley, F. (1978). "The Case History." In *Diagnostic Methods in Speech Pathology*, ed. F. Darley and D. Spriestersbach (New York, NY: Harper and Row).

Davis, J. S., and Ritchie, H. P. (1922). "Classification of Congenital Clefts of Lip and Palate." *Journal of American Medical Association* 2:1323.

Dworkin, J., and Culatta, R. (1980). *Dworkin-Culatta Oral Mechanism Examination*. Nicholasville, KY: Edgewood Press.

Fletcher, S. (1970). "Theory and Instrumentation for Quantitative Measurement of Nasality." *Journal of Speech and Hearing Disorders* 37:329–346.

Fletcher, S. (1976). "Nasalence vs. Listener Judgments of Nasality." *Cleft Palate Journal* 13:31–44.

Fletcher, S. (1978). *Diagnosing Speech Disorders from Cleft Palate*. New York: Grune and Stratton.

Fox, D., and Johns, D. (1970). "Predicting Velopharyngeal Closure with a Modified Tongue-Anchor Technique." *Journal of Speech and Hearing Disorders* 35:248–251.

Hardy, J. (1965). "Airflow and air pressure studies." *ASHA Reports* 1:141–152.

Harkins, C. S., Berlin, A., Harding, R., Longacre, J., and Snodgrasse, R. (1962). "A Classification of Cleft Lip and Cleft Palate." *Journal of Plastic and Reconstructive Surgery* 29:31.

Heller, J. (1979). "Hearing Loss in Patients with Cleft Palate." In *Communicative Disorders Related to Cleft Lip and Palate*, ed. K. R. Bzoch (Boston, MA: Little, Brown).

Hess, D. A. (1959). "Pitch, Intensity and Cleft Palate Voice Quality." *Journal of Speech and Hearing Research* 2:113–125.

Hess, D. A. (1971). "Effects of Certain Variables on Speech of Cleft Palate Persons." *Cleft Palate Journal* 8:387–398.

Hess, D. A. (1976). "A New Experimental Approach to Assessment of Velopharyngeal Adequacy: Nasal Manometric Bleed Testing."

Journal of Speech and Hearing Disorders 41: 427–443.

Jacobs, R. J., Philips, B. J., and Harrison, R. J. (1970). "A Stimulability Test for Cleft Palate Children." *Journal of Speech and Hearing Disorders* 35:354–360.

Karnell, M., Ibuki, K., Morris, H., and Van Demark, D. (1983). "Reliability of the Nasopharyngeal Fiberscope (NPF) for Assessing Velopharyngeal Function: Analysis by Judgment." *Cleft Palate Journal* 20:200–208.

Kernahan, D. A., and Stark, M. D. (1958). "A New Classification for Cleft Lip and Cleft Palate." *Journal of Plastic and Reconstructive Surgery* 22:435–441.

Kline, P. (1983). "Sex Differences in Communication: A Therapy Framework for the Male to Female Transsexual Client." Paper presented at the annual convention of the American Speech-Language-Hearing Association, Cincinnati, OH.

Kuehn, D. (1982). "Assessment of Resonance Disorders." In *Speech, Language and Hearing*, Vol. 11, *Pathologies of Speech and Language*, ed. N. Lass, L. McReynolds, J. Northern, and D. Yoder (Philadelphia, PA: W. B. Saunders).

Lintz, L. B., and Sherman, D. (1961). "Phonetic Elements and Perception of Nasality." *Journal of Speech and Hearing Research* 4:381–396.

Lippmann, R. P. (1981). "Detecting Nasalization Using a Low-Cost Miniature Accelerometer." *Journal of Speech and Hearing Research* 24: 314–317.

McCabe, R., and Bradley D. (1973). "Pre- and Post-Articulation Therapy Assessment." *Language, Speech, and Hearing Services in Schools* 4:13–32.

McDonald, E. T., and Koepp-Baker, H. (1951). "Cleft Palate Speech: An Integration of Research and Clinical Observation." *Journal of Speech and Hearing Disorders* 16:9–19.

McWilliams, B. J., Bluestone, C. D., and Musgrave, R. D. (1969). "Diagnostic Implication of Vocal Cord Nodules in Children with Cleft Palate." *Laryngoscope* 79:2072–2080.

McWilliams, B. J., and Philips, B. (1979). *Velopharyngeal Incompetence: Audio Seminars in Speech Pathology*. Philadelphia, PA: W. B. Saunders.

Mason, R. (1969). "Improving the Efficiency of the Intra-Oral Examination." *Journal of the Tennessee Speech and Hearing Association* 14:4–10.

Mason, R., and Simon, C. (1977). "An Orofacial Examination Checklist." *Language, Speech, and Hearing Services in Schools* 8:155–163.

Mason, R. M., and Grandstaff, H. L. (1971). "Evaluating the Velopharyngeal Mechanism in Hypernasal Speakers." *Language, Speech, and Hearing Services in Schools* 2:53–61.

Mason, R. M., and Riski, J. E. (1982). "The Team Approach in Orofacial Management." *Annals of Plastic Surgery* 8:71–78.

Minifie, F. D. (1973). "Speech Acoustics." In *Normal Aspects of Speech, Hearing, and Language*, ed. F. D. Minifie, T. J. Hixon, and F. Williams (Englewood Cliffs, NJ: Prentice Hall).

Moll, K. (1968). "Speech Characteristics of Individuals with Cleft Lip and Palate." In *Cleft Palate and Communication*, ed. D. Spriestersbach and D. Sherman (New York: Academic Press).

Moll, K. L. (1964). "Objective Measures of Nasality." *Cleft Palate Journal* 1:371–374.

Moon, J. B. (1993). "Evaluation of Velopharyngeal Function." In *Cleft Palate: Interdisciplinary Issues and Treatment*, ed. K. T. Moller and C. D. Starr (Austin, TX: Pro-Ed).

Morris, H. (1962). "Communication Skills of Children with Cleft Lips and Palates." *Journal of Speech and Hearing Research* 5:79–90.

Morris, H. (1966). "The Oral Manometer as a Diagnostic Tool in Clinical Speech Pathology." *Journal of Speech and Hearing Disorders* 31:362–369.

Morris, H. (1979). "Evaluation of Abnormal Articulation Patterns." In *Communicative Disorders Related to Cleft Lip and Palate*, ed. K. Bzoch (Boston, MA: Little, Brown).

Morris, H. L., and Smith, J. K. (1962). "A Multiple Approach for Evaluating Velopharyngeal Competency." *Journal of Speech and Hearing Disorders* 27:218–226.

Nation, J. (1970). "Vocabulary Comprehension and Usage in Preschool Cleft Palate and Normal Children." *Cleft Palate Journal* 7:639–644.

Osberg, P., and Witzel, M. A. (1981). "The Physiologic Basis for Hypernasality during Connected Speech in Cleft Palate Patients: A Nasoendoscopic Study." *Plastic and Reconstructive Surgery* 67, no. 1:1–5.

Pannbacker, M. (1976). "Indications and Contraindications for Speech Therapy in Cleft

Palate." *Journal of National Student Speech and Hearing Association* (December 4): 40–47.

Peterson, H., and Marquardt, T. (1981). *Appraisal and Diagnosis of Speech and Language Disorders.* Englewood Cliffs, NJ: Prentice Hall.

Peterson, S. (1975). "Nasal Emission as a Component of the Misarticulation of Sibilants and Affricates." *Journal of Speech and Hearing Disorders* 40:106–114.

Peterson-Falzone, S. (1982). "Resonance Disorders in Structural Defects." In *Speech, Language and Hearing* Vol. 2, *Pathologies of Speech and Language,* ed. N. Lass, L. McReynolds, J. Northern, and D. Yoder (Philadelphia, PA: W. B. Saunders).

Peterson-Falzone, S. (1994). "Cleft Palate." In *Diagnosis in Speech-Language Pathology,* ed. J. B. Tomblin, H. L. Morris, and D. C. Spriestersbach (San Diego, CA: Singular Publishing).

Pigott, R. W. (1980). "Assessment of Velopharyngeal Function." In *Advances in the Management of Cleft Palate,* ed. M. Edwards and A. Watson (New York: Churchill Livingstone).

Pindzola, R. H. (1987). *A Voice Assessment Protocol for Children and Adults.* Austin, TX: Pro-Ed.

Prather, R. J., and Swift, R. W. (1984). *Manual of Voice Therapy.* Boston, MA: Little, Brown.

Prather, W., and Kos, C. (1968). "Audiological and Otological Considerations." In *Cleft Palate and Communication,* ed. D. Spriestersbach and D. Sherman (New York: Academic Press).

Pryor, A. P., and Scott, C. S. (1983). "*Communication Therapy for the Male Transsexual.*" Paper presented at the annual convention of the American Speech-Language-Hearing Association, Cincinnati, OH.

Rampp, D., and Counihan, D. (1970). "Vocal Pitch-Intensity Relationships in Cleft Palate Speakers." *Cleft Palate Journal* 7:846–857.

Rampp, D. L., Pannbacker, M., and Kinnebrew, M. C. (1984). *VPI Velopharyngeal Incompetency: A Practical Guide for Evaluation and Management.* Austin, TX: Pro-Ed.

Randall, P., Whitaker, L. A., Noone, R. B., and Jones, W. D. (1978). "The Case for the Inferiorly Based Posterior Pharyngeal Flap." *Cleft Palate Journal* 15:262–265.

St. Louis, K., and Ruscello, D. (1981). *The Oral Speech Mechanism Examination.* Baltimore, MD: University Park Press.

Saunders, L. (1972). *Procedure Guides for Evaluation of Speech and Language Disorders in Children.* Danville, IL: Interstate.

Shelton, R. L., Brooks, A. R., and Youngstrom, K. A. (1965). "Clinical Assessment of Palatopharyngeal Closure." *Journal of Speech and Hearing Disorders* 30:37–43.

Shelton, R. L., Hahn, E., and Morris, H. L. (1968). "Diagnosis and Therapy." In *Cleft Palate and Communication,* ed. D. C. Spriestersbach and D. Sherman (New York: Academic Press).

Sherman, D. (1954). "The Merits of Backward Playing of Connected Speech in the Scaling of Voice Quality Disorders." *Journal of Speech and Hearing Disorders* 19:312–321.

Shprintzen, R. J., McCall, G. N., and Skolnick, M. L. (1975). "A New Therapeutic Technique for the Treatment of Velopharyngeal Incompetence." *Journal of Speech and Hearing Disorders* 40:69–83.

Shupe, L. K. (1968). "Speech Intelligibility Measures of Cleft Palate Speakers before and after Pharyngeal Flap Surgery." Unpublished doctoral dissertation, State University of New York at Buffalo.

Smith, R., and McWilliams, B. (1968). "Psycholinguistic Abilities of Children with Clefts." *Cleft Palate Journal* 5:238–249.

Spriestersbach, D. (1955). "Assessing Nasal Quality in Cleft Palate Speech of Children." *Journal of Speech and Hearing Disorders* 20:266–270.

Spriestersbach, D., Dickson, D., Fraser, F., Horowitz, S., McWilliams, B., Paradise, J., and Randall, P. (1973). "Clinical Research in Cleft Lip and Cleft Palate: The State of the Art." *Cleft Palate Journal* 10:113–163.

Subtelny, J., and Subtelny, F. (1959). "Intelligibility and Associated Factors of Cleft Palate Speech." *Journal of Speech and Hearing Research* 2:353–360.

Subtelny, J., Van Hattum, R., and Myers, B. (1972). "Ratings and Measures of Cleft Palate Speech." *Cleft Palate Journal* 8:18–27.

Templin, M., and Darley, F. (1969). *The Templin-Darley Tests of Articulation.* 2nd ed. Iowa City: University of Iowa Bureau of Educational Research and Service.

Trost, J. E. (1981). "Articulatory Additions to the Classical Description of the Speech of Persons with Cleft Palate." *Cleft Palate Journal* 18: 193–203.

Trost-Cardamone, J. E. (1987) *Cleft Palate Misarticulations: A Teaching Tape*. Northridge: Instructional Media Center, California State University.

Trost-Cardamone, J. E., and Bernthal, J. E. (1993). "Articulation Assessment Procedures and Treatment Decisions." In *Cleft Palate: Interdisciplinary Issues and Treatments*, ed. K. T. Moller and C. D. Starr (Austin, TX: Pro-Ed).

Vanderas, A. P. (1987). "Incidence of Cleft Lip, Cleft Palate, and Cleft Lip and Palate Among Races: A Review." *Cleft Palate Journal* 24: 216–225.

Van Demark, D. (1964). "Misarticulations and Listener Judgments of the Speech of Individuals with Cleft Palates." *Cleft Palate Journal* 1: 232–245.

Van Demark, D. (1966). "A Factor Analysis of the Speech of Children with Cleft Palate." *Cleft Palate Journal* 3:159–170.

Van Demark, D. (1971). "Clinical Research Methodology in Evaluating the Therapeutic Process." *Cleft Palate Journal* 8:26–35.

Van Demark, D. (1974). "Assessment of Velopharyngeal Competency for Children with Cleft Palate." *Cleft Palate Journal* 11:310–316.

Van Demark, D. R., and Swickard, S. L. (1980). "A Pre-School Articulation Test to Assess Velopharyngeal Competency: Normative Data." *Cleft Palate Journal* 17:175–181.

Veau, V. (1931). *Division Palatine*. Paris: Masson et Cie.

Warren, D. W. (1979). "PERCI: A Method for Rating Palatal Efficiency." *Cleft Palate Journal* 16:279–285.

Weiss, C. (1974). "The Speech Pathologist's Role in Dealing with Obturator-Wearing School Children." *Journal of Speech and Hearing Disorders* 39:153–162.

Wells, C. (1971). *Cleft Palate and Its Associated Speech Disorders*. New York: McGraw-Hill.

Westlake, H. (1968). "Speech Learning in Cleft Palate Children." In *Cleft Palate Habilitation*, ed. R. Lencione (Syracuse, NY: Syracuse University Press).

Wilson, D. K. (1987). *Voice Problems in Children*. 3rd ed. Baltimore, MD: Williams and Wilkins.

Wilson, F., and Rice, M. (1977). *A Programmed Approach to Voice Therapy*. Austin, TX: Learning Concepts.

Zemlin, W., and Fant, G. (1972). "The Effect of a Velopharyngeal Shunt upon Vocal Tract Damping Times: An Analogue Study." *Speech Transmission Laboratory Quarterly Report* 4:6–10.

Chapter 13

The Diagnostic Report

Only one very important phase of the evaluation remains to be considered: the preparation of the diagnostic report. Put the clinical situation, the interview, testing methods, results, and impressions in writing as soon as possible. Never trust a memory. Commit it to paper while the facial characteristics and voice inflections can still be remembered. Make the report "alive" so that others can experience what occurred just by reading about it. The raw data are of limited value to the clinician or other workers until they are assembled in a clear, precise, and orderly fashion.

A *diagnostic report* is a written record that summarizes the relevant information a clinician obtained—and how he/she obtained it—in his/her professional interaction with a client. It serves the following functions: (1) It acts as a guide for further services to the client—providing a clear statement of how the person was functioning at a given point in time, so that the clinician can document change or lack of change. (2) It communicates the clinician's findings to other professional workers; it provides answers to a number of clinical questions, including: Does the person have a problem? Will treatment be helpful? Will referrals be necessary? (3) It serves as a document for research purposes.

The importance of the first function should be obvious: Intelligent clinical plans evolve naturally from carefully prepared reports. The second purpose of diagnostic reports is to answer questions about clients so that other professionals can plan and provide appropriate services. In addition to transmitting necessary information, a carefully prepared examination report will also tend to establish the credibility of the SLP in the eyes of other workers. To state it another way, a written document is an extension of the diagnostician, and even minor errors in spelling or grammar may cast doubt upon the accuracy and attention to detail with respect to substantive material. Although the clinician may be highly skilled in testing and interviewing, competence may be evaluated by the clinician's written communications. Clinical reports are the principal way in which a clinician relates to other professionals.

Format

There are several ways to organize a diagnostic report (Darley and Spriestersbach 1978; Flower 1984; Hollis and Dunn 1979; Hutchinson, Hanson, and Mecham 1979; Knepflar 1976; Middleton et al. 1992; Peterson and Marquardt 1990). Because reports may vary, depending on the intended reader, no single schema is appropriate for all circumstances; in many instances, the format will be dictated by the agency the clinician serves. We will provide two examples: formats for reports in medical settings and in the public schools.

Clinicians in a medical setting may record their findings in a "problem-oriented" format (Kent and Chabon 1980). Problem-oriented medical records (POMR) feature a carefully defined and "documented list of problems which encompass all the significant difficulties a patient is experiencing" (Enelow and Swisher 1972, 69). The list includes the presenting complaint as well as those problems identified by the members of the treatment team. For example, a patient who suffered a CVA might have right hemiparesis and aphasia leading to problems with daily activities (e.g., feeding, dressing), locomotion, language, intelligibility, and the like. Ideally placed at the front of the patient's file, this list of problems generated by the multidisciplinary team points to areas needing further assessment and/or intervention. All available information about the person is then organized under the four headings shown in Figure 13.1 (Bouchard and Shane 1977). The four headings of information form the acronym SOAP. Daily chart documentations, as well as diagnostic reports, can be written by using the SOAP format. Progress notes need to be concise. The SOAP format is an excellent tool for guiding the clinician toward brevity while ensuring that key information on the day's session is recorded. All that is necessary is a brief statement on the patient's level of cooperation, motivation, or frustration (subjective), a citation of what tasks were attempted and at what levels of stimulation or cueing (objectives), levels of accuracy to which tasks were performed (assessments), and logical next steps in the rehabilitation program (plan).

In recent years, there has been a growing trend in the health care industry toward the use of "functional outcome measures," in which the patient's behaviors are assessed categorically relative to levels of function. The Functional Communication Measures, a component of ASHA's Program Evaluation System, have a broad range of clinical applicability. A format for using the Functional Communication Measures in diagnostic reporting and treatment planning in speech-language pathology has been developed (Tonkovich 1989).

FIGURE 13.1   The SOAP Format for Medical Reports

Subjective	Objective	Assessment	Plan
Interview and case history	Test results	Collation of subjective and objective information	Additional testing Treatment options

Another example is the Functional Independence Measure (FIM) (Research Foundation 1990). The FIM rates patient dependence-independence on a seven-level scale; the ratings are made by a multidisciplinary team on various categories, such as communication, social cognition, locomotion, self-care, and the like. Some facilities have used FIM levels to aid in patient selection and discharge decisions, as well as to track progress over time. The brevity of the FIM has led some agencies to more in-depth descriptors, such as a Pathways record.

A Pathway format typically organizes patient information in columns representing phases or changes over time. Phase 1 entries critique the patient's status at the time of admission, often using FIM levels (1–7 ratings). A stroke Pathway might include items in medical/nursing, nutrition, swallowing, mobility, self-care, cognition, communication, and others completed by the team. Pathways tracking also includes discharge planning and community reentry skills. Detailed Pathways can be appended by specific health care professionals for each area, as would be the case for a communication assessment by an SLP.

In addition, we would like to mention that technology has finally come to the aid of busy clinicians who are often inundated by clinical documentation. A large vocabulary voice recognition system with software specifically developed for generating diagnostic reports, treatment plans, progress notes, and discharge reports has been developed and field-tested at a large hospital (Tonkovich et al. 1990). This system allows clinicians to generate printed reports by speaking aloud a set of words normally used in dictation. This practical application of voice recognition offers an attractive and cost-effective alternative to traditional reporting methods.

Public school clinicians use specialized report formats with components mandated by law (i.e., PL 94-142 and PL 99-457). Following the evaluation of a communicatively impaired student, the SLP prepares a diagnostic report, usually in the generic format described in this chapter. The clinician then condenses the diagnostic findings and suggested areas of intervention into a record called an Individualized Education Program (IEP). The IEP is a student-focused plan devised by a team—teachers, school administrators, special educators (including the SLP), and others, particularly the parents. The plan is a composite of findings and recommendations from all team members to ensure appropriate, integrated services for the total child. The plan is spelled out in response to very specific questions:

1. *What* is the problem(s)?
2. *Where* is the student now?
3. *Who* will do *what* with the student and *how often?*
4. *When* and *how* will progress be measured?

The IEP is a working document; the IEP team—including the parents—can make alterations or eliminate goals, as appropriate. Figure 13.2 displays a portion of an IEP prepared for a child with a phonological disorder.

The SLP in the schools is also responsible for writing the Individualized Family Service Plan (IFSP). The assessment of infants and toddlers (birth to three) presents special considerations in terms of record keeping and evaluation procedures.

FIGURE 13.2 Individualized Educational Program

Student: <u>David Grabowski</u>   Birthdate: <u>1/7/78</u>   Address: <u>224 Orchard</u>

Parents: <u>Gerard and Julie</u>   District/School: <u>Beaver Grove Schools</u>

Grade: <u>First</u>   District of residency: <u>Marquette County</u>

IEP conference date: <u>9/12/83</u>   Projected IEP review date: <u>9/10/84</u>

Eligibility Statement: (What decision/description requires this service?)

David has difficulty with frictional manner of articulation production resulting in several substitutional errors: th/s, th/z, s/sh, ts/ch, dz/dj.

Current Eductional Level: (Where is child currently functioning?)

David is enrolled in a developmental first-grade classroom.

Special Services		
Goals	Objectives	Service description
1. David will produce *s, z* correctly at the word and sentence level. 2. David will produce *sh* correctly at the word and sentence level. 3. Progress reports will be sent to parents and teacher twice a year.	1. David will discriminate target sounds from other sounds with 90% accuracy. 2. David will produce target sounds at the beginning, middle, and end of single words with 90% accuracy. 3. David will correctly produce target sounds within sentences with 80% success.	Speech therapy

Dates of Services		Time in Programs	Reponsible Individuals
Start	End	Daily	
9/19/83	6/1/84	Within small-group 20-minute sessions 2 times a week	Speech-language clinician

Evaluation Plan: (How is it planned to ascertain that goals have been reached?)

1. Goldman-Fristoe Test of Articulation
2. Pre- and post-therapy word list containing target sounds
3. Five-minute sample of spontaneous speech

IEP Committee Members:

Name	Position
Ellen Mattson	Teacher
Roy Brown, Jr.	Principal
Rebecca Clark	Speech-language clinician
Gerard and Julie Grabowski	Parents

Clearly, the family as well as the child are targets of assessment and possible intervention. Public Law 99-457 requires a multidisciplinary team approach to assessment of this population, since no single agency or discipline can meet the diverse needs of infants, toddlers, and their families. After assessment, the team is required by law to generate an IFSP that has the following components:

1. A statement of the child's present levels of development (cognitive, speech-language, hearing, motor, self-help, social)
2. A statement of the family's strengths and needs related to enhancing the child's development
3. A statement of major outcomes expected to be achieved for the child and family
4. The criteria, procedures, and time lines for determing progress
5. The specific early intervention services necessary to meet the unique needs of the child and family, including the method, frequency, and intensity of services
6. The projected dates for the initiation of service and the projected duration
7. The name of the case manager
8. The procedures for transition from early intervention into the preschool

One can readily see that the format of the IFSP has clear implications for assessment. First, it mandates family assessment that forces the SLP to focus on the child's total environmental system. Second, it requires that judgments be made in a variety of areas that need multidisciplinary cooperation (e.g., cognitive, social, language, motor, hearing). Third, it requires the practitioner to recommend evaluation procedures to be used to determine progress. The clinician needs to be prepared to address the issues included in the IFSP when he/she participates in staff meetings with other professionals subsequent to his/her evaluations of these children.

Regardless of the format employed, a diagnostic report should be organized for easy retrieval of information (Pannbacker 1975) and prepared in a manner that reflects high professional standards. Here are additonal criteria that the clinician should use to judge a diagnostic report: Is it accurate? Is it complete? Is it efficiently written (clearly and with an economy of words)? Was it prepared promptly?

Figure 13.3 provides a generic format—one that we have found quite effective and that we recommend to the beginning clinician. It contains several major sections which we will discuss; these sections can be stored as a template in a word-processing program for ease of writing and editing. Of course, reports can continue to be written in longhand for later typing.

Routine Information

In this section, we present basic identifying information—client's name, sex, address, date of birth, telephone number, parent's name where relevant, and of course the date of the examination; an undated report is of very little use. In addition to these routine data, we generally identify the referral source (parent, teacher, physician) and the evaluator. If the client is a school-aged child, we note the name and location of his/her school and the names of the teacher and the principal. The keystone of this initial section of the report is meticulous attention to accuracy.

FIGURE 13.3   Format for Diagnostic Report

I. Routine information

Name: File no.:

Sex: Date:

Address: Phone no.:

Birth date: Age at Evaluation:

Parents: Referred by:

Evaluated by: Address:

II. Statement of the Problem

III. Historical Information

IV. Evaluation

V. Clinical Impressions

VI. Summary

VII. Recommendations

_____

Clinician

_____

Supervisor

Statement of the Problem

In this section, we include a succinct statement of the presenting problem. What is the complaint and who is making it? Be sure to distinguish between the client's complaint and the problem stated by the referral source. In most instances, the reason for referral is stated in the client's (or parent's) own words—always indicated by quotation marks.

Historical Information

Before seeing a client for evaluation, many clinicians request that the individual fill out a brief case history form. Alternately, this information can be gathered in a face-to-face interview. Rather than present a generic example of a case history form, we refer the reader to the case history forms cited in all the preceding chapters. Different information needs to be collected with specific disorders.

Information obtained from referral letters, the case history, and the intake interview are included in this section of the diagnostic report. Material regarding the client's development (general and speech and language); medical, educational, and familial history; and estimates of psychosocial and behavioral adjustments are summarized. Only the most pertinent items are included in the diagnostic report. Because most of the historical information is obtained by questioning the client, a parent, or other informants, we suggest that the clinician briefly describe the interview situation—type of rapport established, the frankness and completeness of the respondent's answers, and any other pertinent observations.

Evaluation

The results of the various tests and examinations are delineated in this section. Before describing the assessment procedures and results, however, we include an opening statement that describes how the client approached the clinical setting and the tasks used to evaluate the communication abilities: Was the client apprehensive, bored, fatigued, cooperative? The name of each test, an explanation of what it does and how it was administered, and the results obtained should be included. Should the clinician include statements about communication skills that are within normal limits at the time of the evaluation? Knepflar (1976) believes that a complete diagnostic report should mention, even if briefly, all aspects of a client's speech, hearing, and language performance so that subsequent assessments can utilize the information as baseline observations. The information is simply presented, not interpreted, in this section of the report.

Clinical Impressions

In this section, we summarize our impressions of the individual and the communication impairment. What type of speech or language problem does the client have? How severe is it? What caused it? What factors seem to be perpetuating it? What impact has it had on the client and the client's family? How much does it interfere with everyday functioning? What are the prospects for treatment? Although we can offer interpretations here, we must still be able to support our impressions with information obtained during the interview or testing. Speculations based on previous clinical experience, such as similarity between the client and other cases the diagnostician has examined, should be clearly labeled as such.

Summary

The summary should be a concise (not more than a short paragraph) statement abstracting the salient features of the whole report. What is the communication disorder? What are the primary features of the disorder? What is the probable cause of the disorder? What is the prognosis (and general estimate of the predicted time frame) for recovery?

Recommendations

This is perhaps the most crucial portion of the report. We must now translate our findings into apporpriate suggestions or directions that will help the client solve communication and related problems. Do we recommend further speech and language evaluations? Is a medical referral necessary? Is treatment indicated? What direction should be taken? By whom, and when? The task, then, is to crystallize all the disparate interactions we have had with the individual, collate all the data, and then provide a flexible blueprint for further action. We must attempt to answer the question: What happens now—where do we go from here? Try to make the recommendations specific and brief. Suggestions for treatment or a more lengthy plan of therapy can be outlined in a letter or follow-up report. One final warning: Do not recommend *specific* evaluations or remediation procedures to workers in other professions. It is improper, for example, to recommend a client for electroencephalography to a neurologist, or for dental braces to an orthodontist; the speech clinician would be chagrined if a physician referred a child and recommended the administration of the ITPA. Be sure that your referrals for additional assessment are based on sound evidence; it is expensive, time consuming, and stressful to the client to make recommendations for comprehensive medical or psychiatric evaluation without serious and compelling reasons:

> *Early in the diagnostic session with five-year-old Mark we suspected the possibility of brain injury. Mindful of the family's limited finances, we wanted to document carefully all signs of apparent cerebral dysfunction before making a referral for a complete pediatric neurological evaluation. Observation revealed a number of serious symptoms: difficulty with motor coordination; labile emotions; rapid and slurred speech; perseveration; and blanking out spells. The necessity for referral was then obvious.*

We would like to close this discussion of component parts to the report by suggesting that the clinician or the employing agency audit a sample number of diagnostic reports for format compliance. Patient care audits (PCAs) are part of the national health care monitoring system for quality assurance. Patient care audits may focus on the quality of care provided patients through a variety of channels, including thoroughness of evaluation and diagnosis, treatment procedures, and audits of patient outcomes. The first is pertinent to this chapter: Files can be retrospectively analyzed to see whether or not routine components are present in the diagnostic report. Before doing a patient care audit of "quality of reports," the clinician or agency must have specified minimal requirements beforehand—such things as inclusion of the client's date of birth; mention of referral source, chart number, and date of evaluation; and performance of a hearing test, oral peripheral examination, and the like. Presetting some desired level of compliance is also necessary (e.g., "At least 90% of the audited reports will have . . ."). We recommend patient care audits, even if self-administered, as a good spot check of compliance with professional standards of information collection and reporting. When deficiencies are found, the clinician can target specific areas for needed improvement and/or can adjust clinical procedures and expectations.

Confidentiality

In our view, confidentiality is basic to any helping profession. All reports and records should be kept secure so that no harm or embarrassment comes to the persons we serve. When a diagnostic report is released, we prefer to mail it to a specific person rather than to the agency itself. Before releasing any information about a client, however, we must secure the client's permission in writing; most speech and hearing centers have permission forms, which are completed prior to or during the diagnostic session.

Because clients and parents have a legal right (Public Law 93-380, Family Educational Rights and Privacy Act of 1974) to read any report containing information about them, we often find it useful to send them a copy of the diagnostic findings. Before mailing the report, however, we always review our findings and recommendations with them. By going over the report with the clients or parents, we can be sure that they understand its contents.

Style

An extended discussion of prose style for report writing is not possible within the scope of this text. The reader will want to consult several of the following sources for more definitive statements about common modes of report writing: Huber (1961), Jerger (1962), Moore (1969), Good (1970), Fishbein (1972), Haynes and Hartman (1975), Pannbacker (1975), Knepflar (1976), Hollis and Dunn (1979), and Tallent (1980). In the interest of brevity, then, we shall simply enumerate several principles of style that we have found useful.

1. Make your presentation straightforward and objective, using a topical outline. Use simple, brief but complete sentences. It is often helpful to write for a specific reader; picture the reader in your mind—the classroom teacher, physician, speech clinician—and then simply tell the story of what you observed and recommend regarding a particular client. When in doubt about a reader's level of understanding, it is better to err on the side of simplicity.

2. Use an impersonal style. Some clinicians use the first person when writing diagnostic reports, but in our view it is preferable to keep the "I" out of it; a reference to "the clinician" or "the examiner" is more in keeping with professional reports. We prefer to individualize the client described in the report, not the writer. Furthermore, we believe that not only does an impersonal style help to minimize the writer's verbal idiosyncracies, but it also tends to encourage objectivity.

3. Edit the report carefully to make certain that spelling and use of tenses, grammar, and punctuation are accurate. Errors, even trivial ones, undermine the confidence of the reader in the diagnostician. Remember, competence is judged to a great extent by the precision of your reporting.

4. Watch your semantics. Be wary of overused or nebulous words such as "nice," "hopefully," "good," and the like. Avoid pet expressions or stereotyped ways of phrasing information. One clinician used the phrase "in terms of" thirteen times in a two-page diagnostic report. Another laced his reports with currently popular words like "input," "interface," and "scenario." Some writers use the word "feel" inappropriately in statements like "The clinician felt the client understood the diagnostic task"; we believe (not feel!) that the word should be reserved for discussing emotions or tactile sensations. Use abbreviations sparingly. Avoid superlatives unless they are clearly indicated.

5. Avoid preparing an "Aunt Fanny" report (Sunberg and Tyler 1962)—a bland written statement that could represent anyone or is so filled with qualifications ("perhaps," "apparently," "tends to") that it reveals nothing—nothing, that is, except a timid diagnostician.

6. Make the report "tight." Do not leave gaps or ambiguity where it is possible to read between the lines. If findings in certain areas are unremarkable, always state this explicitly. Do not leave the reader to guess whether you have investigated all possible aspects.

7. A diagnostic report is no place to display your learning or to parade a large vocabulary. Pedantic reports are misunderstood or unread.

8. Stay close to the data until you wish to draw the observations together and make some interpretations. For example, tell the reader which sounds were in error instead of simply stating that the child sounds infantile.

9. The very essence of good style is the willingness to take the time and energy to write and rewrite the report until it communicates what the clinician did and what the clinician found in the diagnostic session.

The Writing Process

Many students have difficulty writing reports. Most of them have found the task onerous, and a few are threatened and overwhelmed by the prospect of a blank sheet of paper in the typewriter. It has been our experience, however, that rather than have a writing deficiency, most of these students have a writing bias—they do not think they can do it. There are, of course, no quick and simple solutions; but we offer the following suggestions that have proven helpful to more than one beginning report writer.

Write on a daily basis. Each night—before retiring, for example—sit down and write a descriptive paragraph concerning something that happened to you that day. It may be easier for you to tap into your own creative power by starting with material that arouses strong feelings (see Macrorie 1968, 1970). At first it may be halting and difficult; as in any new task, your writing "muscles" will be sore. Do not wait for an inspiration, for that magic moment when, suddenly, it will come to you. Go to it. At the end of the week, review the writing you have done; edit, revise, ask yourself what you meant by each word or phrase. The best way to learn to write, in our opinion, is to write.

Get the message out and revise it later. It is especially important in writing reports to begin as soon as possible while the material is still fresh in your mind. A common error that some beginning writers make is to attempt to produce perfect writing in the initial draft. It does not matter how it looks at this point; you can always edit or have someone help you edit. When you meet barriers or mental blocks, do not linger; jump over them and go on with the rest of the report. When you come back later, you will find that your mind has filled in the blank spots.

It is helpful to have someone read and comment on the initial draft of your report. Although it is difficult to submit one's prose for dissection, ask the reader to be frank and honest in his/her editing. So many times, a phrase that seems clear to the writer who conceived it is vague or obscure to an objective reader. If writing continues to be a problem, consult the work of Strunk and White (1959) and others (Berke 1972; Ferguson 1959; Jones and Faulkner 1971; Kelly, Roth, and Altshuler 1969; Leggett, Mead, and Charvat 1974; Mayes 1972; Wubben 1971).

Follow-Up

The clinician's responsibilities do not end when the diagnostic report is finished and filed. A complete evaluation includes one final important task: a careful follow-up. It is the examiner's professional obligation to determine that the diagnostic activities and recommendations are translated into action; it is useless, perhaps even harmful, to identify and describe problems unless the individual is seen for further testing or treatment as soon as possible. When the diagnostician is also the clinician, the follow-up can be handled directly and with a minimum of paperwork. In an agency such as ours, however (a university speech and hearing clinic), we regularly refer clients to other workers for further assessment or treatment. We use the following questions as guidelines in implementing a follow-up program:

1. Did the intended readers receive the report? The best of secretaries occasionally misfiles a document, so we generally call the referral source within a week after the diagnostic to determine if the report has arrived.
2. Does the reader understand the contents of the report? What questions did it raise, if any, about the client? We always log these phone calls in the client's folder.
3. What is the disposition of the client? Is the client being seen for further testing? Is the client on a waiting list or being seen for treatment?
4. How is the client responding to treatment? We call the local worker, usually on a monthly basis, to assess how the client is doing in treatment relative to our recommendations. Not only does this convey our interest and assistance, it also helps the diagnostic team evaluate the efficacy of its work.

Bibliography

Berke, J. (1972). *Twenty Questions for the Writer.* San Diego, CA: Harcourt Brace Jovanovich.

Bouchard, M., and Shane, H. (1977). "Use of the Problem-Oriented Medical Record in the Speech and Hearing Profession." *Journal of the American Speech and Hearing Association* 19:157–159.

Darley, F., and Spriestersbach, D. (1978). *Diagnostic Methods in Speech Pathology.* 2nd ed. New York: Harper and Row.

Enelow, A., and Swisher, S. (1972). *Interviewing and Patient Care.* New York: Oxford University Press.

Ferguson, C. (1959). *Say It with Words*. New York: Knopf.

Fishbein, M. (1972). *Medical Writing*. Springfield, IL: Charles C Thomas.

Flower, R. (1984). *Delivery of Speech-Language Pathology and Audiology Services*. Baltimore: William and Wilkins.

Good, R. (1970). "The Written Language of Rehabilitation Medicine: Meaning and Usages." *Archives of Physical Medicine and Rehabilitation* 51:29–36.

Haynes, W. O., and Hartman, D. (1975). "The Agony of Report Writing." *Journal of the National Student Speech-Language-Hearing Association* 3:7–15.

Hollis, J., and Dunn, P. (1979). *Psychological Report Writing*. Muncie, IN.: Accelerated Development.

Huber, J. (1961). *Report Writing in Psychology and Psychiatry*. New York: Harper and Row.

Hutchinson, B., Hanson, M., and Mecham, M. (1979). *Diagnostic Handbook of Speech Pathology*. Baltimore, MD: Williams and Wilkins.

Jerger, J. (1962). "Scientific Writing Can Be Readable." *Journal of the American Speech and Hearing Association* 4:101–104.

Jones, A., and Faulkner, C. (1971). *Writing Good Prose*. New York: Scribner's.

Kelly, M., Roth, A., and Altshuler, T. (1969). *Writing Step by Step*. Boston: Houghton Mifflin.

Kent, L., and Chabon, S. (1980). "Problem-Oriented Records in a University Speech and Hearing Clinic." *Journal of the American Speech and Hearing Association* 22:151–158.

Knepflar, K. (1976). *Report Writing*. Danville, IL: Interstate Printers and Publishers.

Leggett, G., Mead C., and Charvat W. (1974). *Handbook for Writers*. 6th ed. Englewood Cliffs, NJ: Prentice Hall.

Macrorie, K. (1968). *Writing to Be Read*. Rochelle Park, NJ: Hayden.

Macrorie, K. (1970). *Uptaught*. Rochelle Park, NJ: Hayden.

Mayes, J. (1972). *Writing and Rewriting*. New York: Macmillan.

Middleton, G. F., Pannbacker, M. H., Vekovious, M. S., Puett, V., and Sanders, K. L. (1992). *Report Writing for Speech-Language Pathologists*. Tucson, AZ: Communication Skill Builders.

Moore, M. (1969). "Pathological Writing." *Journal of the American Speech and Hearing Association* 11:535–538.

Pannbacker, M. (1975). "Diagnostic Report Writing." *Journal of Speech and Hearing Disorders* 40:367–379.

Peterson, H., and Marquardt, T. (1990). *Appraisal and Diagnosis of Speech and Language Disorders*. 2nd ed. Englewood Cliffs, NJ: Prentice Hall.

Research Foundation (1990). *Guide for Use of the Uniform Data Set for Medical Rehabilitation*. Buffalo: Research Foundation, State University of New York.

Strunk, W., and White, E. B. (1959). *The Elements of Style*. New York: Macmillan.

Sunberg, N., and Tyler, L. (1962). *Clinical Psychology*. Englewood Cliffs, NJ: Prentice Hall.

Tallent, N. (1980). *Psychological Report Writing*. Englewood Cliffs, NJ: Prentice Hall.

Tonkovich, J. D. (1989). "Using Functional Outcome Measures in Diagnostic Reporting and Treatment Planning." Paper presented to the convention of the American Speech-Language-Hearing Association, St. Louis, MO.

Tonkovich, J. D., Horowitz, D. M., Gans, B. M., and Matlock, M. C. (1990). "Automating Speech-Language Pathology Documentation with Voice Recognition." Paper presented to the convention of the American Speech-Language-Hearing Association, Seattle, WA.

Wubben, J. (1971). *Guided Writing*. New York: Random House.

Early Child Language Assessment Interview Protocol

General Information

Pertinent History

- Referral source:
- Parent's statement of the problem:
- History of prior assessments:
- History of prior treatments:
- Parental treatment attempts:
- Daycare/Preschool status:
- Number and relationships of people living at home:

Biological Prerequisites for Communication Development

Birth and general health

- Pregnancy:
- Birth:
- History of child illnesses:
- Present state of child's health:

Auditory status

- History of frequent colds:

- History of earaches and ear infections:

- Parent's estimation of hearing acuity:

Neurological status

- Concussions/Unconsciousness:

- Seizures:

- Has the child been seen by a neurologist? For what condition?

- Does the child evidence any motor difficulties?:

General Development

- Concern about self-help skills?

- Concern about fine and gross motor development?

- Concern about social development?

- Concern about communication development?

Social Prerequisites for Communication Development

- Approximate time spent in social interaction on typical day:

- Who are the persons the child frequently interacts with?

- What are the activities associated with social interactions?

- Does the child exhibit any antisocial or socially inappropriate behaviors (avoiding interactions, consistent playing alone?)

- Does the child exhibit any self-stimulating behaviors (eg. rocking, flapping arms, etc.)?

- Does the child maintain eye contact?

- Does the child regulate your behavior nonverbally through gestures or physical manipulation?

- Does the child use objects or repeat actions to get your attention?

- Does the child vocalize during his/her social interactions?

- Does the child joint reference with the caretaker?

- Describe the child's typical day in detail:

Cognitive Prerequisites to Communication Development

Does the child exhibit play routines and behavior which would indicate the following attainments (specify example activity):

- Object permanence:
- Means-End:
- Immediate imitation:
- Functional Use of Objects:
- Deferred imitation:
- Symbolic play with own body:
- Symbolic play with objects:
- Symbolic play with surrogate objects:
- Distal Pointing:
- Combining more than one object at a time in play:
- What are the child's most frequent play activities?

Communication Development

- Does the child exhibit phonetically consistent forms?
- Parent estimation of the number of single words used expressively?
- Parent estimation of MLU?
- Reports of presyntactic devices?
- Parent's report of semantic relation types?
- Parent's estimate of language comprehension?
- Parent estimate of child's intelligibility?

Coding Sheet for Early Multiword Analysis

Child Utterance	Semantic Relation	Function	Initiation	Post Stage I Element
Pushing car	Action + Object	Regulate action	Child Initiated	-ing
Push it	Action + Object	Regulate action	Child Initiated	
Car going	Instrument + Action	Label/comment	Child Initiated	-ing
More car	Recurrence + X	Regulate action	Child Initiated	
Car allgone?	X + Disappearance	Questioning	Child Initiated	
Juice up there	Entity + Locative	Elicited Imitation	Adult Initiated	
Gimme juice	Action + Object	Regulating action	Child Initiated	
That truck	Nomination + X	Answering	Adult Initiated	
Ball	Personal/Social	Label/comment	Child Initiated	
Me ball	Possessor+Possession	Protest	Child Initiated	
No	Personal/Social	Protest	Child Initiated	
Mommy throw	Action + Object	Regulating action	Child Initiated	
Throw it	Action + Locative	Regulating action	Child Initiated	
Go there	Action + Object	Answering	Adult Initiated	
Horsie	General Nominal	Answering	Adult Initiated	
Big horsie	Attribute + Entity	Spontaneous Imit.	Child Initiated	
Me riding	Agent + Action	Label/Comment	Child Initiated	-ing
More ride	Recurrence + X	Questioning	Child Initiated	
Please	Personal/Social	Regulating action	Child Initiated	
Put on table	Action + Locative	Regulating action	Child Initiated	on

Summary Sheet for Early Multiword Analysis

Child: _____ Age: ___ Birth Date: _____ Sample Date: _____

Context of Sample (Include people and objects present):

Length of Sample in Time:

Activities Performed during Sample:

Mean Length of Utterance (Column 1 of Coding Sheet):

Total Number of Child Utterances (Column 1 of Coding Sheet):

Longest Utterance in Morphemes (Column 1 of Coding Sheet):

Number of Single Word Responses (Column 1 of Coding Sheet):

Semantic Relations Evident in Sample (Column 2 of Coding Sheet):

Functions Evident in Sample (Column 3 of Coding Sheet):

Percentages of Child and Adult Initiated Utterances (Column 4 of Coding Sheet):

Post Stage I Elements Noted (Column 5 of Coding Sheet):

Semantic Relations Missing from Sample:

Functions Missing from Sample:

Data Consolidation in Limited Language Evaluations

Identifying Information

Name: Address:
Telephone: Parents:
Date of Evaluation: Date of Birth: Age:

Data Obtained in Evaluation

- ❏ case history
- ❏ reports from professionals
- ❏ hearing screening
- ❏ oral peripheral
- ❏ behavioral observation of caretaker-child
- ❏ behavioral observation of clinician-child
- ❏ parental checklist (lexicon)
- ❏ adaptive behavior scale
- ❏ general developmental battery
- ❏ spontaneous communication sample
- ❏ nonstandardized tasks
- ❏ cognitive scale
- ❏ comprehension test
- ❏ language battery
- ❏ other

Analyses Performed on Data

- ❏ MLU
- ❏ distributional analysis
- ❏ early multiword analysis (semantic relations/functions)
- ❏ communicative gesture analysis
- ❏ cognitive analysis of play
- ❏ vocalization analysis
- ❏ phonetic inventory
- ❏ phonological analysis
- ❏ caretaker-child interaction analysis
- ❏ scoring of standardized measurements
- ❏ analysis of social behavior (e.g., turntaking, joint referencing)
- ❏ scoring of nonstandardized procedures
- ❏ other

Areas of Strength (+) and Concern (–)

Biological		*Cognitive*		*Social*	
Hearing	_____	Play level	_____	Reciprocity	_____
Neurological	_____	SM Substage	_____	Play partner	_____
Medical	_____	Symbolic Play	_____		
Anatomical	_____				

Adaptive Behavior		*Communicative Intent*		*Single Words*	
Self Help	_____	Imperatives	_____	Number	_____
Gross motor	_____	Declaratives	_____	Variety	_____
Fine motor	_____	Level	_____	Functions	_____
Social	_____	Rate	_____		

Early Multiword Combinations		*Phonology*		*Caretaker Strategies*	
Variety	_____	Phonetic Inv.	_____	Joint Referencing	_____
Productivity	_____	Processes	_____	Model	_____
MLU	_____				

Recommendations

Referrals: Further Testing by SLP: Prognosis:

Treatment Directions:

Selected Language Assessment Instruments for Syntax Level Children

Instrument/Author/Source*	Age Range
Analysis of the Language of Learning (Blodgett, E. and E. Cooper; Linguisystems)	5–9
Adolescent Language Screening Test (Morgan, D. and A. Guilford; Communication Skill Builders)	11–17
Assessment of Children's Language Comprehension (Foster, R., Giddan, J. and J. Stark; Consulting Psyc. Press)	3–6.11
Assessing Semantic Skills Through Everyday Themes (Barrett, N., Zachman, L. and Huisingh, R.; Linguisystems)	3–9
Auditory-Visual Single Word Picture Vocabulary Test-Adolescent (Gardner, M.; Slosson)	12–17
Bankson Language Screening Test-2 (Bankson, N.; Pro-Ed)	4–7
Basic School Skills Inventory-Diagnostic (Hammill, D. and Leigh, J.; Pro-Ed)	4–7.5
Basic School Skills Inventory-Screen (Hammill, D. and Leigh, J.; Pro-Ed)	4–6.11
Bilingual Syntax Measure 1 and 2 (Bkurt, M., Dulay, H. and Chavez, E.; Psychological Corp.)	5–12

Boehm Test of Basic Concepts-Preschool Version
(Boehm, A.; Psychological Corp.)   3–5

Boehm Test of Basic Concepts-Revised
(Boehm, A.; Psychological Corp.)   5–7

Bracken Basic Concept Scale
(Bracken, B.; Psychological Corp.)   2.6–8

Carolina Picture Vocabulary Test
(Layton, T. and Holmes, D.; United Educ. Services)   4–11.5

Carrow Elicited Language Inventory
(Carrow, E.; Learning Concepts)   3–7

Clark-Madison Test of Oral Language
(Clark, J. and Madison, C.; Pro-Ed)   4–8

Classroom Communication Screening Procedure for Early Adolescents
(Simon, C.; Interstate)   9–14

Clinical Evaluation of Language Fundamentals-Revised
(Semel, E., Wiig, E. and W. Secord; Psychological Corp.)   5–16

Clinical Evaluation of Language Functions
(Semel, E. and Wiig, E.; Merrill)   5–9

Cognitive Abilities Scale
(Bradley-Johnson, S.; Pro-Ed)   2–3

Comprehensive Receptive and Expressive Vocabulary Test
(Wallace, G. and Hammill, D.; Linguisystems)   4–17

Communication Abilities Diagnostic Test
(Johnston, E. and Johnston, A.; Riverside)   3–9

Del Rio Language Screening Test: English/Spanish
(Toronto, A. et al; National Education Laboratory Pubs.)   3–6

Detroit Tests of Learning Aptitude-3
(Hammill, D.; Pro-Ed)   6–17

Detroit Tests of Learning Aptitude-Primary
(Hammill, D. and Bryant, B.; Pro-Ed)   3–9

Diagnostic Achievement Battery
(Newcomer, P. and Curtis, D.; Pro-Ed)   6–14

Diagnostic Screening Test: Language
(Gnagey, T. and Gnagey, P.; Slosson)   6–13

Dos Amigos Verbal Language Scales
(Critchlow, D.; United Educ. Services)   5–13.5

Early School Inventory
   (Nurss, J. and McGauvran, M.; Psychological Corp.)   5–6

Evaluating Acquired Skills in Communication
   (Riley, A.; Communication Skill Builders)   < 1–8

Early School Inventory-Preliteracy
   (Nurss, J. and McGauvran, M.; Psychological Corp.)   5–6

Evaluating Communicative Competence:
A Functional Pragmatic Procedure
   (Simon, C.; Communication Skill Builders)   9–17

Expressive One Word Picture Vocabulary Test-Revised
   (Gardner, M.; Academic Communication Associates)   2–12

Expressive One Word Picture Vocabulary Test: Upper Extension
   (Gardner, M.; Slosson)   12–15

Fluharty Preschool Speech & Language Screening Test
   (Fluharty, N.; Pro-Ed)   2–6

Full Range Picture Vocabulary Test
   (Ammons, R. and Ammons, H.; Psychological Test Specialists)   2–21

Fullerton Language Test for Adolescents
   (Thorum, A.; Slosson)   11–18

Grammatical Analysis of Elicited Language
   (Moog, J., Kozak, V. and Geers, A.; Cent. Inst. Deaf)   3–6

Illinois Test of Psycholinguistic Abilities
   (Kirk, S., McCarthy, J. and Kirk, W.; Slosson)   2–10

Joliet 3 Minute Speech and Language Screen
   (Kinzler, M. and Johnson, C.; Communication Skill Builders)   5–10

Kindergarten Language Screening Test
   (Fauthier, S. and Madison, C.; Pro-Ed)   4–5

Let's Talk Inventory for Adolescents
   (Wiig, E.; Psychological Corp.)   9–18

Let's Talk Inventory for Children
   (Bray, C. and Wiig, E.; Psychological Corp.)   4–8

Language Processing Test
   (Richard, G. and Hanner, M.; Linguisystems)   5–11

Language Inventory for Teachers
   (Cooper, A. and School, B.; United Educ. Services)   4–12

Language Structured Auditory Retention Span Test
  (Carlson, L.; United Educ. Services)   3–21

The Listening Test
  (Bowers, L. et al; Linguisystems)   6–11

MAP: The Miller Assessment for Preschoolers
  (Miller, L.; AGS)   3–6

Miller-Yoder Language Comprehension Test
  (Miller, J. and D. Yoder; Slosson)   4–8

Multilevel Informal Language Inventory
  (Merrill)   5–11

Northwestern Syntax Screening Test
  (Lee, L.; Northwestern University Press)   3–7

Oral Language Sentence Imitation Diagnostic Inventory
  (Zachman, L. et al; Linguisystems)   none

Patterned Elicitation Syntax Test-Revised
  (Young, E. and Perachio, J.; United Educ. Services)   3–7

Peabody Picture Vocabulary Test-Revised
  (Dunn, L. and Dunn, L.; AGS)   2.5–21

Picture Story Language Test
  (Myklebust, H.; WPS)   7–12

Porch Index of Communicative Ability in Children
  (Porch, B.; Consulting Psychologists Press)   4–12

Preschool Language Assessment Instrument
  (Blank, M., Rose, S. and Berlin, L.; Linguisystems)   3–6

Pragmatics Screening Test
  (Prinz, P., and Weiner, F.; Psychological Corp.)   3–8

Preschool Language Scale-3
  (Zimmerman, I., Stiener, V. and Pond, R.; Merrill)   1.5–7

Psycholinguistic Rating Scale
  (Hobby, K.; WPS)   5–9

Rhode Island Test of Language Structure
  (Engen, E. and T. Engen; United Educ. Services)   3–6

Receptive-Expressive Emergent Language Test-2
  (Bzoch, K. and League, R.; Pro-Ed)   Preschool

Receptive One Word Picture Vocabulary Test: Upper Extension
  (Brownell, R.; Slosson)   12–16

Reynell Developmental Language Scale
   (Reynell, J.; WPS)   1–7

Screening Test of Adolescent Language
   (Prather, E., et al; United Educ. Services)   12–18

Screening Kit of Language Development
   (Bliss, L. and Allen, D.; Slosson)   2–5

Screening Children for Related Early Educational Needs
   (Hresko, W. et al; Pro-Ed)   3–7

Sequenced Inventory of Communication Development-R
   (Hedrick, E., Prather, and Tobin, A.; Pro-Ed)   <1–4

Slosson Articulation Language Test with Phonology
   (Tade, W.; Slosson)   3–6

Spanish Language Assessment Procedures:
A Communication Skills Inventory
   (Mattes, L.; Academic Communication Associates)   5–8

Structured Photographic Language Test 2
   (Werner, E. and Kresheck, J.; Janele Publications)   4–9

Test of Auditory Comprehension of Language-Revised
   (Carrow-Woolfolk, E.; DLM)   3–9

Test of Childrens Language
   (Barenbaum, E. and Newcomer, P.;
   Academic Communication Associates)   5–9

Test of Language Competence-Expanded Edition
   (Wiig, E. and Second, W.; Psychological Corp.)   5–18

Test of Early Language Development-2
   (Hresko, W., Reid, K. and Hammill D.; ACYS)   2–7

Test of Adolescent Language 3
   (Hammill, D., et al; AGS)   12–24

Test of Adolescent/Adult Word Finding
   (German, D.; Academic Communication Associates)   12–80

Test of Language Development: Primary 2
   (Newcomer, P. and Hammill, D.; AGS)   4–8

Tell of Language Development: Intermediate 2
   (Newcomer, P. and Hammill, D.; AGS)   8–12

Test de Vocabulario en Imagenes Peabody
   (Dunn, L. et al; AGS)   2.5–18

Test of Relational Concepts
   (Edmonston, N. and Thane, N.; Pro-Ed)   3–8

Test for Examining Expressive Morphology
   (Shipley, K., Stone, T. and Sue, M.;
   Communication Skill Builders)   3–8

Test of Pragmatic Language
   (Phelps-Terasaki, D. and Phelps-Gunn, L; Pro-Ed)   5–13

Test of Pragmatic Skills
   (Shulman, B.; Communication Skill Builders)   3–8

Test of Problem Solving Revised: Elementary
   (Bowers, L. et al; Linguisystems)   6–11

Test of Problem Solving Revised: Adolescent
   (Bowers, L. et al; Linguisystems)   12–17

Test of Word Finding
   (German, D.; DLM)   6–12

Test of Word Finding in Discourse
   (German, D.; Riverside)   6–12

Test of Word Knowledge
   (Wiig, E. & Secord, W.; Harcourt, Brace Jovanovich   8–17

Test of Written Language-3
   (Hammil, D. and Larsen, S.;
   Academic Communication Associates)   7–17

Test Of Language Development-3
   (Mecham, M. and Jones, D.; Pro-Ed)   3–11

Thought and Language Inventory
   (Markoff, A.; Academic Communication Associates)   6

Token Test for Children
   (Disimoni, F.; Teaching Resources Corp.)   3–12

The Word Test-R Elementary
   (Barrett, M. et al; Linguisystems)   7–11

Utah Test of Language Development-3
   (Mecham, M. and Jones, D.;
   Academic Communication Associates)   3–11

Writing Process Test
   (Warden, M. and Hutchinson, T.; Riverside)   7–18

The Word Test-R Adolescent
   (Barrett, M. et al; Linguisystems)   12–17

*Addresses of major sources are listed below. In some cases, a general supplier (e.g. United Educational Services, Inc.) is listed because we did not have access to the the original test instrument or specific catalogue.

Academic Communication Associates, Publications Division, Department 4, PO Box 6294, Oceanside, CA 92056

American Guidance Service (AGS), Publisher's Building, Circle Pines, MN 55014-1796

Central Institute for the Deaf, 818 South Euclid, St. Louis, MO 63110

Charles E. Merrill Publishing Co., 1300 Alum Creek Drive, Box 508, Columbus, OH 43216

Communication Skill Builders, 3830 E. Bellevue, PO Box 42050E, Tucson, AZ 85733

DLM Teaching Resources, One DLM Park, PO Box 4000, Allen, TX 75002

Interstate Printers and Publishers, Inc., PO Box 50, Danville, IL 61834

Janele

LinguiSystems, Inc., Department ABCD, 3100 4th Avenue, PO Box 747, East Moline, IL 61244

Pro-Ed, 8700 Shoal Creek, Austin, Texas 78758-6897

Psychological Corporation, Harcourt Brace Jovanovich, PO Box 9954, San Antonio, TX 78204

Riverside

Slosson Educational Publications, Inc., PO Box 280, East Aurora, NY 14052

United Educational Services, Inc., PO Box 605, East Aurora, NY 14052

Western Psychological Services, 12031 Wilshire Boulevard, Los Angeles, CA 90025

Index

of one sound for another, 173, 194, 195
Summary probe, 45
Support, providing, 50–51, 351
Swallowing disorders, 307–14
Swift, R.W., 379, 382, 389, 397
Swisher, L., 72–74, 75
Syllables, in esophageal speech, 367
Symbolic play, 104
Symbolic prompts, 276
Symptoms
    interviewing client about physical, 43
    of language disorder in older students, 134–35
Syndromes, 122
Syntactic class of word, 181
Syntactic structures, eliciting particular, 139
Syntax
    assessment using analysis packages, 149–55
    assessment using elicited imitation, 147–49
    cultural differences in, 164
    misarticulation and complexity of, 181
    nonstandardized testing, 139
    standardized testing, 137–39
Syntax/morphology, 135
Systematic Analysis of Language Transcripts
    (SALT), 153
S/Z ratio, 338

TACL, 83, 146
Tait, N., 337–38
Tape analysis, versus live scoring, 64
Target sound, selection of, 194
Teachers
    interviewing, 182
    referral by, 321
    treatment through, 241
Teeth, examination of, 305
Templin-Darley Tests of Articulation, 184
Tension increase therapy, 342
Tension-struggle features of, 237, 245
Test batteries, 111, 112
Testing
    of aphasic, 261–67, 268
    articulation, 384, 391–93
    with cleft palate, 391–93
    for dysarthria, 299–300
    other tests with articulation disordered
        clients, 206–7
    related of stutterer, 246
    single-word, 180, 386

standardized for aphasia, 264–67
    for stimulability, 185–86
Test of Auditory Comprehension of Language
    (TACL), 83, 146
Test-retest reliability, 66
Tests (assessment devices, instruments)
    aerodynamic, 339–40
    analyzing individual items on, 78–79
    for aphasia, 289
    for apraxia of speech, 289–90
    articulation, 384
    for assessment of covert features of
        stuttering, 238
    for assessment of nonaphasic disorders, 268–69
    for assessment of stuttering, 235
    common types of, 60–61
    criterion-referenced, 60–61, 179
    for discovering phonological processes in
        children, 196–98
    to evaluate phonetic context effects, 187–89
    evaluating standardized, 76–77
    formal (norm-referenced), 58–60, 67–83, 89
    informal, 59–60
    interpretation of, 66–76
    language comprehension, 118–19, 139–40,
        144–47
    with limited-language children, 90, 92–94,
        111–12
    nasal flutter, 382–83
    norm-referenced (formal), 58–60, 67–83, 89
    for oral, nonverbal apraxia, 289, 290
    performance on comprehension, 146
    problems of formal, 58–60
    proliferation of, 90
    reliability of, 59–60, 62–66
    scores, 69–75
    sentence articulation, 384
    single-word articulation, 180, 386
    specialized for aphasic, 267
    specialized for swallowing disorders, 313–14
    for swallowing disorders, 309, 313–14
    with syntax-level children, 137–40
    that focus on language, 111–12
    validity of, 59, 61–62
    variance in, 67–70
    for velopharyngeal function assessment,
        394–96
    for young stutterers, 232
    See also Standardized tests; Testing